SYSTEMS CONSULTATION

THE GUILFORD FAMILY THERAPY SERIES
ALAN S. GURMAN, EDITOR

Systems Consultation: A New Perspective for Family Therapy
Lyman C. Wynne, Susan H. McDaniel, and Timothy T. Weber, *Editors*

Clinical Handbook of Marital Therapy
Neil S. Jacobson and Alan S. Gurman, *Editors*

Marriage and Mental Illness: A Sex-Roles Perspective
R. Julian Hafner

Living through Divorce: A Developmental Approach to Divorce Therapy
Joy K. Rice and David G. Rice

Generation to Generation: Family Process in Church and Synagogue
Edwin H. Friedman

Failures in Family Therapy
Sandra B. Coleman, *Editor*

Casebook of Marital Therapy
Alan S. Gurman, *Editor*

Families and Other Systems: The Macrosystemic Context of Family Therapy
John Schwartzman, *Editor*

The Military Family: Dynamics and Treatment
Florence W. Kaslow and Richard I. Ridenour, *Editors*

Marriage and Divorce: A Contemporary Perspective
Carol C. Nadelson and Derek C. Polonsky, *Editors*

Family Care of Schizophrenia: A Problem-Solving Approach to the Treatment of Mental Illness
Ian R. H. Falloon, Jeffrey L. Boyd, and Christine W. McGill

The Process of Change
Peggy Papp

Family Therapy: Principles of Strategic Practice
Allon Bross, *Editor*

Aesthetics of Change
Bradford P. Keeney

Family Therapy in Schizophrenia
William R. McFarlane, *Editor*

Mastering Resistance: A Practical Guide to Family Therapy
Carol M. Anderson and Susan Stewart

Family Therapy and Family Medicine: Toward the Primary Care of Families
William J. Doherty and Macaran A. Baird

Ethnicity and Family Therapy
Monica McGoldrick, John K. Pearce, and Joseph Giordano, *Editors*

Patterns of Brief Family Therapy: An Ecosystemic Approach
Steve de Shazer

The Family Therapy of Drug Abuse and Addiction
M. Duncan Stanton, Thomas C. Todd, and Associates

From Psyche to System: The Evolving Therapy of Carl Whitaker
John R. Neill and David P. Kniskern, *Editors*

Normal Family Processes
Froma Walsh, *Editor*

Helping Couples Change: A Social Learning Approach to Marital Therapy
Richard B. Stuart

SYSTEMS CONSULTATION

A New Perspective for Family Therapy

Edited by

LYMAN C. WYNNE

University of Rochester
School of Medicine and Dentistry

SUSAN H. McDANIEL

University of Rochester
School of Medicine and Dentistry

and

TIMOTHY T. WEBER

Colorado Center for Psychology

FOREWORD BY SALVADOR MINUCHIN

THE GUILFORD PRESS
New York London

A Division of Guilford Publications, Inc.
200 Park Avenue South, New York, N.Y. 10003

Printed in the United States of America

Library of Congress Cataloging in Publication Data

Systems consultation.

(The Guilford family therapy series)
Bibliography: p.
Includes index.
1. Family psychotherapy. 2. Psychiatric consultation.
I. Wynne, Lyman C., 1923- . II. McDaniel,
Susan H. III. Weber, Timothy T. IV. Series.
RC488.5.S96 1986 616.89'156 86-4778
ISBN 0-89862-068-6
ISBN 0-89862-908-X (pbk.)

To Adele, David, and Misty—
Our most important family consultants

CONTRIBUTORS

HARLENE ANDERSON, PhD, private practice, Boston, Massachusetts; Galveston Family Institute, Galveston, Texas

JOHN BANK, MD, Division of Family Medicine, University of Rochester School of Medicine and Dentistry, Rochester, New York

DONALD A. BLOCH, MD, Ackerman Institute for Family Therapy, New York, New York

IRVING BORWICK, PhD, Management Executive Center, Inc., Boston, Massachusetts

THOMAS CAMPBELL, MD, Division of Family Medicine, University of Rochester School of Medicine and Dentistry, Rochester, New York

GIANFRANCO CECCHIN, MD, Centro per lo Studio della Famiglia, Milan, Italy

MARIE M. COHEN, PhD, private practice, Los Angeles, California

LAWRENCE FISHER, PhD, Veterans Administration Medical Center, Fresno, California; University of California, San Francisco, California

EDWIN H. FRIEDMAN, DD, private practice, Bethesda, Maryland

LAURA FRUGGERI, PhD, Centro per lo Studio della Famiglia, Milan, Italy

HAROLD GOOLISHIAN, PhD, Galveston Family Institute, Galveston, Texas

EVAN IMBER-BLACK, PhD, Department of Psychiatry, University of Calgary, Calgary, Alberta, Canada

JAMES E. JONES, PhD, Department of Psychiatry, University of Rochester School of Medicine and Dentistry, Rochester, New York

FLORENCE W. KASLOW, PhD, Florida Couples and Family Institute, West Palm Beach, Florida

JUDITH LANDAU-STANTON, MD, Department of Psychiatry, University of Rochester School of Medicine and Dentistry, Rochester, New York

JOSEPH MANCINI, MD, Division of Family Medicine, University of Rochester School of Medicine and Dentistry, Rochester, New York

SUSAN H. MCDANIEL, PhD, Department of Psychiatry and Division of Family Medicine, University of Rochester School of Medicine and Dentistry, Rochester, New York

STEPHEN MUNSON, MD, Department of Psychiatry, University of Rochester School of Medicine and Dentistry, Rochester, New York

PEGGY PENN, MSW, Ackerman Institute for Family Therapy, New York, New York

Richard A. Perlmutter, MD, Sheppard and Enoch Pratt Hospital, Towson, Maryland

Marcia Sheinberg, MSS, Ackerman Institute for Family Therapy, New York, New York

Bernard Shore, MD, Division of Family Medicine, University of Rochester School of Medicine and Dentistry, Rochester, New York

Margaret Thaler Singer, PhD, Department of Psychology, University of California, Berkeley, California

Carlos E. Sluzki, MD, Department of Psychiatry, Berkshire Medical Center, Pittsfield, Massachusetts

Thomas C. Todd, PhD, Bristol Hospital, Bristol, Connecticut

Timothy T. Weber, PhD, Colorado Center for Psychology, Colorado Springs, Colorado

David K. Wellisch, PhD, Department of Psychiatry and Biobehavioral Sciences, UCLA School of Medicine, Los Angeles, California

Carl A. Whitaker, MD, Department of Psychiatry, University of Wisconsin Medical School, Madison, Wisconsin

John Charles Wynn, DD, Colgate-Rochester Divinity School, Rochester, New York

Adele R. Wynne, MS, private practice, Pittsford, New York

Lyman C. Wynne, MD, PhD, Department of Psychiatry, University of Rochester School of Medicine and Dentistry, Rochester, New York

FOREWORD

Thirty years ago, when, after half a century, the well of individual psychology showed signs of running dry, iconoclasts on America's east and west coasts began to challenge the fundamental premise of psychodynamic theory, the egocentric completeness of the individual human being. This epistemological challenge to the mental health field became known as family therapy.

With the theoretical challenge came practical concerns. How do you transform a way of thinking into a way of doing? Since most of the young Turks were clinicians, trained as individual therapists, this issue became the center of an innovative fervor.

Today, the practice that evolved shows its richness in a dozen or so schools of family therapy, complex sets of techniques, hundreds of centers of training, and a number of practitioners that must run into the tens of thousands. On the plateau of this success we are beginning to stop and reconnoiter: What is the territory we have conquered?

It's not so big. There are hills, but there is no high ground for miles. When we all gather on the plateau, we feel that success of our numbers; but the original epistemological challenge has been replaced by strategic caucuses. Our circular questioning is gathering more and more information—about smaller and smaller circles.

This book is rooted in this historical moment, posing questions. Is family therapy the best label for what we are doing? Is our concern properly bounded by families, or should we expand to include broader contexts? What units are most appropriate for our inquiry? Should we work with hospitals? Courts? Churches? Universities? Schools?

Carlos Sluzki (1985) suggests: "We treat the family because we see the family and we see the family because we evoke the family with our models and our inquiry. People live . . . in multiple, complex, evolving networks, of which we 'extract' the family by means of asking . . . 'Who is in your family?'" (p. 1).

What if the answer to this question is, "I am the Assistant Vice President of X Corporation, and my life design is governed by my loyalty to X."

Or, to paraphrase Whitaker, what if the woman has married the kitchen, the children, the welfare system, her analyst, her church, or her bridge club? What if the man has married his workplace, the military, his psychoanalyst, the AA, or the golf club (for a nonsexist version, alternate the above genders). What if the couple functions as a confused reconstituted family, each subsystem unable either to integrate or to separate? Do we family therapists tackle the "family" that the members experience, or do we insist that (since the only system we really know is governed by our own concept of family) they divorce their nonparadigmatic partners?

A number of years ago I conducted a workshop in Israel, doing a number of consultations to seasoned family therapists who were stuck with some rather difficult families. The families, the therapists, and I were satisfied with the consultations; and since I had no further feedback, I assumed that I had been helpful. But when I did a follow-up a few years later, I learned that in a significant number of my consultations, I had failed to understand the context of therapist and family. In effect, I had constructed and then proceeded to consult an ideal family in therapy with an ideal therapist, divorced from the social context (the psychiatric hospital, the Israeli mental health system, or the kibbutz) that included these therapeutic systems. To work with a more exapnded focus, I had to consult *with* my "consultees," since I was entering an arena with which they were more familiar. The consultant–consultee system then became more symmetrical, and also more helpful. I now try to include a feedback procedure in my consultations; never again can I be that blissfully ignorant.

I think that family therapy, as we teach it today, is trapped in that same ignorance. It's a one-way street. In this book, Wynne, McDaniel, and Weber are suggesting that we abandon our provincialism, open our windows, learn something about the complexity and idiosyncracy of systems, and soar to meta positions. Do we have the intellectual tools necessary for these explorations? Or will we have to admit that we need new tools?

This carefully quilted volume provides multiple perspectives underlining the need for specific knowledge of the systems that one is consulting— like Kaslow's chapter on the military, the Wynnes' on the family court, or Munson's on the pediatric system. At times, the sequence of the chapters indicates the editors' benevolent intention to confuse, as when the organized five-step procedures of Peggy Penn and Marcia Sheinberg, dealing with the isomorphism of the therapist's family system and the patient–family system, is preceded by the purposefully anarchistic ambiguity of Carl Whitaker's thinking, and followed by the pragmatism of Cecchin and Fruggeri, who lead consultants to design interventions within the Italian mental health system that may or may not be family therapy, without seeing the client. Or when Edwin Friedman provides convincing evidence that the Bowen approach to family therapy contains the basic elements for consultations with business organizations, but in the next chapter Borwick, recommending humility to family therapists, suggests that in working with organizations, family therapists must question the direct application of family therapy techniques to their work.

The diversity of approaches in consultation and the variety of systems considered in this book add to the impact of this volume. We know that the questions raised will have to be addressed by family therapists acting as consultants, therapists, teachers, and supervisors. But as the editors point out, "A consultation model induces a pause before plunging into therapy, and increases the likelihood that family therapy, or whatever services, will be thoughtfully, not automatically, offered and accepted." I strongly agree.

Salvador Minuchin, MD
Family Systems, Inc.
New York, New York

REFERENCE

Sluzki, C. Families, networks, and other strange shapes. *AFTA Newsletter*, No. 19 (Spring), 1985, pp. 1–2.

PREFACE

The ideas for this volume germinated during discussions among the three editors about problems of supervision of family therapists. Specifically, we were impressed with the value of the role of supervisor of supervisors. This role provides the advantages of what has been called a "meta" position by systems-oriented family therapists who were influenced by the late Gregory Bateson. As we tried to understand the complexities of the problems of supervision, we began to realize that similar issues arose in consultant roles that each of us had taken. This led into our questioning what the differences might be between being a supervisor and being a consultant to family therapist colleagues. Our ideas evolved and became more sharply focused as we informally took consultant and consultee roles with one another while discussing a variety of concerns in our work. We soon realized that being a consultant provides a valuable flexibility that permits initiative and autonomy with a colleague. As we reviewed our experiences as consultants and consultees in various settings, such as a department of psychiatry, a division of family medicine, a department of pediatrics, schools, church and community programs, and the courts, we became impressed with the richness of opportunities that seem increasingly available to family therapists as consultants. When we decided to organize these thoughts into book form, we wanted to expand our knowledge and inform our thinking by inviting contributions from colleagues who we knew have special expertise as consultants in a variety of contexts.

Still another idea that evolved out of these discussions was our conceptualization of families not only as clients of consultee-therapists, but as consultees planning their own future. What made this notion seem especially exciting was that it fit in with the widespread, growing desire of family therapists to recognize more fully the healthy, responsible functioning and resources of families. We realized that the process of respectfully collaborating with families to select options for action may be better described as consultation than as therapy.

Another result of our discussions as editors, and of later readings of the contributions by the authors of this volume, was that we became aware of differences between consultation oriented to families and consultation with businesses and other organizations in the community. We have included some discussion of these matters, although the main focus of the volume remains on the family therapist who is also functioning as a consultant in health care settings.

In planning the contributions by the various authors, we were influenced by the model set forth by Alan Gurman and David Kniskern in the *Handbook of Family Therapy*. They outlined a series of issues and questions that they then asked the authors to consider in their chapters. We did in fact prepare such a set of guidelines, and some of the contributors alleged that they were useful. The questions that formed these initial guidelines have been elaborated and revised and now compose the basis of our checklist for consultation (see Chapter 3). In addition, the contributors were encouraged to provide case examples to illustrate their consultations and to describe successes and opportunities, as well as mistakes and failures.

The volume includes the formulations of the editors in the introductory and concluding sections. These ideas have evolved out of our personal experiences and extensive discussions with each other, but they have also been influenced by the contributions of the other authors, to whom we are grateful. In the introductory section (Chapters 1–4), we develop our concept of systems consultation and differentiate this process from other activities in which family therapists take part. The major portion of the book (Chapters 5–25) consists of the chapters by our contributors, who describe systems consultation in a variety of settings. These chapters are arranged in a somewhat arbitrary fashion but do reflect in general four main contexts in which family therapists have served as consultants: (1) mental health systems; (2) medical settings; (3) community groups and services; and (4) military and business organizations. In Chapter 26 and in the commentaries about each section, we discuss some of the ways in which the contributors' ideas compare with our own and with each other. Finally, in Chapter 27 we turn to a discussion of unanswered questions and future directions for the family therapist as systems consultant.

The editors wish to acknowledge the encouragement and support given to us in this venture by Alan Gurman, editor of The Guilford Family Therapy Series. Most important, we express appreciation to Margaret L. Toohey for her invaluable assistance in many forms, without which the volume would have been impossible to write or to complete. Her contributions included extensive stylistic editing and commentary on the content, both of which helped clarify our writing and our ideas. We wish to thank Cynthia O'Keefe and Cherie Rynerson for their dedicated, cheerful responsiveness and patient, hard work at the word processor, which enabled us to feel easy about the numerous revisions that we believed would improve our presentation. We also wish to acknowledge the support and the forums for discussion of our ideas provided by the Department of Psychiatry and the Division of Family Medicine at the University of Rochester School of Medicine and Dentistry, and by the Colorado Center for Psychology. Finally, we thank our families and close friends for their endurance, honest criticism, and abiding support for this project and our work in general.

The Editors

CONTENTS

I

PRINCIPLES OF SYSTEMS CONSULTATION

1

THE ROAD FROM FAMILY THERAPY TO SYSTEMS CONSULTATION

LYMAN C. WYNNE

TIMOTHY T. WEBER

SUSAN H. McDANIEL

University of Rochester School of Medicine and Dentistry[1]
Rochester, New York

As family therapists, we function as clinicians, teachers, supervisors, researchers, and administrators. In this volume, we have described our experiences when taking the role of consultant, a role that may be either a prologue or an alternative to these other functions. We believe that in many circumstances professionals who are based in such diverse fields as psychotherapy, education, community services, and business can be most effective if they work from the perspective of consultation rather than immediately and automatically engaging in, for example, therapy or teaching.

Our entry into the field of consultation has been guided and informed, sometimes explicitly, sometimes implicitly, by the overarching conceptual framework of systems theory. We use the concept of "systems consultation" to refer to the application of systems concepts and principles in consultation not only with families but also with other systems such as medical programs, the courts, and community networks. Because of the systems perspective of family therapy, family therapists can bring special skills to consultation in multiple contexts. At this point in history, we believe that it is timely to sharpen awareness of the rapidly increasing opportunities for consultative roles by family therapists and other systems-oriented health care professionals. An important goal of this book is to provide models and guidelines for proceeding with such consultative ventures. Although we see

1. The editors began work on this volume while they all were on the faculty of the University of Rochester; Timothy T. Weber is now on the staff of the Colorado Center for Psychology, Colorado Springs, Colorado.

the field of systems consultation as having rich potentialities, we also are keenly aware that these can be realized only by attending to the risks and pitfalls that may be encountered.

Systems theory has been regarded with varying degrees of enthusiasm by professionals from different disciplines. For example, in medicine a biopsychosocial model has been recognized in recent years as a comprehensive, systems-oriented basis for integrating factors in health and illness that range from society to molecular biology (Engel, 1977, 1980). The biopsychosocial model has constituted a vigorous attack upon the more conventional biotechnical medical model in which personality, the family, and other psychosocial systems are ignored or are viewed reductionistically as mere aggregates of biologic systems. However, most physicians, including psychiatrists, have accepted only grudgingly and inconsistently the concept of biopsychosocial systems.

In contrast, family therapists have embraced systems theory enthusiastically and often uncritically. The concept of the family as a system level that is distinctively different from the personality and the biology of the individual person has been almost universally accepted by family therapists. Because recurrent family patterns can be readily observed during family therapy, family therapists have taken as axiomatic the principle that the family unit is a system that is more than its individual members. Indeed, some family therapists have fallen into a family-level version of the reductionistic trap that has ensnared those who use a narrow biotechnical medical model; for these family therapists, the term "system" means the family and little or nothing more. More commonly, however, family therapists have struggled to apply a concept of the family as a subsystem within the context of larger, shifting systems, such as transgenerational family patterns and social networks. For family therapists, the family also represents a context for component subsystems, such as the marital pair, the offspring, mother–daughter or father–son alliances, as well as for the behavioral, intrapsychic, and biological systems of individuals. In short, the "family *is* context and *has* context" (Bloch, 1980).

In addition, a widely accepted tenet of family therapy has been the concept of the therapeutic system—the therapist together with the patient or family in a transactional unit that evolves its own distinctive patterns and rules. The family therapeutic system has become the primary unit for clinical study and research by family therapists. The patterns and rules of the family therapeutic system tend to be similar to those of the family itself; that is, the patterns of the therapeutic system and the family tend to be "isomorphic" (Bertalanffy, 1968). Such systematic formulations have strengthened the conceptual framework for the family field, but the complexity of interwoven and overlapping systems has uncovered unresolved difficulties for assessment and treatment.

The more clearly that we have recognized those difficulties, the more fully and painfully have we come to realize that discrepancies between our theory and our practice continue. Surely, part of the difficulty is the complexity of systems concepts (Simon, Stierlin, & Wynne, 1985). Furthermore, the language of systems theory was not built into our initial professional education and is by no means consistently used in professional discussions and publications of family therapists. As we have discussed these discrepancies between theory and practice, we have become disquietingly aware that the very term "family therapy," the heart of our professional identities, carries implications that may be at odds with our avowed systems concepts and principles for treatment.

The term "therapy" means the "healing, curing, and treatment of illness or disability" (*The American Heritage Dictionary of the English Language,* 1981). The concept of illness or disability is clearly based upon medical tradition. When family therapy began, the idea of curing an illness of the family was carried over from this tradition. "Psychotherapy" is defined as the "psychological treatment of mental, emotional, and neurosis *disorders* [italics added]" (*The American Heritage Dictionary of the English Language,* 1981). The analogous concept that family therapy is the treatment of family disorders leaves family therapists uneasy. Nevertheless, the term "family therapy" is embraced with ever-increasing enthusiasm. We suggest that family therapists pause and examine more fully whether all that they are doing is best regarded as "therapy." Therapy of what, for whom? We shall argue that the loose, even promiscuous, use of this term in the family field tends to confuse and mislead both the public and professional colleagues about our intentions and actual functioning. Furthermore, we ourselves sometimes blur, overextend, or misdirect our theorizing and our practice by inadequate examination of the implications of the concept of family therapy.

Family therapists for some years have been more vigorous in their complaints about the inadequacy of psychiatric classifications than they have been active in formulating an appropriate alternative. The current nomenclature of the American Psychiatric Association's *Diagnostic and Statistical Manual of Mental Disorders* (DSM-III) (1980) specifies that "each of the mental disorders is conceptualized as a clinically significant behavioral or psychological syndrome or pattern that occurs in an *individual* [italics added]" (p. 6). All family therapists find this exclusionary definition at odds with the concept that dysfunction can also occur at family and relational levels. Many family therapists have argued that a typology of "family pathologies" should be delineated and could be used in combination with psychiatric and medical classifications. At present, however, family therapists and researchers are very far from reaching accord on any family typology system (Fisher, 1977; Wynne, in press). The idea that a family is "sick," "pathologic," or "pathogenic" and therefore needs therapy is rejected by many family self-help advocates on the grounds that such terms are accusatory and blaming, and undermine family confidence and competence (Bernheim, Lewine, & Beale, 1982). A profile of functions and dysfunctions on a series of family dimensions may be a more appropriate research approach for describing what family therapy treats. However, some family therapists believe that no classification schema can be conceptually adequate to embrace the principles of systems theory, both across and within system levels. At present, the narrative description of family problems and contexts seems more widely used and accepted as a clinical starting point for family therapy.

At this point, we are not attempting to resolve these dilemmas about classification. Rather, we are proposing a different kind of approach, another way of thinking about health care issues and the role of helping professionals in relation to them. In observing how we and our colleagues have struggled and tried to cope with the concept of therapy and the role of therapist, we have concluded that an alternative way of thinking, another language, is needed in our repertory. We believe that the concept of *consultation* can help fill this need. This term has been available for many years, of course, but we believe it deserves a more central place in the thinking and vocabulary of helping professionals. What we shall call "systems consultation" provides a strategic and appropriate framework for identifying problems and considering options for action in a great many health care and mental health activities as well as other endeavors in business, education, and human services. This volume constitutes an effort to explore some of the challenges and rewards, as well as the hazards and limitations of a systems consultation framework.

THE CAPLAN CONCEPT OF MENTAL HEALTH CONSULTATION

As we began to organize our ideas about consultation, we returned to the literature in this field, and particularly to the literature in the field of mental health consultation. Here the work of Gerald Caplan (1963, 1970) is seminal. Caplan's conceptualization of consultation has much in common with our formulation (especially see Caplan, 1970, Chap. 2). Unquestionably, many of the ideas introduced by Caplan and expanded by such other authors as Altrocchi (1972), Bindman (1966), Gallessich (1982), and Greenblatt (1980) have been important to the history of consultation endeavors. On the other hand, Caplan's well-known classification of four major types of mental health consultation strikes us as cumbersome and static, and carries implications that we regard as unfortunate. Caplan's categories were: (1) client-centered case consultation; (2) program-centered administrative consultation; (3) consultee-centered case consultation; and (4) consultee-centered administrative consultation. Although we are aware that the body of consultation literature organized around this classification has for many years been prescribed reading in the educational courses of psychologists, psychiatrists, social workers, and other mental health professionals, we have found it conceptually arid and quite unsatisfactory for our use in systems-oriented consultations.

For example, we are dissatisfied with Caplan's distinction between *consultee*-centered consultation and *client*-centered consultation: The consultee and the client are regarded as separate "targets" for the consultation. In contrast to this compartmentalized and lineal approach to consultation, we have found it more helpful if the consultee and client (and the "concerns" or "problem") are viewed as inextricably functioning within the same system. Similarly, the distinction between *consultee*-centered consultation and *program*-centered consultation seems to us to separate out unrealistically the programs of the consultee from the functioning of the consultee as a person. In addition, the concept of *administrative* consultation seems far too ambiguous for the various kinds of consultative situations in which we have found ourselves. Administrative considerations involve a highly varied set of roles and functions, for example, those of teachers, psychotherapy supervisors, seminar leaders, fiscal officers, and so on, as well as those who are ordinarily thought of as executives or administrators. A considerably greater diversity of consultative relationships exists than is implied by these categories of the traditional mental health consultation literature. Most important, in the traditional formulation of consultation, the role of the consultant as a necessary participant in the consultation system is given far too little attention.

One of the more recent contributions to the consultation literature is June Gallessich's book, *The Profession and Practice of Consultation* (1982). Her orientation differs from our own (and Caplan's) in that she describes consultation as a profession in its own right, whereas we shall be discussing consultation as only one of the functions contributing to professional identity. A psychologist or family therapist who takes on a consultant role does not give up his or her professional identity as a psychologist or family therapist. Galessich describes her work in the "profession of consultation" as beginning with Caplan's approach toward mental health consultation, but she has added concepts of organizational development and group relations theory. She correctly notes that these latter theories have developed parallel to each other, with very little cross-referencing between them in the literature of each approach.

THE ESSENTIAL INGREDIENTS OF SYSTEMS CONSULTATION

Three primary components of consultation systems can be differentiated. We shall use the term "consultation" to denote the process in which a *consultee* seeks assistance from a *consultant* in order to identify or clarify a *concern* or problem and to consider the options available for problem resolution.

THE CONSULTEE

The consultee retains primary responsibility to take action and implement ideas stemming from the consultation. Not only does the consultee have the legal, ethical, and administrative responsibility for initiative and action, but he or she also has the right and responsibility to accept or reject the recommendations and ideas that have emerged during the consultation process. Although the traditional consultation literature describes consultees as professionals seeking help with work problems (Caplan, 1970), consultation also may take place with nonprofessional consultees: any individual, couple, family, or group of persons who has not yet decided upon a course of action, such as entering therapy, and who seeks a consultant's assistance in making a plan or reaching a decision.

THE CONSULTEE'S CONCERN

Initially, the consultee may believe that the central problem or issue for consultation is located internally (the subject of concern for a consultee couple may be "Something's wrong with our marriage"); the problem may be viewed as external (a businessman may request a consultation because "My employees are feuding with each other"); or the consultee may be concerned about a relational difficulty with a client, family, or organization (a family therapist may say "My relationship with the Smith family has gone sour"). Although most problems that become the subject of consultation are difficulties or dysfunctions, consultation also may be requested because of issues generated by positive growth or success and by the wish to embark on new ventures.

THE CONSULTANT

The consultant takes a comprehensive, "meta" view of the consultee's concern, including the consultee–client relationship and whatever other system contexts are relevant to the problem and its resolution. The consultant becomes a component of a new consultation system (composed of consultant, consultee, and client or problem) in which the consultant does not take responsibility from the consultee for decisions or actions.

Although consultants are often sought because they are thought to have a particular kind of expertise, skill, or competence, there are situations in which it is the distinctive role and perspective of the consultant, meta to the consultee and the consultee's concern, that make the consultant potentially useful. For example, a family therapist who is serving as a consultant to a family therapist colleague may be able to help by bringing a fresh viewpoint to a clinical problem in which the consultee is enmeshed, and yet not necessarily be a more experienced or skillfull therapist. A distinctive feature of *systems* consultation is that the consultant explicitly attempts to consider the multiple contexts or systems of the presenting problem.

THE ADVANTAGES OF THE CONCEPT OF SYSTEMS CONSULTATION

The appeal to us of the concept of systems consultation can be described under a number of closely related headings:

1. *In consultation, the nature of the problem is not prejudged.* While the role relationship of "therapist" and "patient" implies that the problem involves a disorder or illness that needs to be cured, the concept of a consultation system leaves open for exploration whether a significant problem can be identified, and who is able and willing to take responsiblity for further action (if any). A primary task in systems consultation is to identify the nature of the presenting concern or problem in the context of multiple relevant systems, and to consider the options for what should take place next and who should participate. The concept of therapy implies that the mode of intervention already has been identified.

2. *The consultant can advantageously take a meta position from which systemic relationships and patterns can be assessed.* Other roles, such as

that of the therapist, place the professional much more fully and immediately within the therapeutic system, in which expectations and constraints requiring "curative" action are assumed. Starting as an observer, the consultant has more freedom to assess relationships and interactions, for example, among a therapist, family, and referring person. A consultant is in an advantageous position to step back from the fragments of a problem and to view the situation in context. Nevertheless, the consultant as observer is part of the "observing system" (Foerster, 1981) or, as we call it, the consultation system, but may begin from a position that is more fully meta to the problem than is possible for more enmeshed participants.

3. *Consultation facilitates the reframing of problems.* Family therapists have widely adopted the technique of reframing problems as a central feature of their treatment approaches. We believe that the label "therapist" often handicaps the professional and constricts the range of options for reframing the presenting problem or situation in terms that may not call for therapy. Especially with complex and chronic problems, it may be highly advantageous to examine the situation from a radically new perspective, to open up new options, and to facilitate the creation of new patterns of interaction. Someone who is initially identified as a "therapist" is constrained by the expectation that he or she will "depathologize" a problem that has been regarded as an illness or disorder, even though it may be more usefully framed in different terms.

4. *Consultation can readily give emphasis to health, strengths, and positive resources.* A consultant can more naturally and easily focus attention on the assets and healthy resources that a family is able to mobilize. To put this in another way, the consultant is usually in a more flexible position to contextualize problems in a fresh manner. Closely related to the issue of reframing is the approach, given much greater recognition in recent years, of drawing upon and recognizing the healthy resources of families and individuals even where dysfunction has dominated attention.

5. *Collaborative relationships between consultant and consultee can be readily established.* The role relationships of therapist–patient, supervisor–supervisee, teacher–student, and administrator–employee imply a complementarity in which one of the participants is one-up and the other is one-down. However, there are many situations in which collaboration between peers in exploring problems and implementing solutions is appropriate and desirable for the task and the situation. We believe that consultation maximizes opportunities for such collaborative relationships.

6. *A consultant role provides a base for flexible shifts to alternative professional roles.* The role of a consultant is not a fixed or permanent form of professional functioning and can be a self-defined base from which the professional can move into other roles. In contrast, once a person has taken

on a therapist role, it is much more difficult to move to other roles, such as being a consultant or a teacher. We also find useful a distinction between consultation in which someone has been explicitly sought out to serve as a consultant versus the more common situation in which the consultant role is self-defined. Defining oneself as a consultant can become a strategy for proceeding with maximal options and flexibility in health care and other professional relationships. In many professional relationships it is conceptually clarifying to think of oneself as a consultant, but it may be unnecessary to label oneself as such with clients or colleagues. In other situations, making the label explicit may help shape a desired direction for the relationship.

AN EXAMPLE OF SYSTEMS CONSULTATION

Throughout this volume we shall intersperse case examples to illustrate theoretical points being presented. Our first case example illustrates an ordinary, less than optimal consultative situation in which multiple systems needed to be considered in order to resolve a seemingly straightforward presenting problem. This example may also show why we find that consultation from a systems perspective is not adequately characterized by constricting terms such as "consultee-centered case consultation."

Where is the problem? A case example. A psychologist, Dr. Matthew, requested consultation from a family therapist about a problem in her therapy with Ted Ross, a 19-year-old male with whom she had been working for several months.[2] Because of an incident in which Ted had drunkenly threatened to assault a relative, he had been taken into temporary custody and then referred to the court system. As part of his probation plan, he was required to have a psychological evaluation. Because Dr. Matthew became very concerned during this evaluation about Ted's susceptibility to alcohol, she wanted to take a definite position about treatment for this problem. Specifically, she considered suggesting that Ted enroll in an educational class at the local alcoholism treatment center. She was very distressed that he was not taking any action on his own about his problem with alcohol, and she wanted him to receive some specialized assistance. Ted, however, did not agree that he had a problem with alcohol.

Faced with her "intractable" patient, Dr. Matthew came to the consultant with this question: "Should I suggest to Ted that he get involved with this alcohol treatment program, or should I call his probation officer and get her to put pressure on him to participate in the program?" Dr. Matthew began the consultation by

2. All names used in case examples in this volume are pseudonyms.

expressing her concern that she had been "rescuing" her patients and that she wanted some ideas on how not to rescue them when they began to have problems. Dr. Matthew wanted Ted to take more action, but at the same time she did not want to take responsibility for getting him to do so because the more she actively made suggestions, the more he seemed to resist those suggestions in a quiet way.

With the goal of helping Dr. Matthew set more realistic limits regarding her responsibility, the consultant discussed with her how it was important to put more responsibility back onto Ted as to what he was going to do about his difficulty with alcohol. It also seemed to the consultant that Dr. Matthew was about to triangulate the probation officer so that she, as the therapist, would not have to deal directly with the patient in this sensitive matter. On several other occasions, when faced with a difficult issue with one of her patients, Dr. Matthew had attempted to bring in other family members or other therapists to assist her. Having seen this pattern in Dr. Matthew's therapy in two prior consultations, the consultant suggested that she deal with this patient directly, rather than using the probation offfcer for leverage.

After hearing the suggestion that she go to her patient directly about the alcohol issue, Dr. Matthew told the consultant that her supervisor at the agency where she saw this patient had suggested a different course of action, saying, "It is not appropriate for you to be in the role of a critical parent." Consequently, the supervisor had explicitly suggested that Dr. Matthew ask the probation office to apply leverage to the patient to participate in the alcohol treatment program.

At this point, the therapist was hearing two incongruent messages: Her supervisor was telling her to go to the probation officer and to get that officer to apply pressure, while the consultant was telling her that she should go directly to the patient and not triangulate the probation officer in an issue in which she *could* take responsibility. Upon hearing that Dr. Matthew's supervisor had suggested a different course of action, the consultant quickly took a "time out" and discussed with Dr. Matthew her experience of having to deal with conflicting messages from two people who were advising her. As the consultant discussed with her this process of triangulation and subsequent immobility, Dr. Matthew realized that this same pattern existed between herself and the patient, and between the patient and his supervisors at work. The pattern in the therapist–patient–work system triangle was the following: The patient had been under a great deal of stress at work recently and was working overtime far beyond the number of hours he could tolerate. Seeing his exhaustion, Dr. Matthew was attempting to get the patient to reduce his workload, to take more time off from work, and not to work overtime. The more she suggested that he do this to reduce his stress, the less he seemed to want to take any action. The therapist was labeling the patient as being "passive–aggressive" and was wondering how to deal with this personality deficit. She then reported that Ted's supervisors at work had been encouraging him to establish a good work history, to work overtime, and to climb the success ladder in the organization. The patient's mentors at work were giving him a message directly opposite to that of his therapist. The therapist was saying, "slow down," while his mentors at work were saying, "speed up." Faced with these incongruous messages, the patient was paralyzed.

As the consultant discussed these isomorphic predicaments, Dr. Matthew also began to realize that for many years Ted had been caught in a triangle with his embattled parents. Having been the responsible child in the family, Ted felt that he had to be loyal to both parents who over the years had given him opposite and conflicting messages. For example, his father often went drinking and would invite Ted to go along with him to bars. At the same time, his mother encouraged Ted to avoid this "evil habit" and to stay healthy. This was only one among many examples of incongruous messages that Ted's parents had given him. Feeling a deep loyalty to both parents, Ted had become immobilized.

Seen from a larger systems perspective, the consultation system included a number of complicated triangles. The first involved the consultee who was stuck in the position of having to listen and be loyal to the messages of both her consultant and her supervisor. The second triangle was comprised of the patient receiving conflicting messages from his therapist and his mentors at work. A third triangle included the patient and his father and mother. The consultation problem was that the triangle between the consultant, the consultee, and her supervisor was both mirroring and possibly exacerbating or reactivating the similar triangles in the rest of the consulting context. Systemically, the object of concern was not simply the patient, and the problem could not be usefully located within the patient. Rather, a perspective about the context of interlocking systems appeared crucial in identifying the factors that were helping to perpetuate this systemic problem.

To conclude this example, the consultant's immediate strategy was to detriangulate himself by sending Dr. Matthew back to her supervisor to work out the dilemma of how to manage the problem between herself, the probation officer, and the patient. The supervisor, not the consultant, was directly responsible for Dr. Matthew's conduct of the case. The major impact of this consultation session was that both consultant and consultee gained a fresh perspective on how internal problems (such as the "passive-aggressive deficit") must be seen within a larger context. Reframing the problem in this systems perspective afforded both the consultant and the consultee a new vision of their own functioning and alternative solutions to the presenting problem.

This example emphasizes the importance of clearly conceptualizing the consultant role. We believe it is timely and important that consultation processes be reexamined in both a scholarly and empirically relevant manner that uses systems theory as the conceptual framework. The present volume is a preliminary effort in this direction, but it by no means exhausts the topic. As we have reviewed our own experiences and those of the contributing authors to this volume, we have steadily revised our own thinking and repeatedly have been impressed by the ways in which these formulations have strengthened our work, not only in consultation per se, but also in sharpening our understanding of our teaching, supervisory, and other roles.

We recognize that our current experience or thinking does not enable us to encompass or even to understand all versions of consultative theory and practice. However, we believe that the principles of systems consultation that are discussed and illustrated in this volume provide a broader and more flexible approach to consultative issues than do most current models of consultation with which we are familiar. It remains for the future to evaluate whether "systems consultation" is in fact relevant beyond the types of examples that are illustrated in this volume. For the moment, we are content to propose that family therapists and perhaps others who have a similar theoretical orientation will profit from thoughtfully applying systems principles to their consultative activities, either as consultants or as consultees. Thus, we return to our starting point—our role as family therapists. From this role we have derived our actual clinical experience, and this role gives substance to our conceptual formulations.

REFERENCES

Altrocchi, J. Mental health consultation. In S. E. Golann & C. Eisdorfer (Eds.), *Handbook of community mental health.* New York: Appleton-Century-Crofts, 1972.

The American heritage dictionary of the English language. Boston: Houghton Mifflin, 1981.

American Psychiatric Association. *Diagnostic and statistical manual of mental disorders* (3rd ed.; DSM-III). Washington, DC: Author, 1980.

Bernheim, K. F., Lewine, R. R. J., & Beale, C. T. *The caring family: Living with chronic mental illness.* New York: Random House, 1982.

Bertalanffy, L. von. *General systems theory.* New York: Braziller, 1968.

Bindman, A. J. The clinical psychologist as a mental health consultant. In L. E. Abt & B. F. Reiss (Eds.), *Progress in clincial psychology.* New York: Grune & Stratton, 1966.

Bloch, D. A. The future of family therapy. In M. Andolfi & I. Zwerling (Eds.), *Dimensions of family therapy.* New York: Guilford, 1980.

Caplan, G. Types of mental health consultation. *American Journal of Orthopsychiatry,* 1963, *33,* 470–481.

Caplan, G. *The theory of practice of mental health consultation.* New York: Basic Books, 1970.

Engel, G. L. The need for a new medical model: A challenge for biomedicine. *Science,* 1977, *196,* 129–136.

Engel, G. L. The clinical application of the biopsychosocial model. *American Journal of Psychiatry,* 1980, *137,* 535–544.

Fisher, L. On the classification of families: A progress report. *Archives of General Psychiatry,* 1977, *34,* 424–433.

Foerster, H. von. *Observing systems.* Seaside, CA: Intersystems Publications, 1981.

Gallessich, J. *The profession and practice of consultation.* San Francisco: Jossey-Bass, 1982.

Greenblatt, M. Mental health consultation. In H. I. Kaplan, A. M. Freedman, & B. J. Sadock (Eds.), *Comprehensive textbook of psychiatry.* Baltimore: Williams & Wilkins, 1980.

Simon, F., Stierlin, H., & Wynne, L. C. *The language of family therapy: A systemic vocabulary and sourcebook*. New York: Family Process Press, 1985.

Wynne, L. C. A preliminary proposal for strengthening the multiaxial approach of DSM-III: Possible family-oriented revisions. In G. L. Tischler (Ed.), *Diagnosis and classification in psychiatry*. Cambridge, UK: Cambridge University Press, in press.

2

THE TERRITORY OF SYSTEMS CONSULTATION

SUSAN H. McDANIEL

LYMAN C. WYNNE

TIMOTHY T. WEBER

University of Rochester School of Medicine and Dentistry
Rochester, New York

Of central importance in our study of consultation has been the issue of role clarity. One of the recurrent problems underlying requests for consultation is confusion about what role the consultee and, in turn, the consultant should assume in dealing with a given problem. Lack of role clarity will compromise a consultant's effectiveness in assisting the consultee's efforts at role definition. With these issues in mind, we shall begin with an overall discussion of the problems posed by the continua between consultation and psychotherapy, supervision, teaching, and administration.

THE THERAPY-CONSULTATION CONTINUUM

At present, developments within the field of psychotherapy, including family therapy, blur the distinctions between therapy and consultation. A major current trend in both family therapy and individual psychotherapy is the emphasis on a brief, problem-centered approach. One of the conceptual and pragmatic consequences of this trend is that therapy and consultation have become increasingly similar, but, as we shall argue, significant differences remain in the core assumptions associated with each field.

Traditionally, the role of therapist implies the complementary role of patient. When family therapy was introduced, the formulation that the family is the patient was widely and vigorously advocated and is still taught as a concept in some training programs. A patient seeks, or is given, diagnosis and treatment for discomfort or dysfunction that is defined, in the medically derived tradition, as a disorder. Family "counselors," in contrast, work with "clients," a term also favored by therapists who dislike the implications of the term "patients" (who by definition have "disorders"). These clinicians nevertheless retain the politically and economically advantageous label "therapist." These terminologic differences are not simply semantic, but have both subtle and explicit consequences for role functioning. The term "consultation" avoids many of these problems.

We propose that prior to a decision to engage in family therapy (and perhaps individual psychotherapy as well) a consultation phase in which *the family is the consultee* is advantageous. Initially, when individuals or families contact mental health professionals, they are usually unclear, or cannot agree about the nature and scope of their concerns and problems. Consultation provides a relationship in which the family and the consultant can collaboratively delineate the problem and consider options for resolution. The decision may be that no further help is needed or that something other than therapy is needed or desired. Consultation with the family as consultee thus explicitly taps the family's responsible decision making and builds upon its healthy resources and competences. Therapy, as has often been noted, begins with consideration of difficulties and failings, and, at least subtly, tends to downplay capabilities for self-direction and autonomy.

Another implication of the traditional concept of therapy is that patients, having accepted the possibility of illness or disorder, are expected to allow infringements of customary privacy in order to facilitate diagnosis and treatment. In turn, the therapist is expected to act in a trustworthy manner and to accept an appropriate degree of care-taking responsibility usually without time limits. In contrast, the consultant's role is time limited and focuses upon the consultee's presenting concerns. The consultant may want to contextualize and reframe the area of concern, but the consultee retains responsibility for determining the scope of the consultation. In short, the therapist takes direct and primary responsibility for facilitating change, whereas the consultee, not the consultant, retains explicit responsibility for change.

Furthermore, the consultee is understood to be free to accept or to reject the consultative advice. In therapy there is an acknowledged pressure to accept the interpretations, limit setting, or directives in order for the therapy to be effective. The notion of transference in therapy implies a quasi-coercive pressure to carry out the therapist's expectations. In typical consultative roles, the consultant expects the consultee to take seriously the proposals that are made, but at the same time to remain free to accept or reject the advice that is given.

Between consultant and consultee, a relationship of colleagues is commonly sought or expected. Consultants who arrogate to themselves a one-up status are usually criticized for doing so, especially in medical consultations. Therapy, in contrast, implies a hierarchical helper–"helpee" (or is it helpless?) relationship, or a relationship between caretaker and someone who is ill or disabled.

The educational component in consultation is more explicit than in most therapy. Education is not "up front" in insight-oriented psychotherapy for the family or individual, although one can make a case that there is a significant, usually unacknowledged component of education in all psychotherapy, including strategic and growth-oriented, experiential family therapy (Wynne, 1981). However, the primary, avowed goal of traditional psychotherapy is to modify a form of disorder or dysfunction in the individual or family and only secondarily to educate the person or family to become more knowledgeable or skilled in handling similar problems in the future. In its emphasis on the latter goals, consultation can more readily and explicitly be oriented to *health and assets* than can therapy, which by definition is a concept that is oriented to healing pathology.

In recent years, some forms of family therapy have become similar to a consultation model. For example, they include a psychoeducational component in which time is set aside to give information about a disorder or about a problem such as a serious mental illness or a physical illness (Anderson, Hogarty, & Reiss, 1980). This approach can be effective in establishing a trusting relationship and in some cases is all that the family needs or wishes at that time. The implication is that the family is qualified to take the ball, to take responsibility for their own future activities and destiny, and that the continuing involvement of a therapist is not necessary. Such psychoeducational programs are often not viewed, or paid for, as part of "therapy," but can be quite readily accepted as "consultations." Families of schizophrenics, for example, often are reluctant to take part in "therapy" because this implies to them that they are "sick" or blameworthy.

Traditionally, a major difference between consultation and psychotherapy has been that in consultation, advice giving has been thought to be a central feature, while in psychotherapy, especially when it is insight-oriented, advice is explicitly avoided. Nevertheless, directives and prescriptions in psychotherapy certainly can be regarded as forms of advice, and information about how to proceed in the patient role within the therapy setting, if not outside, is minimally necessary. In addition, as discussed in Chapter 26, systems consultants differ in the extent to which they focus on advice or information-giving aspects of the process of the consultation. Thus, the difference between psychotherapy and consultation with respect to advice giving seems neither clear-cut nor generalizable. In this and other respects, therapy and consultation appear to overlap along a series of dimensions or continua.

Consultation, from the beginning, must take stock of multiple systems of interaction. Traditional psychotherapy, particularly in the psychoanalytically oriented mode, has been more content to work with the system of persons in the room, whether this is with an individual or with the nuclear family. The assumption is that if there are other systems involved, they will be affected indirectly through the impact upon the persons who are present. The consultant, however, can more readily and expectedly be concerned with transactions across several systems, both inside and outside the consulting room.

A consultation-like orientation is especially obvious in family therapy with a problem-focused or problem-oriented emphasis, often within a time-limited framework. If the number of sessions is not specified, it is understood that therapy will terminate with the resolution of a specific identified problem. Although renegotiation of the contract to continue on a time- or session limited basis or to work on a newly specified problem may take place, therapy is now much less open-ended than it once was and less ambitious to work toward resolution of *all* the major dysfunctions that the individual or family may have. Similarly, the consultative mode is primarily oriented to clarifying salient issues, solving specific problems, and identifying strengths and resources, not only within the family itself, but also in the extended family, the social network, or the agencies that will be relevant to future plans.

Furthermore, family therapy has moved toward a greater emphasis on changes in observable behavior rather than primarily, or only, changes in subjective experience. Certainly, family therapists differ greatly in their emphasis upon what Whitaker has called the experiential–symbolic approach (Whitaker & Keith, 1981). However, even in the work of Whitaker there is great attention to changes that are observable. These various features of present-day family therapy have moved much more toward a consultation model than we believe has been generally recognized. Thus, some of these contrasts are becoming less striking with respect to much present-day family therapy, as well as to brief forms of individual psychotherapy, in comparison to consultation. Although therapy with individuals or families is moving toward a more consultative model, the terminology of therapy often muddles the thinking of therapists and constitutes a handicap in communicating with clients, families, and nonfamily therapy colleagues.

Later chapters will illustrate how work can shift from consultation to therapy, from consultation to teaching, and from consultation to supervision, or may move in a reverse direction with somewhat greater difficulty. Consultation can serve as a stock-taking stage in which a decision can be sensibly made about what kind of relationship is appropriate thereafter. It may be apparent that the family and consultee are able to proceed without further professional intervention or action. On the other hand, it may be appropriate to shift to an explicit therapeutic, supervisory, or teaching relationship. The following example indicates the importance of role clarification when consultation is added to therapy.

Consultant or cotherapist? A case example. A therapist who was bogged down in therapy with a contentious couple proposed that a colleague with whom he had often worked as a cotherapist be called in as a consultant. He suggested the consultation very much in the manner that a physician might call in another colleague for a second opinion about treatment that is in difficulty. In this instance, the first session with the consultant present became intensely involved and confusing, and neither the primary therapist nor the consultant adequately defined the consultant's role. Without discussion, consultation quickly evolved into cotherapy. Only later, after further sessions, did the woman in the couple start to object strenuously that this was not the therapy that she had bargained for; the "new person" was still here even though she had understood, correctly, that this was supposed to be a consultation, which implied to her a temporary and advisory function. By that time, the alignments between the four participants were too complicated to be reshaped as either therapy or consultation. An unsatisfactory termination soon followed. Some of the difficulties that emerged could be directly attributed to a failure to define and maintain a meta role for the consultant or, alternatively, to establish clearly a new phase of therapy with a cotherapist.

THE TEACHING-CONSULTATION CONTINUUM

Just as consultation may flow into therapy, and vice versa, so teaching and consultation have some commonalities and may flow into each other. A discussion of the similarities and difference between teaching and consultation will provide a basis for an examination of the interface between these two activities. There are some fundamental similarities in that both consultant and teacher may provide educational functions and both may facilitate learning and growth.

The differences between teaching and consultation are many. The traditional teacher chooses the information to be taught and decides upon the syllabus and teaching format. In consultation, it is the consultee who requests the information that he or she believes would be helpful. In teaching, the focus is broadly or narrowly based upon the topic to be taught. In consultation, the consultant focuses upon the problem presented by the consultee. Traditional teaching is content-oriented; consultation uses the content as a vehicle for a process orientation. Focus upon the process by the consultant allows the consultant to support the consultee's competence and the consultee's eventual ability to handle the problem on his or her own. This differs from didactic teaching in which the goal is acquisition of knowledge by the student.

Another significant difference that occurs between teaching and consultation lies in the kind of relationship that exists between the teacher–student and the consultant–consultee. In a teaching relationship, the hierarchy is clear: The teacher usually is senior to and more knowledgeable than the student. The consultation role grows out of a relationship between colleagues, a relationship of peers, in which one colleague is requesting information from another colleague who has some expertise in a well-defined area. The consultant is a resource and adviser for the colleague requesting the consultation, whereas the teacher has some supraordinate responsibility for helping the student to learn.

Because consultation involves a symmetrical relationship but teaching involves a complementary relationship, the student and the consultee may use the information generated by these two roles in quite a different fashion. The consultee can reject or modify the consultant's input. Traditionally, the student is expected to accept the teacher's advice and acknowledge the teacher's greater expertise without excessive protest. In addition, teaching is organized by the teacher within an institutional system in advance of the course taking place. Consultation, on the other hand, occurs in an ad hoc way with the time and content determined by the consultee and his or her needs. Most important, the teacher evaluates the student's performance both formally and informally. In consultation, it is the consultee who evaluates the consultant, deciding whether to accept the consultant's recommendations. Also, the consultee ultimately may decide whether to seek a consultation again when another problem arises.

While there are many specific differences between these two roles, the boundaries between them are often fluid. It is at the interface of these boundaries where it is very important for the individual to negotiate explicitly the role that is appropriate to the context and to the problem. Part of what makes negotiating these roles difficult is that teaching may occur within the context of consultation and consultation may occur within the context of teaching.

Learning a lesson: A case example. An example of confusion between these roles occurred when a medical faculty group requested that a family therapist "teach" a group interested in medical care and family systems theory. However, the family therapist did not adequately clarify this contract and entered the group as a traditional teacher, determining what the "students" needed to learn about family systems theory as well as sharing her expertise about the particular cases that were discussed. Despite her knowledge about systems principles and her attempts to be helpful, she perceived dissatisfaction and conflict about her role from the other group members. Among colleagues, the teaching approach was destined to fail because the teaching role implied more of a one-up position than was appropriate for this group. She had moved into a teaching role prematurely without recognizing the history of peer relationships that characterized the group.

After about 6 weeks, the therapist realized that a less expansive, consultation approach was more appropriate for her position in this group. She shifted gears and renegotiated her role. In this new framework, she focused on what the faculty defined as their needs. She requested feedback from other group members and was able to develop relationships of more mutuality and exchange. The group took a more case-oriented approach in which all members could express their particular perspectives. Moving to this way of functioning as a colleague was much more effective in meeting the goals of teaching and exchanging ideas about family systems theory as well as facilitating the group process.

Confusion in the other direction can occur when consultation is part of a larger teaching framework. For example, in the medical context, residents often approach faculty with "consult requests" in which it is unclear whether teaching or consultation is more appropriate. For a faculty member to respond as if this request is pure "consultation" may be premature. At that stage, the teaching role usually should be supraordinate.

Another situation in which teaching and consultation overlap occurs when a faculty person uses case consultation for illustrative purposes as part of teaching within the context of a seminar. Still another instance of overlap is found when a seminar format grows out of a larger consultation framework after the consultee has requested a specific package of information. In the latter situation, the consultation differs from teaching in that no formal evaluation is given by the consultant, and the material that is taught is oriented toward the consultee's particular needs or problems.

Ministering to their needs: A case example. A consultant was working with a number of ministers individually on specific problem cases in their congregations. He found that all of these ministers were dealing with problems involving family systems issues. A few of the ministers requested a more formal teaching format around family systems principles, and the consultant organized a 10-week seminar that focused upon working with families. In this situation, the teaching seminar was an extension of the case-consultation format. The seminar was limited in time and content, with the curriculum based on the specific questions and problems of the ministers. There was no evaluation of the participants by the consultant.

It is interesting to note that more modern approaches to teaching move closer to a consultative model. In these newer teaching approaches, teachers often request evaluations by students and solicit input from students regarding course content. As alluded to earlier, the use of a consultative format in a large teaching framework respects and supports students' autonomy. Regardless of which role is chosen, clarifying the roles of the consultant and the teacher will increase the potential for the family and therapist to succeed at their tasks.

THE SUPERVISION-CONSULTATION CONTINUUM

The relationship between a supervisor and a supervisee is in many ways analogous to the relationship between a teacher and a student, both structurally and functionally. The supervisor is hierarchically superior to the supervisee and brings to the supervisory relationship expertise in some area. While the term "supervisor" is sometimes used more loosely to imply only an advisory role, ordinarily the supervisor is legally and administratively responsible for the supervisee's cases. Neither the teacher nor the consultant have this kind of responsibility for a case. Hence, the supervisor will carefully follow the case, while the teacher and consultant will relate to cases on a more ad hoc and tangential basis. In supervision, the supervisor usually takes initiative; in consultation the consultee has this responsibility. As in teaching, in a supervisory relationship the supervisor is responsible for setting the agenda, determining which cases will be reviewed, when supervision will take place, and when supervision will terminate. In consultation, the consultee is responsible for taking the initiative, deciding which cases will be reviewed, and if and how the consultant's advice will be incorporated into case management.

Occasionally the supervisory relationship may turn into consultation or a consultative relationship may turn into supervision. In these cases, it is crucial to be very clear about the particular role that has been negotiated and to make the role explicit rather than implicit. Implicit roles open the possibility for confusion and resistance.

Becoming colleagues: A case example. Supervision turned into consultation with Dr. S when he moved from being a psychiatric resident to become a junior faculty member. During his residency, he had been working as a supervisee with a senior faculty member. When he joined the faculty, the relationship was renegotiated. Instead of the prior arrangement of meeting on a regular weekly basis with evaluation being done by the supervisor, the relationship was continued on a consultative basis. As a new faculty member, Dr. S decided when and if the senior person would be sought out as a consultant. The key point is that, as the consultee, the former trainee now had primary responsibility for the management of cases. Previously, the supervisor had been the one who "signed off" on clinical records and had primary responsibility. These functions were taken over by the junior faculty member in his role as consultee.

When role changes take place within a training program, a period of consultation may facilitate renegotiating a contract or understanding. Within a supervisory framework, it is possible to use a consultation format in order to stimulate the supervisee to achieve a greater degree of autonomy while the supervisor still retains primary responsibility. This kind of modification usually occurs with more advanced trainees and can be a useful intermediate step toward a true consultative relationship. There is a risk in this kind of transition. Specifically, if a supervisor prematurely shifts to a consultation relationship when the consultee is not ready to assume primary responsibility for the case, the result may be poor therapy and inadequate supervision. However, when well-timed and used in a responsible way by the supervisor, this strategy can be effective in furthering the growth and independent skills of trainees.

Because of the similarity between supervision and consultation, it is easy for the participants to become confused about their specific roles and the contract between them. Role confusion between consultant and consultee may isomorphically reflect or engender a role confusion among family members in a case-oriented family therapy consultation.

The enthusiastic consultant: A case example. A clergyman called a family therapist to inquire about a possible referral for a couple that was experiencing marital difficulty. The clergyman had been working with this couple for several months, but, within the last few weeks, had become increasingly frustrated with the lack of progress in the case. The therapist suggested that instead of accepting the referral he should function as a consultant to the clergyman. The consultation took place at the clergyman's office.

After observing one session with the couple, the consultant, without being asked by the consultee, began to give the consultee advice on the case, directing him to take certain steps if this case were to be managed properly; in effect, he took over the primary responsibility for working with the couple. Stimulated by the case, the consultant taught the clergyman about certain principles regarding couple systems and began to set a course of treatment. As the consultant began to function like a supervisor, difficulties arose in his relationship with the clergyman. There were a number of logistical problems regarding when the next session would take place, who would be at the session, what time the session would occur, who would be responsible for leading the session, and so on. In an effort to manage this confusion, the consultant took even greater charge of the case and discussed how the couple was expected to behave in view of the intervention made by the consultant in previous sessions. Predictably, as the consultant took more responsibility, the consultee became even more elusive and resistant to subsequent work.

The role confusion between consultant and consultee was isomorphic to role confusion of the couple. This immature couple had been struggling with the issue of who was really in charge of the marriage. The husband, who previously had dominated his wife, suddenly found himself in the position of being puzzled but deferential to her about major new activities she was undertaking outside of the marriage.

The consultant began to realize that the confusion between him and the consultee was actually mirroring and exacerbating the role confusion between the couple. When he noticed this pattern, the consultant sought to clarify the extent of his responsibility in the case. He called the consultee and renegotiated the contract, stating very clearly that he would be available to the consultee but that the consultee was really in charge of the case and could use the consultant when necessary. The consultant also began to ask for the consultee's opinion about how the case could be more effectively managed. Shifting more to a relationship between colleagues empowered the consultee, who began to resume charge of the case.

In this example the consultee clearly had primary responsibility for the case; the context did not permit the consultant to assume primary responsibility for it. In order to function as a supervisor, a supervisor must be delegated authority from an individual or organization. For these reasons, senior family therapists working with more junior clinicians in private practice, outside an organizational framework, may have difficulties in obtaining compliance with supervisory instructions. Usually consultation offers a more appropriate model for that kind of relationship because the private practitioner has the right and responsibility to decide whether to reject or accept the suggestions made by the consultant.

Therefore, it is necessary to be very clear about the roles of supervisor–supervisee and consultant–consultee. When there is a confusion in the roles and in the nature of the contract, the confusion can result in frustration and mismanagement not only for the professionals involved but also for the clients who expect to be the beneficiaries of clinical expertise. Thus, in the above case, there was an initial referral to a therapist. The therapist turned the referral into a consultation, yet began to act like a supervisor without the authority to implement this role. This unilateral role shift resulted in confusion not only with the consultee but also with the couple. After the consultant had clarified his role, his relationship with the consultee improved and, in turn, this had a positive effect upon work with the couple.

THE ADMINISTRATION-CONSULTATION CONTINUUM

Supervision and consultation overlap along a continuum in the assessment and treatment of specific cases. There is a parallel continuum that can be found between administration and consultation in the management of programs and agencies. Here the consultant may be hired by an agency, clinic, or program that is, in turn, a subsystem of a larger organization. Such consultations require a systems orientation that goes beyond the family even more than is necessary in the kinds of consultations that we have discussed above. However, the same kinds of principles are involved. The difference is that specific patients and families are more focally involved in case consultations and larger systems are involved in program consultations.

The line between administration and program consultation is especially ambiguous and may create difficulties. For example, an administrator, such as a departmental chairperson, may be an in-house consultant. The chairperson may believe that it would be useful to become familiar with the clinical functioning of various staff members and may decide to be a consultant to their work. This arrangement is fraught with difficulties if the chairperson does not clearly allow the staff to retain responsibility for case management. If that person implicitly or explicitly overrides the staff's judgment, he or she is not usually serving as a consultant but, rather, is still operating within the administrative role. The latter role may be appropriate under certain circumstances, but it is preferable that it not be confused or obscured by expectations that ordinarily are associated with consultation.

Even more problematic is a situation in which a program consultant becomes important in an organization and starts to take over administrative functions. This may take place quietly and covertly when the consultant has considerable prestige and the formal administrator is not so highly regarded by staff members. Under such circumstances, the consultant can easily undermine the formal organization of whatever structure remains. This may result in a major policy fight and the consultant may be unceremoniously fired.

Challenging the boss: A case example. Problems occurred in a setting in which a departmental chairman was a member of a faculty T-group that was meeting with an organizational consultant. The staff members used the T-group to express their dissatisfaction and undercut the formal authority of the departmental chairman. Despite the consultant's efforts to contain this rebellion within the setting of the consultation workshop, the chairman felt that his position had been inappropriately challenged and that this continuing consultation was disruptive. The consultant was therefore dismissed. Although the staff members had been invited by the consultant to speak their minds, it is questionable whether this could have happened in a constructive fashion. The consultant did not have a contract with the chairman that would enable him to negate the usual hierarchy and to work with the organization, including the chairman, as if it were a peer group.

Such problems in the distinction between administration and consultation will arise if the consultant shifts from working with one consultee, such as the chairman, to another, such as the staff, without explicitly renegotiating the consultation contract. Informal contracts during extended consultations can shift in subtle ways and need to be reviewed regularly.

Also, a consultant working with a divisional or component program needs to understand the overall administrative structure and to obtain support from the upper level director. For example, family therapists working as consultants with members of a staff oriented only to individual therapy, or to pharmacotherapy, may find that the consultation is viewed by the overall administration as not helpful or, worse, as subversive. Especially in instances of repeated case consultations, an alertness to organizational issues is a concern that systems consultants must always have in mind.

Figure 2-1 schematizes the pattern of relationship between the various systems that relate to family consultations. It should be noted that not only is there a continuum between family therapy and family consultation, between supervision and consultation, and so on, but also that there are clear differences between therapy and supervision, teaching and administration, and so on. The general point that we wish to emphasize is that the lines are easily blurred and that roles are often transformed during the course of ongoing relationships. We believe that the renegotiation of roles will facilitate productive work in this field, and that the clear recognition of the role of a systems consultant is an alternative that needs to be initially considered and regularly reconsidered.

FIGURE 2-1. Systems consultations and other roles in the helping professions.

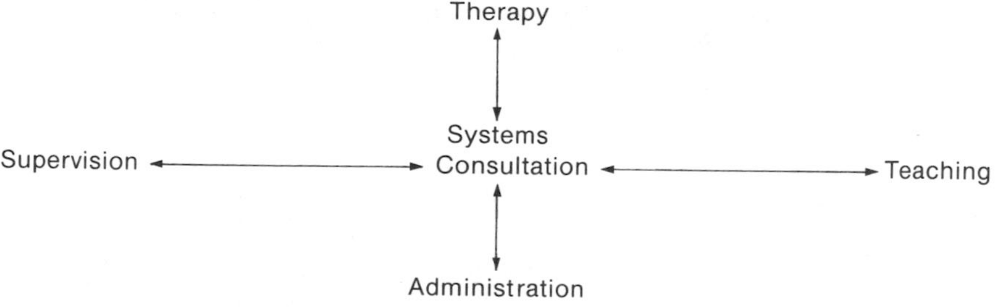

REFERENCES

Anderson, C. M., Hogarty, G. E., & Reiss, D. J. Family treatment of adult schizophrenic patients: A psychoeducational approach. *Schizophrenia Bulletin*, 1980, *6*, 490–505.

Whitaker, C. A., & Keith, D. V. Symbolic–experiential family therapy. In A. Gurman & D. Kniskern (Eds)., *Handbook of family therapy*. New York: Brunner/Mazel, 1981.

Wynne, L. C. *The educational component in family therapy: New directions and opportunities*. Paper presented at American Association for Marriage and Family Therapy meeting, Rochester, NY, May 16, 1981.

3

SIGNPOSTS FOR A SYSTEMS CONSULTATION

TIMOTHY T. WEBER

SUSAN H. McDANIEL

LYMAN C. WYNNE

University of Rochester School of Medicine and Dentistry
Rochester, New York

Consultants are like hikers in uncharted woods. The terrain of consultation can be confusing and its boundaries ambiguous, and there is no map to guide the consultant's behavior. As we have indicated, maps automatically transposed from therapy, teaching, supervision, or administration simply will not suffice. Although concepts from family therapy, for example, may help one to understand the territory of consultation and to implement changes, the two territories, consultation and therapy, have different terrains, requiring consultants to use a map somewhat different from the one they would use as therapists.

We are not proposing a specific map for consultation, that is, a fixed set of directions as to how to proceed, what turns to make, or how far to go down the path before changing course. That kind of map fixes a consultant on a too narrow, preconceived route that impairs recognition of the unique contours and alternative pathways in the terrain of a specific consultation. Consultants who are focused on their own agenda rather than on the unique problems and needs of the consultee's territory are on a perilous course. Caplan (1970) commented that the consultant's "conceptual map must indicate the limits of his professional domain. Although his role may not be obviously prestructured, he is not in fact free to do anything that comes into his head or to respond completely to all requests from would-be consultees" (p. 31).

We shall present here a set of questions, a checklist that can be thought of as signposts to assist the consultant in mapping the territory distinctive for each consultation. These questions are intended to heighten the consultant's sensitivity to the consultee's terrain and to sharpen the consultant's inquiry, formulation, and implementation. Although the answers to these questions are highly diversified, as illustrated in the chapters that follow, the questions themselves and the order in which they are presented constitute a guide that will help organize the consultant's thoughts and behaviors. We present these signposts as a practical guide for beginners learning consultation skills in training programs and as a reminder for more experienced consultants. (For detailed descriptions of the procedures of traditional forms of consultation, see Gallesich, 1982, and Parsons & Meyers, 1984.) This checklist has been constructed with the consultant in mind. Consultees will want to consider a complementary series of questions that need to be asked when a consultation is requested and carried out.

Our questions can be grouped in relation to seven processes of consultation: (1) exploring the possibility of consultation; (2) contracting; (3) connecting; (4) assessing; (5) implementing; (6) evaluating; and (7) leaving. We prefer to use the term "processes" instead of "stages" in order to highlight their fluidity and overlap. "Stage" connotes a fixed progression from one step to the next, whereas "process" more accurately describes how these steps intertwine in the consultant's actual work. For example, during the connecting process, the consultant is also assessing the structure of the organization. It should also be noted that consultants may work with only one individual as the consultee, for example, with a family therapist who is seeking consultation about a family in treatment. More commonly, the consultation takes place with organizations in which there may be subcontracts with specific groups or individuals. Later, a consultant may terminate his or her work with one part of the organization while concurrently revising the consultation contract and connecting with another part of the organization. Thus, the processes overlap, even though there is a general sequential order that the consultant follows from entry to exit.

CHECKLIST FOR A CONSULTANT

A. Exploring
1. Who is the person making the request? That is, who is the potential consultee? Is the potential consultee another *professional* who has responsibility for therapy, teaching, and so on, with a client or organization, or is the consultee a *nonprofessional* person, family, or group that wants assistance in making decisions about the future?
2. How is the problem initially described? How explicit is the request for consultation?

3. How did the request come about? Is the person who makes the request doing so on behalf of someone else? If the person making the request is a member of a work organization or a family, what role does he or she have?
4. Is a consultant role appropriate for this particular request? May another role be more appropriate?
5. What are the political ramifications of this potential consultation?
6. Why were you, rather than someone else, asked to consult?
7. What personal or professional investment do you have in the success or failure of this consultation?

B. Contracting
1. What are the initial target problems and goals that the consultee and you as the consultant have agreed to consider?
2. What services do you agree to provide?
3. What services does the consultee agree to provide?
4. What procedures will be used for sharing information during the consultation?
5. Who will participate directly and indirectly in the consultation?
6. Who are the other professionals working with the consultee? Are there supervisors, administrators, or other consultants who have an impact or influence upon the consultee?
7. Where will the consultation take place?
8. What are the fee arrangements?
9. Have the initial, minimal conditions for proceeding with an effective consultation been met?
10. What are the potential risks and consequences of this consultation?

C. Connecting
1. Given the consultation context, what joining techniques can you use with the consultee, including various subsystems of the organization? How formal or informal should the joining process be with this consultee?
2. Who are the key members of the consultation system and how will they be involved in shaping the goals and methods of the consultation?

D. Assessing
1. What methods can you use to gather information and educate yourself about the system?
2. What are the important hierarchies, coalitions, triangles, and boundary problems in the organization?
3. How are you perceived by the consultee, the different subsystems, and key individuals within the organization?

4. What stage of the "life cycle" is the system in? How does this stage shape the consultation request and your task?
5. What recent events have prompted the consultation request?
6. What attempts have been made to solve the target problems in the past, either internally or by using an outside consultant? What have been the results of these attempted solutions?
7. What are the explicit and implicit belief systems of the consultee?
8. What are the implicit requests of the consultee?

E. Implementing
1. What are the particular methods chosen by you and the consultee for meeting the consultation request?
2. How can the recommendations of the consultation be framed to be consistent with the organization's belief system?
3. Is education and information giving explicitly incorporated into the consultation? If so, how?
4. Will you continue to collaborate with the consultee in implementing the consultation plan? If so, how?
5. What procedures, if any, are used to insure the durability of change after termination of the consultation?
6. Have new goals arisen during the consultation? How are they to be addressed?

F. Evaluating
1. What assessment procedures will be used to evaluate the consultation? Who should participate in the evaluation?
2. What changes have occurred in the organization during the period of the consultation both from your perspective and from that of the consultee?
3. What goals were not met by the consultation, and why?
4. What are the plans for follow-up evaluation?
5. What have you learned through this consultation that will be applicable in the future? What role do you feel you have played in the successes and failures of the consultation?

G. Leaving
1. Under what circumstances may it be appropriate to renegotiate a consultation contract for a new problem, or for a new relationship and another role?
2. How can you best conclude your relationship with the consultee and leave the consultation system?

Consultation usually begins with a preliminary phase in which the potential consultant and consultee explore, formally or informally, the possibility of a consultation. For example, when the potential consultee is another professional, the contact may be as informal as a luncheon conversation about a case that poses problems, or it may involve a formal request from an organization for consultation with an outside expert. In our view, it is important for the person whose services are requested to think clearly about the role he or she is being asked to assume. The variations could involve the referral or transfer of a case for treatment or discussion. The possibility of consultation should be considered even though a request has been made for another kind of service, such as supervision or teaching.

Many consultations occur at a time of upheaval in individuals, families, or organizations. It is important during the exploratory phase to be alert to the implicit requests and political ramifications of the proposed consultation. It is possible to be caught up in various power maneuvers before one is able to establish a clear position as a consultant. Becoming an unwitting agent to one side in a power struggle is incompatible with effective consultation.

We wish to emphasize that the process of contracting involves reciprocal transactions between consultant and consultee. It should not be a matter of only accepting or rejecting a contract; there should be a period of negotiating that sets the tone for the give-and-take characteristic of a good consultation. At the same time one must be alert to conditions that could tie one's hands, for example, the withholding of relevant information. Written contracts clarify the responsibilities and conditions necessary for the consultation to proceed effectively.

Effective implementation of the consultation is dependent on how one connects with various parts of the system. It is especially important to connect with those members of the system who are powerful and central to determining how decisions are implemented in the system. Both formal and informal settings provide opportunities for solidifying the joining process.

Often because of turmoil in systems, consultees may press for quick solutions to complex problems. It is important for the consultant to allow plenty of time for connecting, observing, questioning, and general assessment. Just as diagnosis and treatment intertwine and overlap in therapy, so assessment and implementation phases of consultation are intimately connected. Because consultation is often requested during a period of turmoil for a person or organization, much of the assessment process involves coming to understand what is fueling the turmoil and how the problem may be resolved. The consultant may be able to understand these problems quite early as a result of explicit request, but often the specific assessment process is complex and ongoing throughout the consultation.

Central to the role of the consultant is his or her position meta to the system; the consultant does not have primary responsibility for deciding which recommendations will be accepted or implemented. Other roles, such as therapist, supervisor, or administrator, require one to assume direct responsibility within the system.

Both informal and formal methods of evaluation can provide data not only for renegotiation or continuation of the consultation contract but also for future similar consultations. The consultant should include his or her own role in the consultation as part of the evaluation. Although the consultant needs to give primary attention to an evaluation of whether the original goals were achieved, unanticipated consequences—both positive and negative—should not be overlooked in the evaluation.

As in therapy, terminating a consultation may be difficult. The gratifications of the consultative relationship may tempt all participants to continue beyond resolution of the problem stipulated in the original contract. Consultative relationships that have a long-standing or renewed time frame need to be reviewed periodically and considered as to whether termination is overdue. Many temptations exist in every consultation for the consultant to view himself or herself as indispensable. In an ideal consultation, the system prospers and grows after the consultant's departure.

REFERENCES

Caplan, G. *The theory of practice of mental health consultation.* New York: Basic Books, 1970.

Galessich, J. *The profession and practice of consultation.* San Francisco: Jossey-Bass, 1982.

Parsons, R. D., & Meyers, J. *Developing consultation skills: A guide to training, development, and assessment for human services professionals.* San Francisco: Jossey-Bass, 1984.

4

LOSING YOUR WAY AS A CONSULTANT

TIMOTHY T. WEBER

LYMAN C. WYNNE

SUSAN H. McDANIEL

University of Rochester School of Medicine and Dentistry
Rochester, New York

The previous chapters have outlined the primary principles and tasks of systems consultation. Such outlines can be deceptively simple. The reader may have the illusion that by following this approach, a successful outcome is assured. Life is seldom so tidy, especially in systems consultation where the complexity of the field affords ample opportunities for failure.

Our conceptualization of systems consultation has become clearer to us the more we have examined our failures; these failures have helped us to refine our methods, strategies, and techniques. What follows are seven brief case examples that illustrate typical failures we have encountered in systems consultation and exemplify the issues and principles that we believe were involved. Each of these examples illustrates failures that have occurred across one or more of the phases of consultation discussed in Chapter 3.

FAILURE #1: LOOK BEFORE YOU LEAP

With much enthusiasm the Family Clinic at Southern Hospital opened its doors to the public. The clinic's mandate was not only to provide clinical services to patients within the hospital and the community, but also to offer educational resources to organizations in the area and to other services within the hospital. The clinic's first major thrust beyond its own borders was to further a working relationship with other hospital services, partly to increase its service to the hospital and partly to enlarge its referral base. Ms. Melinda Gray, a nurse in the Oncology Clinic, had expressed an interest in working more closely with the Family Clinic and had mentioned the possibility of involving the staff of the Family Clinic in future research projects and in clinical case consultations.

One afternoon Ms. Gray called one of the family therapists in the Family Clinic to request specific help with a patient and her family. The Oncology Clinic had been following 18-year-old Tracy Boston, an attractive college freshman who had developed a brain tumor 5 years before. During much of the 5 years, the oncology staff believed that treatment might be successful. The staff had taken great pride in their professional expertise and had admired Tracy's zest for life. Likewise, Tracy's family had become close to the clinic staff, especially in the early years when Tracy's pain was great and the prognosis was uncertain.

Within the last 6 months, the tumor had begun growing again, and was now to the point where the clinic staff rapidly was losing hope for Tracy's recovery. They were becoming highly distressed not only for Tracy but also for Tracy's family, which was having trouble coping with the possibility that she was going to die. Despite the staff members' awareness that Tracy's condition was bleak, they seemed to be frozen in their ability to work with Tracy and her family about the problem of her impending death.

Ms. Gray was close to desperation when she called the Family Clinic one afternoon. As she spoke to a family therapist in the clinic, she phrased her request as follows: "I am working with a family that is having trouble accepting their daughter's imminent death. Can you help us?" Ms. Gray elaborated the details of Tracy's condition and mentioned that she was having difficulty broaching the subject of Tracy's serious condition with the family. Tracy's parents had been concerned that their daughter should not lose hope despite the prospect of her dying; they wanted to avoid talking about it among themselves and with Tracy. Ms. Gray was uncertain how to proceed with this family and requested the family therapist's assistance.

As Ms. Gray continued to talk about the case, the family therapist realized that this could be the ideal entering point for the Family Clinic to establish its credibility with the Oncology Clinic. Without considering the benefits of assuming the meta position of a consultant in this case, the family therapist immediately accepted what seemed to be a referral. He invited Ms. Gray to participate as a cotherapist, sensing that he would need some assistance with this problem, and asked her to invite the entire family for the first interview.

The first session with the entire family (Tracy, her parents, and her siblings) moved very slowly and at times seemed to be at the point of a quick termination even before the session concluded. Mrs. Boston, Tracy's mother, moved restlessly in her seat throughout the session as she periodically glanced in disgust at the family therapist and Ms. Gray. Occasionally she commented that it was important for people to have hope and that it was unfortunate that hope could be taken away so easily. All the family members and Ms. Gray seemed to stray far afield from the topic of concern: Tracy's serious condition.

Because the session seemed stuck, the family therapist retreated to a private discussion with Ms. Gray in another room. Only at this point did he find out why the referral for therapy had been made. He learned that Dr. Stone, the attending physician in the Oncology Clinic who had diagnosed Tracy as terminally ill, had refused to talk to Tracy and her family about her dying. Consequently the responsibility (and anxiety) for work with Tracy and her family had been passed to Ms. Gray who, in desperation, had passed on the anxiety and responsibility to the Family Clinic, specifically, to the family therapist. While the family therapist was well aware that this family had difficulty facing Tracy's imminent death, he had not inquired about complications within the clinic staff and was unaware of how he had welcomed the clinic's anxiety with open arms. The family therapist and Ms. Gray returned to the family and brought the session to a swift conclusion. The family therapist then shifted to a consulting role and worked with both the clinic staff and the Boston family. Seven weeks later, Tracy died.

The major problem in this case was that the family therapist had prematurely assumed the role of therapist, surrendering the meta position of a consultant. Instead of looking over the system to determine what role would be best for the particular problem, he quickly leaped into the specific role of family therapist, taking both the responsibility and anxiety for dealing with this family. Had he taken the role of a consultant instead of immediately accepting this referral for therapy, he would have met with Ms. Gray and other staff in the Oncology Clinic to discuss the dimensions of the problem, their attempts to solve the problem, and what could have been done within their own program, realizing that therapy might become indicated at a later time. The pressing problem was between the Boston family and the Oncology Clinic. Members of this system were denying the imminence of Tracy's death and the implications of failure. This crisis within the oncology staff, mixed with the feelings of a desperate family, prompted everyone to look for someone else to bear the burden. The family therapist, intent on helping those who needed help, was a likely candidate.

It is wise to look before leaping, *to define oneself in a consultant role and to retain this role until it is clear what is being specifically requested* and how the particular needs of the system can best be addressed. Starting from the meta position of a consultant makes it easier to reach a consensus about appropriate later roles.

FAILURE #2: A CASE OF MISTAKEN IDENTITY

"I need your help, James. I think you'd be real good with the problem I'm working on now. Do you have a moment to talk?" Beth Dercum's request was sufficiently attractive to lure James Hastings into a brief meeting. Beth and James were both family therapists on the staff of the Family Service Center, a community agency within a large metropolitan area. They had been on the staff of the Family Service Center for several years now and had collaborated on a number of educational projects. James had several more years of experience than Beth and, in addition, had received extensive training in family therapy at well-known training institutes. Beth respected James's therapeutic skills and thought that he might be just the person to help her.

Beth explained her predicament to James: "A few weeks ago I began to teach a small class of university students who wanted to gain more exposure to family therapy during this quarter. I thought it would be valuable for them to see a live session with a family, and so I invited the students to come over next week to observe a family session from behind a one-way mirror. My problem is that I would like to sit behind the mirror with the students and comment on someone else working with the family. When I thought of the person who could best show these students how to work with a family, I thought of you."

James's curiosity peaked as he thought about the proposed interview. He asked Beth to continue. "What's interesting, James, is that a family I worked with about 2 years ago just called me and requested to return to therapy. Ed and Ruth Smith are the parents, and they have two children: Tom is 17 years old and Ann is 14. Ruth Smith called me the other day and said that they were having problems with Tom again, and they thought they needed some help."

James asked Beth about her work with the Smith family 2 years ago. With an undertone of frustration, Beth told James that her work with the Smith family had not gone as well as she had hoped: "The first time they came in, the parents were having problems with both Tom and Ann who were unruly, weren't interested in helping around the house, and had poor grades at school. It seemed to me that the parents, Ed and Ruth, were having a very difficult time talking with each other. After meeting with the family for a few sessions and with Tom and Ann, I suggested to the parents that we meet together and work out difficulties that they were having with each other. They came to a few sessions together, and then the wife came alone for a few more sessions; but she failed to continue. I had a lot of trouble trying to get the family to come to the meetings and finally I couldn't even get the parents to come in. I really don't understand why they want to come back to see me now. But they did call, and we've made the first appointment for next week."

It was agreed that during the demonstration family interview Beth would comment on James's work with the Smith family and, after the interview, James and Beth would meet and discuss the interview with the students. James stipulated that Beth first get the consent of the Smith family to be interviewed in front of the university students. Beth immediately called the Smith family and got their consent.

In the days before the interview with the Smith family, James thought about what he wanted to accomplish in this exercise. He thought of himself as a consultant to Beth. He wanted to help her get a fresh start with the Smith family and to avoid some of the pitfalls that had impeded treatment in the past. He knew that it would be important to frame the problem in such a way that the parents would not feel blamed for the problems of their children, especially because Beth had seemed to underscore their marital difficulty prematurely in the first round of therapy two years ago. It also seemed useful to relabel the family's difficulties as a developmental crisis around Tom's leaving home for a distant college. Besides serving as a consultant to Beth, James envisioned his role to the university students as that of a teacher who would demonstrate some basic principles of engaging the family, interviewing the family, and diagnosing the problem from a systems orientation in a nonblaming manner.

Because the Smiths had already consented to be interviewed in front of the university students, little time was spent before the interview in discussing the procedural arrangements. James and the Smiths walked into the interview room, and Beth and her university students went into the room behind the one-way mirror. The interview progressed as James had expected. He engaged the family, asked for a specific definition of the problem by all family members, supported each family member when he could, and gently nudged them toward viewing the problem as a developmental one, with the challenge of reorganizing themselves in new ways. He conducted the interview with only mild intensity, hoping to link the family back into therapy while demonstrating to the university students some of the basic principles of family interviewing. He thought that some of the more subtle notions of how he viewed the problem and some possible treatment strategies could be communicated to Beth at a later point.

As James was concluding the interview, he told the Smiths that he would be consulting with Mrs. Dercum about the interview. He wished the Smith family success in their work with Mrs. Dercum and said that he hoped that they would be able to pursue the goals that they had identified in this consultation interview. Before James was finished, Mrs. Smith abruptly interrupted him: "Hold it! Aren't *you* going to be our therapist?" Mr. Smith then reinforced his wife's claim on James: "We thought you were going to continue to work with us! Now that we have something started, we'd like to continue with you." James was flattered, but bewildered. He thought Beth had explained to the Smith family that he was a consultant to Beth and also was demonstrating how to interview a family to the university students. What had Beth told the Smith family about this interview? James excused himself and retreated behind the one-way mirror. After a discussion with Beth, James agreed to continue with the Smith family in therapy. However, a high price had been paid for this first interview. Instead of therapy beginning with clarity, it commenced with confusion.

The problem in this case is that the contract was not clear. James thought that he was serving as a consultant to Beth and secondarily was demonstrating interviewing techniques to the university students. Beth had assumed that James was going to conduct the demonstration interview in a teaching format and implicitly hoped that she might interest James in assuming the role of therapist for this family. When she approached James with her consultation request, she essentially had masked an important part of the request; "Take this problem off my hands." James's emotional investment in demonstrating his interviewing skills undoubtedly undermined his ability to identify Beth's underlying agenda. The Smith family thought that James was going to serve as their therapist. They had agreed to be interviewed in front of the university students only because they wanted to start afresh with someone other than Beth.

In summary, there were contractual misunderstandings between the consultant, the consultee, and the family. James had not clarified what Beth wanted. Furthermore, had James and Beth met with the Smith family prior to the interview and discussed with them the contract more clearly, the Smiths would not have continued with the assumption throughout the interview that James was their new therapist. This case illustrates the crucial importance of *clarifying the consultation contract, specifying the goals of consultation, determining who will do what, and communicating that understanding to the key people in the system*, including those who provide and those who are provided with the consultation.

FAILURE #3: SECRETS

A family therapist in the community received a call from Mrs. Bonnie Smith, a supervisor at Western Travel Agency. Mrs. Smith had heard this family therapist give an interesting talk on family communication at a workshop in the community several weeks before. She had thought about how his expertise could be useful to the personnel at Western Travel Agency, and she had called him to request his assistance in helping her colleagues with what she described as "communication problems." Mrs. Smith met with the family therapist/consultant at lunch one day to discuss these problems.

Mrs. Smith explained that she recently had noticed that the 20 employees of the agency had been lagging in their performance. She described how employees seemed to be disgruntled with each other and not as enthusiastic about their work as they had been. Furthermore, conflicts between certain key employees who had been there for a number of years were creating an atmosphere that made it difficult for the employees to serve the customers. Mrs. Smith was interested in having the employees learn how to cooperate rather than compete. She thought that if the employees were to have a better sense of themselves as individuals and greater clarity about their personal goals, their values, and their career interests, they would find more energy for their work.

After his conversation with Mrs. Smith, the consultant began to prepare an elaborate 2-day consultation that emphasized communication skills, self-awareness, life-work planning, and so on. The workshop was planned for Friday night and all day Saturday. As preparations were made to involve all the employees, some of the key employees requested permission to be absent because of prior commitments, exhaustion, lack of time, and so on. Despite the absence of key employees, the workshop was held. During the workshop, the consultant had a difficult time engaging many of the employees around the goals and procedures. Some employees were overheard during one of the breaks commenting: "The last thing in the world we need is one of these touchy–feelie workshops by a shrink." In spite of the consultant's careful preparation and his preworkshop consultation with Mrs. Smith, he found himself exasperated and puzzled as to why his careful plans were being met with such disdain; perhaps he had not prepared carefully enough, or perhaps he had not joined with the employees at the outset of the workshop.

What had contributed to the failure of the consultation with Western Travel Agency? In this case, the consultant had failed to contract with a person with broad enough authority and also had failed to consider possible implicit agendas behind the consultation request. The explicit request was to "help our employees." Had the consultant examined the system from a broader perspective, he would have found that the implicit request was: "I need to show the new bosses of this business that I know what I'm doing, that I'm sensitive to the employees, and that I want to improve their production."

What the consultant did not know was that Western Travel Agency had recently been acquired by a larger travel agency. This parent corporation had met with the employees of Western Travel Agency and had told them that new roles and positions for employees were under consideration and that those positions would be determined within the next several months. Under the parent corporation's new proposal, several supervisors would now be put under one primary supervisor. The secondary supervisors would be in charge of different tasks within Western Travel Agency, but the primary supervisor would monitor the activities of the secondary supervisors and would communicate directly to corporate executives in the parent corporation.

Knowing that the system was in flux and that the executives of the parent corporation were very carefully looking at all the supervisors, Mrs. Smith decided to seek an "insider's track" by impressing the new management with her organizational sensitivity. Essentially, she was trying to edge out other supervisors for the top spot in the new organization. She had communicated with the parent corporation several times about her interest in bringing in a consultant to help the employees with communication, personal development, and office skills. Rather than having a real interest in any positive outcome of the workshop itself, Mrs. Smith had been more interested in obtaining the consultant's services as a way of establishing her potential expertise in the new organization.

When a consultant is asked to assist an individual or organization in dealing with a problem, the consultant will be tempted to focus only on the explicit presenting problem as defined by the person requesting the consultation. Lurking behind the explicit problem may be a host of implicit agendas that may be kept hidden from the consultant. The consultant will be trapped if he or she responds only to the explicit problem; *implicit agendas should be fully explored.*

FAILURE #4: GOING THROUGH THE MOTIONS

After months of negotiations, the contract had finally been awarded. A special committee of the Department of Psychiatry at Parkview Hospital was delighted that the department would be providing consultation services to the New Life Residential Treatment Center. Directors of the Department of Psychiatry and New Life had agreed that the consultation contract would benefit both organizations. The Department of Psychiatry had been interested in both the potential consultation income and in the opportunity to give psychiatric residents experience in working with a community residential treatment center. The management of New Life was under some pressure to demonstrate its effectiveness as a residential treatment center. It had been awarded several contracts by the state and, as part of the agreement, needed to document that it was receiving consultation services from an outside organization.

Details of the consultation were arranged between the directors of New Life and a special committee of the Department of Psychiatry. The psychiatric residents were assigned to deliver consultation services to the staff at New Life. Although this staff had not participated in defining what type of consultation services were needed, they were given the assignment of welcoming the psychiatric residents and of consulting with them according to the terms of the consultation contract.

The psychiatric residents considered this consultation low on their list of priorities. They were heavily committed to responsibilities at the hospital and with community groups. They had not participated in the contract negotiations and believed that their mentors were only mildly interested in this consultation. There was no faculty coordinator for the consultation and the residents were simply assigned to work with the staff of New Life.

The initial meeting between the residents and the New Life staff was planned and postponed several times. After this tentative beginning, the residents did meet with the New Life staff with the goal of clarifying exactly what help was needed and what resources the residents had to offer. The residents found that the New Life staff members wanted help, but had difficulty describing exactly what their problems were and how they wanted assistance. Staff members described vague problems and highlighted difficulties with the upper management of New Life, which the residents could do nothing about. They also could not help with the staff's criticism of the treatment center, especially that its architecture seemed antiquated and not designed to meet the psychotherapeutic needs of the community. Staff members repeatedly discussed the pressing need for a group room large enough to accommodate the entire population of New Life.

The psychiatric residents had difficulty connecting with the staff. They had little sense of what the problems of the New Life staff were and how they could be of help. Frequently the residents asked themselves why they were there. At the same time, they were reluctant to push the New Life staff to be specific. Exhausted from their other duties at the hospital, the residents fulfilled their consultation obligations by meeting with the New Life staff, but did little else to push for a more effective consultation. Both the New Life team and the team of residents were going through the motions of a consultation. They were fulfilling the consultation obligations without meeting the consultation needs. Each team, however, was looking good to its superiors.

What had kept this consultation from getting off the ground? The initial contracting process was inadequate, with no agreed-upon problems or goals, so the joining process could not be successful. Those who designed the consultation were not the ones who were to implement it. The contract had been arranged by the upper management of both New Life and the Department of Psychiatry, but the staff members of New Life and the psychiatric residents were the ones assigned to carry out the terms of the consultation. There was little if any personal investment in the consultation among those who were to do the primary work. This was a hand-me-down consultation that evoked little interest or creativity. *Organizational consultation must begin with attention to the administrative context so that consultation goals can be meaningfully agreed upon and implemented.*

FAILURE #5: HELP, I'M BEING HELPED

The long nights and uneasy days were gnawing at the Reverend Jacobs. His first 3 years at Grace Church had included the usual disappointments. But in the last 6 months, storms had been gathering at Grace Church, and he had been increasingly buckling under the pressure. Jacobs was at the point where he thought he needed some outside help. Although he was somewhat reluctant to do so because of the implication of failure, he called a family therapist he knew and asked for a consultation because of problems in his congregation and his increasing depression. He arrived for the consultation dressed neatly in a tie and sweater, but his face was etched with the marks of discontent and weariness. He thanked the consultant for setting aside some time for him and, after slouching in his seat, explained the events of the last 6 months.

"There has been a small group of ten dissidents within Grace Church who have been causing a great deal of havoc. They've been complaining to other church members about my leadership. They come to me and tell me that I can't do anything right. A number of them are on the church council and are demanding that I give a very specific accounting of my time, to the point where I can't even do what I'm called to do. These dissidents also have been rude and abrupt to the other members. Some of the people who have supported me are leaving the congregation now because they just can't put up with it. No matter what I've tried to do, nothing seems to work. I've tried to talk to some of these dissidents informally, but they don't seem to want to listen to what I have to say. It's come to the point where my personal life is being affected. I can't sleep at night, my eating is terrible, and I'm losing energy to do almost anything in the church. I come home and I tell my wife about these problems, and I don't even know if she wants to listen to me anymore."

Jacobs appeared to be a kind person who was sensitive to how he displeased others and cautious about facing unpleasant situations. He had been doing what he thought was his best in the congregation, but increasingly was being inundated with a lot of complaints and little support. Jacobs then told the consultant that his current thought was to visit each one of the dissidents in their homes and to gather from them a specific list of their complaints so that he might better understand the problem. In the same breath, Jacobs sighed, as if to say, "I don't have an ounce of energy left for what I want to do."

The consultant was concerned about his client's fatigue and lack of energy. The signs of depression were pronounced. On that basis he told Jacobs that he seriously doubted whether he could or should proceed with his well-intentioned plan. The consultant believed that, as much as Jacobs wanted to understand the problem, any further efforts on his part to deal with these dissidents would only increase his frustration and disappointment. He urged Jacobs to slow down, withdraw, and to nourish himself before charging after others. The clergyman brightened at the consultant's suggestion to abandon his plan for contacting these people. He thought that this was the kind of encouragement he needed to hear, and he left the session as if a weight had been lifted from his shoulders.

The following week, Jacobs called the consultant and immediately apologized for not being able to feel better. He said he had left the consultation feeling encouraged and that the consultant's advice was what he needed to hear. But he added that things were unchanged and that he felt depressed and believed there was nothing he could do to help himself. Jacobs asked the consultant whether he could refer him to a psychiatrist who could prescribe a medication to help him with his depression. Although Jacobs did see a psychiatrist, no medication was prescribed, and the minister returned to the consultant the following week.

What had stymied the Reverend Jacobs? Was it possible that the consultant's advice had served to perpetuate the problem rather than help Jacobs manage his depression? In the following consultation sessions, the answers to these questions became clear. This clergyman was surrounded by supervisors—both formal and informal consultants. The consultant was only one among the many helpers in his life. His wife was one of the informal consultants. Recently she had taken a course on stress and assertiveness and had learned that it was important in stressful situations to charge ahead with action instead of withdrawing. She had been cheerleading her husband to push ahead and not withdraw in disappointment. She told him that if he were more active and assertive and confronted the dissidents, he would feel more competent and less depressed. She encouraged him to confront the dissidents, believing that not to do so was to admit defeat.

The Reverend Jacobs was deeply loyal to his wife, but he also felt obliged to listen to the help of his clergy colleagues with whom he met once a week. From their experience in their own congregations, these colleagues were advising Jacobs not to give any more attention to those dissidents who, they felt, were only steering him away from his ministry in the congregation. "Don't try to placate them because you've already tried that and it hasn't worked. Besides, they'll take advantage of you if you put yourself into their hands."

Other informal consultants besides his wife and his colleagues included some active supporters within Grace Church. Some supporters were saying that he should move ahead and confront the dissidents. Others were telling him not to pay attention to them. Still other supporters were saying, "Watch who you talk to. You can talk to some, but you can't talk to the others." How could Jacobs please all of those who were trying to help him?

What finally confounded the Reverend Jacobs was that his own bishop, acting not as a consultant but as a supervisor, had told him that prior to their next meeting, Jacobs was to visit each dissident and to generate a list of specific complaints that they had about his ministry and the operation of Grace Church. Jacobs had not informed the consultant that his plan to visit the dissidents was, in fact, a demand from the bishop. Unknowingly, the consultant had given Jacobs advice that was directly at odds with the mandate from the bishop.

Although Jacobs was facing the pressure of the dissidents, a greater problem was that he was paralyzed by excessive "support." He was silently crying out, "Help, I'm being helped!" Had all his supporters been giving Jacobs the same message, perhaps he would have been able to proceed with definitive action and his depression might have lifted. Instead of one resounding chorus, the Reverend Jacobs was hearing several conflicting messages that he was not able to reconcile.

A consultant is often only one among the many helpers who are attempting to assist a consultee. There may be several supervisors and a host of both formal and informal consultants who all have taken upon themselves a mission to rescue a consultee from despair. Unintentionally, the helpers may swamp the consultee with contradictory views and competing demands.

It is crucial for the formal consultant to assess how all of the informal consultants are involved with the consultee. Rather than binding the consultee even tighter with one more piece of advice, it will be more helpful if the consultant clarifies the overall context of who is saying what to the consultee before trying to formulate a plan of action. Whatever the plan, it is important to remember that the consultee's biggest bind may not be the problem presented, but the well-intentioned solutions offered by helpers.

FAILURE #6: RISKY BUSINESS

Blue Mountain School was an old, well-established boarding school in the mountains of the Northeast. For decades, it had been one of the premier showcases demonstrating how boarding schools can attend to the full range of academic, physical, and emotional needs of their students. In the past few years, Blue Mountain School had found that the students were manifesting emotional difficulties that the faculty and staff could not handle with their present skills. The headmaster called a psychologist/family therapist and said that the school wanted to have a consultation relationship with someone on whom they could depend. In years past, the school had referred some students to practitioners within the community, but had had little success in developing any close working relationships.

The psychologist began seeing numerous referrals from Blue Mountain School. After several months of psychotherapy with a number of students, she met with the headmaster and the dean of students. At that meeting, she suggested that the school employ a residential counselor who would be a liaison between her and the school, and who could also manage the less critical and more informal counseling needs of the students. The psychologist's aim was not simply to accept referrals, but to help the school by developing a prevention program.

The consultant's proposal was accepted by the executive committee at Blue Mountain School, and the search began for the person who could fill the position as resident counselor. The consultant assisted in the search process and also interviewed members of the faculty and staff as to what kind of person they might want for a resident counselor.

As the school conducted its search over the next few weeks, the students being seen by the psychologist began to present with more complicated and difficult crises. Some students were reluctant to participate in therapy as they had before. Other students mentioned that their advisers were eager to speak with her about problems that the students were having in school. She found that students wanted to take the role of intermediary between herself and the advisers at the school. Several of the students whom the psychologist was seeing were found to have broken school rules and had been brought before the discipline committee, which seemed to take extreme measures to restrict the students' privileges. Although she had had a reasonably good working relationship with the student discipline committee before, she now found herself at odds with their decisions and she quickly registered her concern with the head of the committee.

In the course of several weeks, the crises in these students' lives had multiplied, and the consultant had found herself bristling at the school's response to the students' minor infractions. Moreover, she found herself not nearly as effective in negotiating solutions with the student discipline committee. The consultant finally was given a clue as to what was going on when she made a brief phone call to one of the nurses at Blue Mountain School. The consultant had called to straighten out an upcoming appointment with the nursing staff at the school. In the process of talking to this nurse, she discovered that her suggestion to hire a resident school counselor had had major repercussions among the faculty and staff.

The nurse said, "There has been a lot of change around here lately." The family therapist asked, "What do you mean?" The nurse explained that historically the nurses in the school had been used by the students as informal counselors. Students would come into the infirmary and discuss with the nurses their personal, family, and academic problems. The nurses had always seen themselves as the "school counselors," even though this role was not part of their official job description. The consultant had never considered that there might be informal school counselors. She discovered that the students' advisers had also served as informal counselors for students. Some advisers were more interested in academic guidance, but many of them had regarded themselves as surrogate "aunts" and "uncles" and had taken these roles with the utmost seriousness. The nurse ended the conversation by expressing regret that Blue Mountain School had begun this search for a resident school counselor. An important role for her and others was being taken away.

The consultant had failed to assess the consequences of consultation for the system. Her suggestion that the school employ a full-time resident counselor had been supported by leaders of Blue Mountain School. Their encouragement had reinforced her perspective and limited her perception of other parts of the system, specifically the school nurses and student advisers. Valued roles that they had occupied for many years were now being stripped from them and delegated to a newcomer.

The consultant's failure to assess these risks resulted not only in a lack of support for the consultation proposal, but in the possibility of sabotage by the school nurses and student advisers. More important, those who were affected most directly were the students themselves. Caught between the school nurses and advisers on the one hand, and the family therapist on the other hand, the students found themselves in an atmosphere of increasing tension and mirrored this strife in their academic and personal crises.

Along with the benefits of consultation, there are also risks. The impact of consultation may change an organization in such a way that those who have lived in it for some time find that their roles and responsibilities are significantly shifted in ways that they find undesirable. Any effective consultation not only gives but also takes away. Those who welcome the consultant may soon find themselves packing their bags. *One of the consultant's responsibilities is to assess how consultation will alter the organization of the system and to prepare the system for that change.* Failing to assess these risks of consultation can result in undoing potential benefits of the consultation, or even in its complete failure.

FAILURE #7: THE PERMANENT VISITOR

Advent, Inc. was an innovative, community walk-in service for adolescents who had run away from home and often were caught up in drug abuse and antisocial activities. The staff members were well trained as group therapists and community outreach organizers, but not as family therapists. They had begun to see that many of the adolescents were still deeply involved with their families, though they usually had many negative feelings. Several staff members had begun to wonder how positive resources in these families could be tapped and how contacts with families could be integrated with peer-group, school, and legal systems contacts. They decided to invite a family therapist to consult with them on these aspects of their staff development.

One of the staff members suggested contacting Dr. Paul Andrews, a family therapist whom he had heard speak on families with teenagers who had drug problems. He had been impressed by how Dr. Andrews shared his personal experiences of having grown up in a family where his younger sister had a serious problem with drug abuse. The staff member thought that because of the family therapist's personal experience and his professional expertise with families, he would be an ideal consultant for Advent. The other staff members agreed. Dr. Andrews subsequently met with the staff as a group, and a consultation contract was set up for staff development. The staff requested help in learning how to identify the specific problems of families in this setting, how to examine alternative solutions, and how to organize a group for these families. Dr. Andrews was enthusiastic about this consultation. He helped the staff contact families and quickly established multiple family groups. Staff members were active in the multiple family groups, but Dr. Andrews clearly was the guiding force. As the months continued, the staff became more and more adept at linking with families and in problem solving with them.

Dr. Andrews's role changed little over the subsequent months although staff competence and confidence was growing. Dr. Andrews believed that his consultation with Advent was now an integral part of their functioning. He maintained a central position in staff meetings while continuing to facilitate the multiple family group meetings, as well as conducting workshops on delinquent adolescents and family functioning. A few of the junior staff began to resent Dr. Andrews's position, but they filed no complaints and requested no other consultant because Dr. Andrews was doing such a "fine job." In short, Dr. Andrews and the staff had grown comfortable together at the expense of future staff development.

The problem in this consultation was that Dr. Andrews's position was becoming permanent. He had been asked to consult for staff development in the family area. Instead of maintaining an "outsider" relationship with Advent, he had moved into the organization and was settling down as a permanent resident. Advent was in danger of not developing their own staff to work flexibly in a comprehensive and integrated manner with families, as they had done with the schools and legal system. The staff could fall back on Dr. Andrews rather than pushing themselves into new ventures.

For his part, Dr. Andrews had difficulty distancing himself from Advent, in part because of his emotional ties to the primary concern of the program. From personal experience, Dr. Andrews knew what it was like to live with a drug-abusing teenager. He had a personal commitment, a mission, to help families with these struggles because his own family had never received professional assistance in their long struggle. In some sense, Dr. Andrews wanted more for these families than they wanted for themselves. Consequently, he could not terminate his consultation.

A sign that a consultation has been effective is an absent consultant. A readiness to look for the exit sign should begin with the question: "What needs to happen in order for me to leave this place?" Although the consultant may occasionally visit again, such "visitations" are far different from becoming a permanent resident in the system. A consultant-in-residence implies that the system cannot take care of itself.

II

CONSULTATION IN MENTAL HEALTH SYSTEMS

The diversity of chapters in this section on consultation in mental health systems illustrates the complexity of the concept of systems consultation. The settings in which these family therapists work vary considerably and the mode of their engagement with consultees also differs. Sometimes these consultants interview families directly, sometimes not, but this aspect of technique does not determine who is the consultee. The consultee is the person or group who requests the consultation and to whom the consultant makes a report or recommendation. Because of the many ways that systems consultation may be defined and implemented, the identification of consultee subsystem boundaries becomes a paramount task. At the same time, the boundaries of the systems consultant's other roles, as therapist, teacher, supervisor, and administrator, must be delineated initially and often need to be clarified and modified later on.

The work of Todd illustrates these variations from a vantage point that is commonly experienced by family therapists who become consultants in mental health programs. He works in a setting in which his administrative and supervisory roles have been intertwined with his functioning as a consultant to a family therapist who is also a member of an interdisciplinary team. Whitaker, who perhaps has served as a case consultant with a greater number of family therapists than any other person in the field, engages each family directly in his distinctive personal style. At the same time, he maintains a clear relationship with the family therapist as the consultee. Penn and Sheinberg present an intriguing new method in which a team of co-consultants meets with a family therapist who is stuck because of unidentified thematic resonance between the family in treatment and the personal systems of the therapist. In a carefully planned sequence of interviews, they meet with both the family therapist/consultee and the family in such a way that the therapist's centrality is protected and effectiveness is regained. Cecchin and Fruggeri function in a community-based mental health setting in which the consultee staff members are assisted in carrying out a variety of services other than family therapy. Unlike the other authors in this section, Cecchin and Fruggeri do not meet directly with specific families in their application of systemic principles. Finally, Perlmutter and Jones have served as consultants in an emergency psychiatric service of a teaching hospital. In this setting, they interview families in order to teach principles of family interviewing and to facilitate staff decision making in which the family context is taken into account.

5

FAMILY SYSTEMS CONSULTATION WITH MENTAL HEALTH PROFESSIONALS

THOMAS C. TODD
Bristol Hospital
Bristol, Connecticut

This chapter systematically presents the process of consultation that I have used in consulting with mental health professionals. This experience has evolved in a number of contexts, including the Philadelphia Child Guidance Clinic, the Harlem Valley Psychiatric Center, and the Marriage and Family Therapy Program of the Bristol Hospital. Consultation in each of these contexts has presented a unique set of parameters and unique problems; taken as a whole, these experiences have shown the critical importance of considering the overall context when offering consultation. Underlying my consulting experience is an integrated strutural–strategic model of family therapy (Stanton, 1981a, 1981b; Stanton & Todd, 1982; Todd, 1983).

OVERVIEW OF THE CONSULTATION PROCESS

THE DISTINCTION BETWEEN CONSULTATION AND SUPERVISION

In consulting with fellow mental health professionals, it is often difficult to keep a clear distinction between consultation, supervision, and training. Probably the most crucial issue is case responsibility. In a consulting relationship, it is important to emphasize that the consultant does not assume responsibility for the case, or even for insuring that his or her own recommendations are implemented. By contrast, a supervisory relationship implies that the supervisee is clearly accountable to the supervisor for the conduct of the case, including following the supervisor's recommendations. In both consultation and supervision, the emphasis is clearly upon the case, while in a teaching/training relationship, the primary focus is upon the learning of the students.

My experience has taught me the importance of keeping these distinctions clear. In the several contexts noted above, I have had considerable administrative responsibility and have served in multiple roles; this has made it vital that I clarify what "hat" I was wearing at a given time. To take an extreme example, I frequently have been asked to provide one-shot case consultation for family therapy cases being seen by one of the psychology interns. I was the director of the clinic and also the chief psychologist (therefore, I was ultimately responsible for the internship program, but was not the ongoing, immediate supervisor). These multiple relationships made it imperative that the focus and limitations of the consultation contract be clear. In particular, this meant that the therapist was kept responsible for the outcome of the consultation. If the consultant's recommendations made sense to the therapist, the therapist needed to be prepared to defend them on that basis, rather than saying "Tom told me to do that." While this was a difficult contract to fulfill, the alternatives would have resulted in extreme confusion in the hierarchy of clinical accountability.

OUTLINE OF THE CONSULTATION PROCESS

The model I have employed presupposes that the consultation occurs as a two-stage process. In the first stage, someone involved in the case makes a request for a consultation. At that stage, the goal is to assess the nature of the case and the treatment system in order to make decisions about who should be involved in the consultation session and to determine what additional information should be obtained prior to the session. In the second stage, the consultant interviews the family members, rather than making recommendations solely on the basis of secondary information. The overall goal of consultation is to develop recommendations that will be helpful to the therapist and the family in meeting treatment goals; the recommendations and interventions may take a variety of forms, but they are all intended to address the primary treatment goals.

I have attempted to develop a planning schema to summarize the consultation process. This model, which is presented in Figure 5-1, indicates the sequence of decisions that I make during the consultation process. For each key decision, the model indicates the kinds of information that need to be collected and analyzed at that stage.

FIGURE 5-1. Schema for implementing family therapy consultation from a structural–strategic framework.

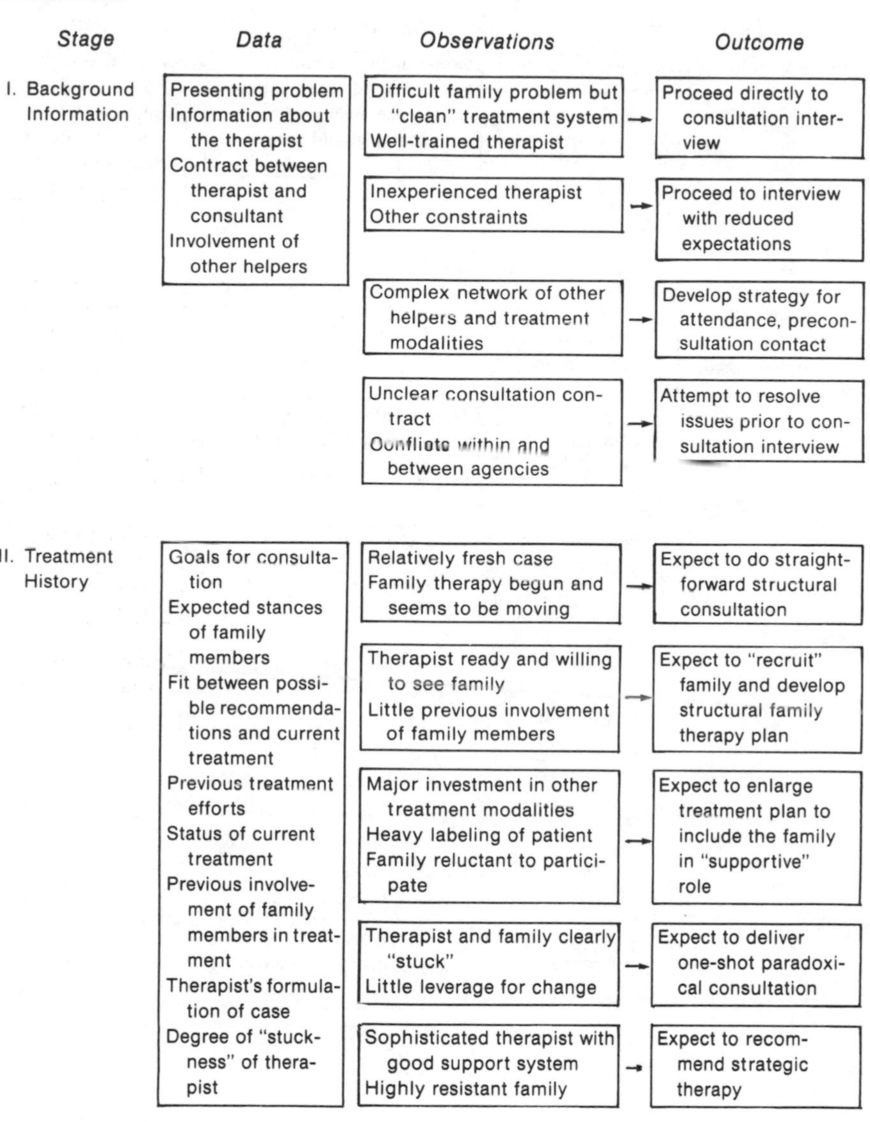

(continued)

FIGURE 5-1. (*Continued*)

Stage	*Data*	*Observations*	*Outcome*
III. Setting the Stage	Organize preliminary data from preconsultation discussions	Generate and revise presession hypotheses concerning case, including roles of therapist and other helpers →	Establish clear "ground rules" for session attendance, roles of therapist, consultant, other helpers
IV. The Formal Consultation Session: Initial Stages	Consultant checks presession hypotheses by observing interaction of family members and therapist to assess the following: • Clarity of family goals; areas of disagreement • Relationship between family and therapist • Rigidity and responsiveness of family system	Family and therapist open to input from the consultant →	Continue to develop straightforward structural interventions
		Goals and contract clear and mutual, but system is "stuck" →	Develop more intense structural intervention to break through impasse
		Strong tendency to keep patient in the spotlight →	Look for framework to relate patient's behavior to the family
		Goals clear, but all change efforts are disqualified and blocked →	Gather material for strategic final intervention
V. Possible Interventions	Consultant tests response of system to stronger interventions based on previous stages	Family continues to respond to straightforward interventions →	Develop outline for structural family therapy
		Focus remains on patient, with emphasis on non-family modalities such medication and hospitalization →	Recommend specific plan to include family in "non-family" treatment
		Family and therapist remain "stuck" →	Develop paradoxical intervention for family *and* therapist
		Therapist able to participate in strategic interventions →	Develop overall strategic plan that therapist can pursue

FIGURE 5-1. (*Continued*)

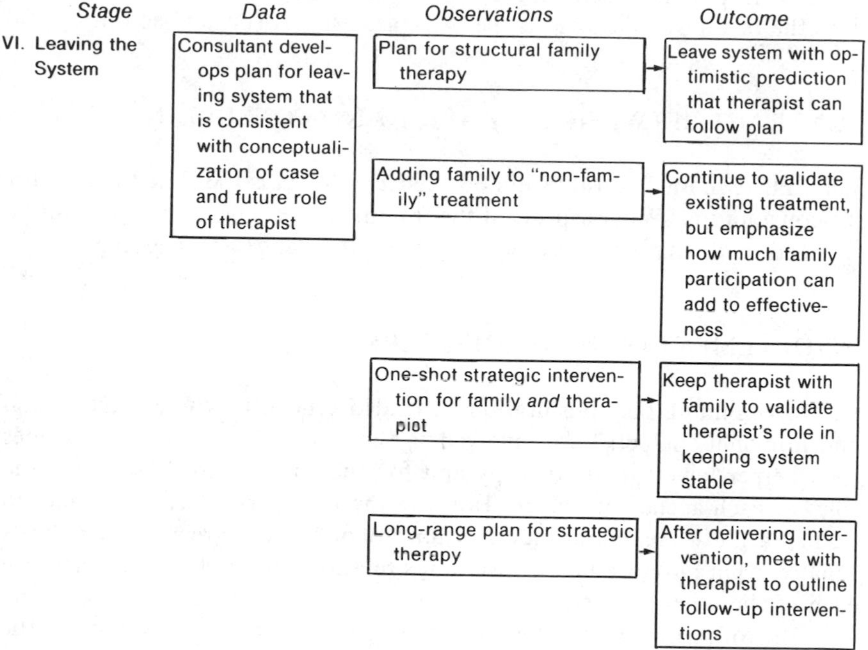

I. BACKGROUND INFORMATION

OBJECTIVES OF THIS STAGE

In collecting background information about the case, the consultant seeks to determine the nature of the consultation contract and the range of options open to the consultant. Information about the therapist and other helpers, and discussion of the consultation contract should make it possible to rule out certain possible recommendations from the consultant, while pointing toward other likely possibilities.

THE THERAPIST

A convenient place for the consultant to begin gathering and organizing information is to summarize what is known about the therapist. What training and experience does the therapist have? What are his or her clinical areas of strength or weakness? To what extent is the therapist committed to family therapy? What is the therapist's role in the agency, that is, what clout does the therapist have, who is the therapist's supervisor, and so on?

CONTRACT BETWEEN THERAPIST AND CONSULTANT

Who has requested consultation on the case? What is the stated reason for the consultation? What aspects of the treatment are "givens" that cannot be changed, and what areas are possibly open to change and negotiation?

INVOLVEMENT OF OTHER HELPERS

Before beginning the consultation, it is also crucial to know what formal and informal "helpers" are involved in the case. What expectations does each helper have for the therapy and for the consultation? What are the roles of each agency or helper? How are these helpers interrelated, and, in particular, how are interagency decisions made and disagreements resolved? Finally, what have been the consultant's relationships and past history with each of the other helpers?

The following case will be presented in some detail as an example of the consultation process. An extremely complicated case has been deliberately chosen because it illustrates many of the considerations that the consultant needs to keep in mind.

A Case Example

Presenting Problem. The consultee presented the following case background. Mike, age 29, was the only child of two elderly parents of German descent. Father, age 74, had retired early from business. He was apparently a heavy drinker and a diabetic with numerous complications. He had discontinued all medication, leading his physician to say, "I don't know how he is still alive." Mother, age 73, had come to America with her husband immediately after World War II; she had had numerous miscarriages in her efforts to have children, with Mike her only live birth. Mike had been hospitalized at the Harlem Valley Psychiatric Center with serious depression coupled with distorted thinking. Although Mike was still an inpatient, he had begun to attend a day hospital program run by Harlem Valley.

Apparently Mike had functioned satisfactorily until he left home to enter college. After two abortive efforts, he returned home. He functioned marginally for several years and had periods of depression. For about 2 years he was a patient in a day treatment program. This program, coupled with numerous crisis visits, had been enough to prevent hospitalization until an attempt was made to have him move away from home and enter a halfway house. He lasted in the halfway house program only one week before seriously cutting his wrists, which led to his hospitalization. On admission, he was diagnosed as having a schizoaffective disorder, because of the combination of severe depressive symptoms and thought disorder.

At the time of the consultation, he had been hospitalized for over 4 months. A month after admission, he had been referred to an intensive day hospital program, while he continued to reside in the inpatient unit. After about a month, he became seriously depressed and expressed suicidal thoughts, so he was removed from the day hospital program for greater security. One month prior to the consultation, he began attending the day hospital again, although his condition had not improved dramatically.

The Therapist. I was approached for a consultation on the case by Glenn Bronley, PhD, a staff psychologist in the day hospital program and the primary outpatient therapist for Mike and his family. Dr. Bronley had had extensive family therapy training but, in the day hospital program where he worked, family therapy was not the major modality; however, it was encouraged as long as it did not jeopardize a patient's participation in the day hospital program.

Contract between Therapist and Consultant. In this case, the therapist who requested consultation had worked extensively with me. Staff members with other roles in the case seemed likely to be supportive of the consultation because the family was generally seen as a difficult one. Nonetheless, there were potential problems related to my role as consultant, because of both current context and past history. At the time of the consultation, I was chief psychologist at Harlem Valley, which meant that I was the supervisor of the psychologist who was Mike's inpatient therapist. My previous role seemed likely to create additional problems. As former director of the agency, I had been the administrative supervisor of the head of the day hospital program, who was now Dr. Bronley's supervisor. More important, this state-funded agency was in direct competition with the county agency that had provided day treatment for Mike and individual therapy for his mother. This conflict was partially offset by my departure from the agency and by the respect for my reputation as a family therapy trainer.

The general outline of the treatment plan was clear and relatively nonnegotiable: Mike was to leave the inpatient service as soon as he had connected well with the day hospital program and as soon as it seemed safe for him to return home. Eventually he would leave the day hospital program to attend the county day treatment program.

Some details of the plan were probably subject to modification. For example, the timetables for the inpatient and the day hospital phases were relatively flexible. Dr. Bronley could continue with the family therapy after Mike was transfered to the county program as long as there was no extreme opposition. (Probably the major determinants of this would be how difficult the case appeared to be and how eager Dr. Bronley was to keep the case; as long as the case seemed difficult and undesirable, he would probably receive little opposition to continuing.)

There was some sentiment on the inpatient unit for having Mike move into a halfway house instead of returning home. Preliminary indications were that neither Mike nor his parents would agree. It did appear that the inpatient team would accept his return home as long as the parents could be engaged in treatment.

Involvement of Other Helpers. The array of other helpers in the case was formidable and a clear source of potential difficulty. Minimally, the list included the inpatient psychologist who had been seeing Mike individually, as well as the other members of the inpatient team. In addition to Dr. Bronley, there were several day hospital staff members who would be seeing Mike individually or in group therapy and might have contact with the parents. County day treatment staff had been involved in the hospitalization, were involved in discharge planning, and would be receiving Mike back into the program. Finally, there was the county psychologist who had been seeing the mother in individual therapy.

On the surface, all of these helpers were moderately supportive of family treatment, especially because all had experienced the difficulty of working with the parents. There were undoubtedly some differences of opinion concerning the relative importance of the family therapy compared to other modalities, and the probability of success. More important, there were clear differences concerning what the approach to the family should be: The inpatient therapist wanted Mike to be more direct with his parents; the inpatient therapist and the day treatment staff wanted him to confront his father on his drinking; and the mother's therapist wanted her to leave the father. Some efforts in each of these directions had been made, but had failed dismally. The most promising way to resolve these differences was to have all of the major players involved in the consultation interview, in the hope that they would recognize the desirability of the recommended plan. Other mechanisms for resolving disagreements, particularly between state and county agencies, seemed fraught with difficulty.

Probable Outcomes. The most likely outcome was that I would recommend that Dr. Bronley conduct family therapy on a regular basis. The exact nature of that therapy was not clear, although early indications seemed to be that the parents would be extremely resistant to having the focus of therapy include their relationship or the father's drinking. It was therefore most likely that the therapy would be ostensibly focused on helping Mike. If parental resistance was extreme, it was possible that I would not recommend formal family therapy and would suggest instead that the parents be involved in Mike's treatment more indirectly.

Preparing for the Consultation Interview. It was clearly important for the other helpers to attend the family consultation session. The list included the inpatient therapist, the mother's therapist, a representative from the county day program, and any day hospital staff members who were interested. The session would be conducted at a time when the psychology interns were learning strategic therapy and consultation, so they would also be in attendance. No decision had been made concerning which helpers would actually sit in on the session and which would watch behind the one-way mirror.

Because of the highly diplomatic nature of the case, an unusual amount of preliminary work went into preparing for the consultation session. It seemed particularly important not to create any appearance of "selling" the consultation interview, so Dr. Bronley mentioned it casually at first in the interagency planning meetings and in day hospital staff meetings. Dr. Bronley met with the mother's therapist and Mike's previous therapist from the day treatment program and was pleased when they brought up the possibility of consultation. He made no promises, other than to attempt to persuade me.

Prior to the consultation, a full-scale meeting was held with all of the professionals who would be involved in the session. After some discussion, it was agreed that Dr. Bronley, the inpatient psychologist, the day treatment therapist, and I would all participate in the session. The mother's therapist was content to watch behind the mirror with the interns.

While the number of participants seemed potentially unwieldly and even overwhelming, it was justified on the basis of the participants' having extensive previous knowledge of Mike and his family; comparatively speaking, Dr. Bronley had had little previous contact with the family and I had none. Because of the well-established relationship between Dr. Bronley and myself, the respect given us by the other professionals, and the comparative inexperience of the other participants, I felt that it would be possible to maintain control of the interview. If the interview went according to plan, the other participants would be likely to lend their support to the ultimate recommendations.

DISCUSSION

This stage of the case is concerned with constraints, leverage, and options. The consultant may be constrained by the nature of the consultation contract, by the therapist's lack of status in the agency, or by interagency problems that cannot be resolved. Changes that theoretically might be possible may not be feasible because of the consultant's lack of leverage (for example, when the consultation is imposed on the therapist or is not highly valued). Finally, the therapist's lack of training and skill may preclude certain options, such as a shift to more strategic treatment, or may even prevent a shift to any formal family therapy.

II. TREATMENT HISTORY

OBJECTIVES OF THIS STAGE

During this stage, the consultant will gather the following information about previous treatment: (1) the goals for consultation; (2) the likely stances and degree of support or resistance of family members; (3) how potential interventions and explanations would be consistent with or depart from the current treatment; (4) the previous efforts at treatment; (5) the status of current treatments; (6) previous involvement of family members in treatment; (7) the therapist's formulation of the case; and (8) the degree to which the therapist is "stuck" with the case and with other members of the treatment team.

Case Example (Continued)

Goals for Consultation. The goals for the consultation were heavily influenced by Dr. Bronley's role in the case and agency. Because the therapist was on the day hospital staff, his primary concern was to develop a treatment plan that included Mike's day hospital stay as a transition from inpatient status to the community. Because the day hospital was a transitional, time-limited program, the assumption was that the plan should include the eventual transition to the county-run continuing-treatment day program. The family was seen as both a possible stressor that could lead to rehospitalization and as a possible source of support. A straightforward means of including the family was sought that could be understood and endorsed by both inpatient and county day treatment staff. Ideally, I felt it should also be a plan that could be continued by the day treatment staff, if Dr. Bronley could not continue to see the family in therapy when Mike went from day hospital to day treatment.

Expected Stances of Family Members. I thought that Mike's mother was likely to support any treatment oriented toward her son because she was so involved with him. Her agenda concerning the father's drinking was unclear. I viewed the father as more difficult to engage, particularly if he "smelled a rat" and expected hidden agendas concerning his drinking and his health. Mike seemed very ambivalent—he was clearly concerned about his father, yet was also very protective of him. For those reasons, I expected him to show considerable ambivalence and anxiety about the family consultation session.

Fit between Possible Recommendations and Current Treatment. At first glance, it seemed consistent with the inpatient plan to have the family come for an interview because some effort had been made to involve the family in inpatient planning. On the other hand, Mike's inpatient therapist had been hinting about the father's drinking, so it was likely that the family might expect this to be a hidden agenda of the family session.

The role of the mother's outpatient therapy was less clear. My conversations with her therapist suggested that he saw her as heavily invested in the individual therapy. One content area of the therapy had been her marriage, with a focus on her asserting herself more toward her husband or possibly leaving him. These considerations suggested that the proposed family therapy might compete with her individual therapy, and that the husband might expect family sessions to focus on the marital relationship.

Previous Efforts at Treatment. The outcome of previous efforts at treatment seemed to justify a considerable degree of pessimism. The most positive indicator was that Mike had never been hospitalized before, although he had an extensive history of involvement in therapy and in structured day programs. The mother had typically been involved in Mike's treatment and had been in therapy herself for over a year. Many professionals, including the day treatment staff, the mother's therapist, and the mobile geriatric team, had attempted to engage the father in treatment, but without success.

Status of Current Treatment. When the consultation was requested, Mike was in his fourth month of inpatient hospitalization. Opinions varied about how close he was to discharge. He was participating satisfactorily in the day hospital program, although he remained depressed and spoke predominantly in metaphors. Dr. Bronley's role was a curious one: He had only seen Mike informally in the program, and Mike's response to him was a mixture of negativity, curiosity, and respect. As yet there had been little effort to involve the family in the day hospital program.

At least in the eyes of the inpatient psychologist, the status of the individual therapy on the inpatient unit was quite different. He had been seeing Mike at least twice a week for the 15 weeks Mike had been hospitalized, and Mike seemed to have a strong connection to him. The inpatient therapist was promoting the possibility of his continuing with Mike on an outpatient basis, although such a role was rarely sanctioned for inpatient staff.

Previous Involvement of Family Members in Treatment. As mentioned above, previous efforts to involve the parents in treatment, particularly as a couple, had been failures. The mother appeared to be willing to involve herself in Mike's treatment, but not with her husband there. On the other hand, it was not clear that anyone had attempted to involve the father in treatment that was clearly focused on the son.

Therapist's Formulation of Case. The therapist, Dr. Bronley, tended to emphasize systemic factors in his case formulations, and Mike's case was no exception. He believed that, on some level, Mike and the mother wanted the father to receive help, although neither was willing to push for it and would probably deny it. He saw the other helpers as playing important roles that probably helped maintain the status quo. As far as individual pathology was concerned, the therapist was quite willing to consider a schizophrenic process, apart from any family factors, as operative in many of the day hospital cases. With Mike, he was less clear that there was real evidence of psychosis; Mike was certainly highly anxious and preoccupied, and frequently spoke metaphorically, yet his thinking did not seem to be psychotic.

Therapist Stuckness. Because Dr. Bronley was newly involved in the case, he was not personally experiencing any significant degree of stuckness. The treatment system as a whole was definitely somewhat stuck; it had been unsuccessful in its efforts to keep Mike out of the hospital and its efforts to involve father in treatment. Previous placement in the halfway house program was nearly disastrous, yet no one was enthusiastic about Mike's returning home. Finally, there was considerable disagreement about the need for continued hospitalization or Mike's ultimate prognosis.

DISCUSSION

At this point, the consultant should at least have some clear ideas of what may be encountered during the consultation session. Hypotheses about the therapist's role in the case are particularly important because they may suggest "ground rules" that the consultant may recommend for the therapist's role within the consultation session itself; they may also provide clues about how radical an intervention may be needed and proposed. There should also be some clear indications of which family members and others (including helpers) should be invited to the session or contacted prior to the session.

III. SETTING THE STAGE

OBJECTIVES OF THIS STAGE

During this stage, the consultant will make two kinds of formulations of the information that has been already gathered: (1) clearly stated presession hypotheses and (2) clearly negotiated ground rules for the session.

PRESESSION HYPOTHESES

By this point, the consultant has begun to accumulate sufficient information to begin to formulate tentative hypotheses concerning the case. What speculations does the consultant have concerning the role of the symptoms? How do the symptoms and the therapy relate to the family system? What roles do the therapist and other helpers seem to play in promoting change or supporting the status quo? What alliances and coalitions appear to exist between helpers and different family members?

These tentative hypotheses may suggest certain avenues for change that appear particularly promising. Similarly, they form the basis for establishing the tentative priorities for the consultation session.

ESTABLISHING GROUND RULES FOR THE SESSION

It is ideal to establish the ground rules for the consultation prior to setting up the consultation session. If this is impossible or impractical, these issues should at least be discussed prior to beginning the session. What will be the role of the therapist during the consultation session? Will the therapist be active or passive? Is the therapist expected to begin the session?

What will be the involvement of other helpers during the consultation session? Who will be present? Will they participate directly or will they observe? What will the patient and family be told about their presence and their possible roles?

Who in the family is expected to come to the consultation session? In cases in which there has been relatively little involvement of the family in the previous treatment, it is wise to develop a specific plan for including them, namely, who will invite them, which family members should be contacted directly, and how any resistance will be handled. How much time will be required for the consultation, including time after the consultation to summarize and plan for the future?

Specific plans are needed to set the stage for the consultation. How will the consultant be introduced? What will be the stated purpose for the consultation?

Case Example (Continued)

Presession Hypotheses. I suspected that Mike's problems were closely related to difficulties in the "leaving home" stage, and that these difficulties were related to the extreme difficulty that the parents had in dealing with each other. Mike seemed concerned with his father's drinking and his health, yet was unwilling to deal with him directly. The mother was similarly unwilling to confront her husband about his drinking.

As far as the treatment system was concerned, it seemed that the various helpers were aggravating the problems inherent in the case. All seemed to side with Mike and his mother, implicitly siding against the father. Secondarily, the helpers seemed to blame the parents for Mike's hospitalization, with a power struggle developing over whether Mike should return home.

Clearly, it would be necessary to have the family experience the consultation session as distinct from previous treatment efforts. Most important, this meant carefully approaching the father about his drinking. Somehow, the father had to be involved because Mike seemed so concerned about him. Part of the consultation, possibly the most important part, was to get the other helpers to "back off," or at least coordinate the various treatment efforts.

Ground Rules for the Session. In the meeting prior to the consultation session, the participants developed a plan that outlined the roles each participant would play during the session. Dr. Bronley's role would be minimized at first, partly because he was relatively new to the case, and partly to avoid competition with the inpatient and outpatient therapists. Dr. Bronley would introduce me, and I would then conduct the remainder of the session, with the helpers in the session prepared to answer questions. The inpatient psychologist was instructed to act as Mike's advocate, especially since Mike was typically so indirect and the therapist knew him so well. On the other hand, the psychologist was warned to take his cues from the consultant (who was also his supervisor) so that the therapists could maintain a "united front." The family would be told that there were other therapists watching behind the mirror, and that they would be asked to provide suggestions during and following the session.

I asked Dr. Bronley to contact the parents concerning attending the consultation session. The purpose would be described as getting the parents' input about Mike's treatment and having them help to develop the plan for future treatment. If Dr. Bronley encountered any resistance concerning attendance, he was to emphasize that they were only committing themselves to come for a single session and to remind them of the special nature of this opportunity for consultation.

The helpers, interns, and other participants allocated two hours for the session, including planning-time prior to the session and debriefing afterwards. Videotaping of the session was planned, but the parents were not to be informed ahead of time, in view of their possible high level of resistance to coming. If they opposed taping, the issue would not be pushed.

DISCUSSION

Usually this stage is relatively quick and straightforward. The most difficult part is establishing contingency plans for any resistance about session attendance and other ground rules. This includes negotiating the "bottom line" position for holding the session at all. The therapist and consultant should agree in advance on what could happen that would be so extreme as to make it necessary to cancel the consultation.

While it is certainly ideal to have the consultant's hypotheses stated explicitly and discussed with the therapist in advance, at times this may be contraindicated. For example, the consultant may suspect overinvolvement or covert alliances with particular family members, yet may wish to gather information from direct observation before revealing this hunch. If there is a possibility that the consultant may later wish to use a paradoxical intervention with the therapist–family system, he or she should consider the advisability of not sharing relevant hypotheses with the therapist at this stage.

IV. THE FORMAL CONSULTATION SESSION: INITIAL STAGES

OBJECTIVES OF THIS STAGE

While the consultant enters the consultation session with clear hypotheses and predictions about the likely course of the session, several key decisions depend upon direct observation of the family interaction and the interaction between the therapist and the family. During this stage, the consultant begins to gather information related to specific hypotheses and to assess (1) the clarity of family goals and areas of disagreement; (2) the relationship between the family and the therapist; and (3) the rigidity and responsiveness of the family system.

Typically the consultation session begins with the introduction of the consultant and completion of any procedural details such as permission to tape the session. After the consultant has joined briefly with each family member, the consultation usually begins with a brief case review, with information provided by the family, the therapist, and any other helpers who attend the session.

FAMILY'S VIEW OF GOALS AND ACCOMPLISHMENTS OF TREATMENT

The questions that should be answered include: What did each family member hope would be accomplished through therapy? To what extent does each member feel that these initial goals have been met? Naturally, the consultant will be alert to disagreements between family members about the nature of the problem, the degree of improvement, and the usefulness of treatment.

RELATIONSHIP BETWEEN FAMILY AND THERAPIST

Similarly, the consultant will be alert to indications of the relationship between the therapist and each family member. (For example, if the father is very skeptical about the value of treatment, while the mother is enthusiastic, it is easy for the therapist to side covertly with the mother if the therapist pushes strongly for therapy.) Does the therapist appear to be overidentified with the patient and aligned against the family? Does the therapist see any particular family member as the "villain"? Are there splits within the family concerning therapy, such as disagreements about the comparative usefulness of different treatment components (medication, individual treatment, family treatment, and so on)?

DEGREE OF STUCKNESS EXPERIENCED BY FAMILY AND BY THERAPIST

The consultant must determine to what extent the family experiences treatment as being bogged down and whether the therapist shares this view? At times, the family feels surprised that the therapist sees a need for consultation when they believed that treatment is proceeding smoothly. Who feels the most stuck? To what do they attribute the stuckness or lack of progress?

TESTING COMPLIANCE AND THE RESPONSIVENESS OF THE SYSTEM

Before making any major interventions, the consultant "tests the water" by ascertaining the degree to which the family is likely to comply with straightforward suggestions. What suggestions has the therapist made in the past, and what has been the response of the family members? How flexible is the system?

Case Example (Continued)

In many ways the session itself was uneventful, compared to the extensive preparation of the treatment system before the session. No one was particularly surprised when the father failed to attend, with no excuse other than not wanting to be involved. I made the strategic decision for the treatment team to see the family anyway, because they were probably unprepared to force the issue with the father. Instead, the strategy was to demonstrate a concern about the father and make it clear that it would be safe for him to come in.

While on the inpatient unit, Mike had been extremely anxious about having the session, and he remained so in the session. His individual therapist tried to get him to talk about his father, but he remained indirect and metaphoric in his speech and seemed clearly to be protecting his father. In order to reduce Mike's anxiety and protectiveness, I talked about my own worries about my mother, who happened to have a similar combination of physical and alcohol-related problems. While I admitted having occasional flashes of anger at my mother, my overall tone was definitely supportive and nonblaming. Following this intervention, Mike and his mother relaxed visibly and began to be able to discuss their concerns about the father much more directly.

Family's View of Goals and Accomplishments. Mike and his mother voiced the predictable goals—that he should leave the inpatient unit and function adequately, which apparently meant functioning in a supportive context such as the day hospital. They were frustrated by his lengthy stay in the hospital but seemed to hold no resentment or to blame anyone for this. They felt that the previous treatment and the hospitalization had provided crucial support for Mike, even though his psychiatric condition had not improved as they had hoped. Because the father was absent, it was difficult to ascertain the degree to which the mother and the father were in agreement about Mike's treatment.

Relationship between Family and Treatment System. Mike seemed to relate relatively well to the inpatient therapist, although not to the extent portrayed by the therapist. There was no indication that Mike would have extreme difficulty separating from him. Nevertheless, there were hints that this therapist and the mother could easily cross swords about what was best for Mike. The mother and Mike both spoke highly of previous treatment efforts and saw the county day treatment staff as very supportive.

Stuckness of the Family. The family, like the professionals, seemed to feel most stuck in two areas—getting Mike stabilized outside the hospital and getting the father to deal with his drinking and health problems.

Compliance and Flexibility. The mother and Mike were unexpectedly compliant after the consultant's strategic use of self-disclosure. The degree of defensiveness and indirectness diminished following that intervention. The father's absence from the session suggested rigid avoidance of therapy on his part, although this needed to be tested more directly. Early indications were that the treatment system showed considerable flexibility and openness to my input.

DISCUSSION

While the consultant will have refrained from making any dramatic interventions during this early portion of the session, there will be many subtle indications of the likely response of the family to various types and avenues of intervention. Similarly, there will be clear indications of ways in which the relationship between the family and the therapist needs to change and of possible means for effecting these changes.

V. POSSIBLE INTERVENTIONS

OBJECTIVES OF THIS STAGE

During this stage, the consultant chooses one or more interventions to test during the consultation session. Possibilities include: (1) major changes in treatment modalities; (2) adding family therapy to existing treatment plan;

(3) including family involvement in non-family treatment; (4) major change in family therapy direction (e.g., shift to strategic therapy); (5) modest change in "basic" family therapy; (6) eliminating involvement of other helpers; (7) clarifying and improving relationships among helpers; and (8) indirect approaches to other helpers.

At this point, which may be halfway into the session, the consultant probably has formed some strong impression of the directions in which treatment needs to go and ideas about how to move the system (including the treatment system) in those directions. There are several major forms that the intervention can take, with the choice of intervention heavily determined by the treatment context and the degree of compliance that is expected.

INCLUDING THE FAMILY IN NON-FAMILY TREATMENT

Often it is obvious that full-fledged family therapy is not indicated. There may be no one with the skill and training to provide it, or there may be no need to add family therapy to the existing treatment regimen. It may also be unlikely that the family would be willing to engage in such therapy.

None of this means that the family cannot be usefully included in a treatment plan that is based predominantly on other modalities, such as inpatient or day treatment. The consultant can recommend ways of including the family in order to support the treatment. For example, there may be ways in which the family can support treatment compliance, such as insuring that the patient take medication or attend the program. They can be asked to provide needed feedback to the therapist and other staff, for example, by observing the occurrence of symptoms. Most important, their role can be identified as helpful and even crucial to the treatment, rather than competitive or undermining.

STRUCTURAL INTERVENTIONS

The above interventions are useful when the family has been virtually excluded from treatment and can be engaged by identifying a simple but helpful role. More commonly, consultation from a family therapist is sought when one or more family members are very actively engaged, and even overinvolved, in the treatment. Other family members may be too distant and uninvolved. Without recommending full-fledged family therapy, the consultant can often offer structural interventions that will improve this situation. For example, an overinvolved father can be given instructions that structure his role more carefully, or certain topics may be defined as off-limits, to be discussed only between the patient and the therapist. An underinvolved parent may become a built-in conduit for information, so that all communication between the family and the treatment program is channeled through that parent. To support the executive role of the parents, they may be given an important voice in treatment decisions. None of these interventions presuppose any sophistication about family therapy on the part of the therapist.

RECOMMENDATIONS OF FAMILY THERAPY

When the resources are available, it may be useful for the consultant to recommend ongoing family therapy, either performed by the current therapist or by a new therapist. This option depends heavily on the therapist's degree of skill and whether this new role as family therapist is consistent with the therapist's previous role in treatment. Recommending family therapy is particularly appropriate when family issues have been identified in the consultation and the family members have experienced some success in dealing with them during the consultation session.

STRATEGIC OR PARADOXICAL INTERVENTIONS

Often the consultant finds that all of the straightforward paths outlined above are blocked. The family may deny a need to be involved in treatment, or may be extremely antagonistic to all recommendations. At least as often, the primary obstacles are in the treatment system itself. Often the therapist lacks the power to carry out what the consultant would recommend. Other helpers may already be well entrenched in the situation, and be unable or unwilling to alter their roles.

Typical examples include situations in which the therapist cannot directly prevent a patient from obtaining prescription drugs, or keep a patient from being rehospitalized against the therapist's wishes. A key family member may have a long-term involvement in a form of therapy that may work counter to the treatment in question. For example, the father may be heavily involved in attending AA meetings, which are helpful to him but prevent his involvement in parental activities. Therapist, patient, and family may have reached an ultrastable position that is difficult to alter. In any of these situations, the consultant may feel that it is impossible to do anything that directly challenges the existing situation, and may instead choose to employ the strategic intervention of urging no change; the expected family resistance to this intervention will usually produce change paradoxically.

In the ultra-stuck therapy situations, where it is obvious that the therapist has become a powerful factor in maintaining the status quo, it is misguided to recommend major changes in the treatment plan. Instead, it is better to validate the therapist and family members in their wisdom in choosing to go so slowly. While some members might be showing signs of impatience, the consultant sees restraint as the prudent course and recommends continued therapy of this type as the best safeguard for insuring that change does not get too rapid. Such an intervention cannot be done sarcastically or tongue-in-cheek; it must be rooted in some appreciation of the factors that make all of the parties involved willing to settle for the status quo because they are fearful of worse alternatives.

DIALOGUE WITH THE THERAPIST

Another effective technique for dealing with resistance is to deliver messages indirectly by offering them to the therapist. Typically, the consultant will take a much tougher stance than the therapist. This can take the form of having the consultant make forceful recommendations and letting the therapist "pick up the pieces" in later sessions. For example, the consultant can express strongly that nothing will happen in the therapy until the father's alcoholism is dealt with, while the therapist can help the family to deal with the difficulties in facing this issue. It is also useful for the therapist and consultant to voice opposite positions on issues about which the family is ambivalent, similar to the "Greek Chorus" technique (Papp, 1980). It is best for the consultant to be the pessimistic spokesman for the status quo and outline all of the reasons why the situation cannot, and probably should not, change. This leaves the therapist free to side with those parts of the family system that support change. All of these techniques will be more effective if the therapist has some advance warning that they may be necessary and is aware that their success requires some dynamic tension between the consultant's position and the therapist's, rather than the maintenance of a united front.

Case Example (Continued)

Assessment of Possible Interventions. At this stage in the interview, there were two or three major interventions that needed to be tested further. First, I hoped that the treatment plan could be simplified considerably by eliminating the inpatient therapist and the mother's individual therapist. It also seemed desirable to find a way for state and county day treatment staff members to work together. Second, it seemed obvious that directly involving the father in treatment was important, although it might prove more realistic to count on communicating with him indirectly. Third, a plan for discharge from inpatient status in the near future seemed appropriate and possible, although everyone was still quite nervous about this possibility.

Interventions. I framed the dilemma of the consultation team as similar to Mike's dilemma—even though the father was not the immediate problem and although he consistently refused help, his condition could not be ignored and had a major impact on Mike. While Mike needed to deal with his own issues and get on with his life, he would find this impossible if he were so worried about father. Similarly, while he needed to make a break and begin to think about living on his own, he could not leave his father and mother stranded. I stated that Mike and his mother would need to continue to express their concern for the father without pressuring him to change. Any contact with therapists would have to be clearly labeled as intended for Mike's benefit and based on the parents' obvious wish to see him better. I recommended that day hospital and county staff should work closely with the parents and with inpatient staff to judge Mike's readiness for discharge. Living outside the home might be possible if the parents agreed that it was a good idea and as long as Mike maintained contact with them.

Response to Interventions. Feedback from Mike and the mother and from the two therapists in the room suggested that we were on the right track but should proceed slowly. No one seemed eager to have either Mike's or his mother's individual therapy suddenly discontinued. Mike's discharge seemed to be agreed upon in general, but with considerable apprehension. Mike and his mother were happy that someone would reach out to the father, but made it clear that they did not want to be part of any confrontation. Above all, everyone was well aware that some of the most important players were absent from the consultation, including the father, the inpatient psychiatrist, and various program directors, and that planning without taking them into account seemed risky.

The Plan. After a private huddle with the team, the consultant proposed a plan with several components: (1) family sessions should be held in the family's home; (2) the two therapists for the family sessions were to be Dr. Bronley and the therapist from the county day treatment program; (3) Mike should be placed in a halfway house program with the parents' blessing and with continued family sessions and day hospital programming; and (4) a letter explaining the plan and enlisting the father's support was to be delivered to him after the session.

The Letter

TO: (Each Member of Mike's Family)
FROM: Mike's Treatment Team
SUBJECT: Proposed Treatment Plan

The team wanted to be sure that each family member gets a written summary from us about what we were proposing and what the "ground rules" would be.

Two therapists—one from Day Hospital and one from the County program—are willing to come weekly to meet with the family and discuss Mike's treatment. Many issues were not resolved today, including when Mike will be discharged and what would be the backup plan if the halfway house says "No."

The team feels that it is very important for Mike that both parents be involved in his treatment. We should be clear that the therapists are *not* doctors and we are not coming primarily to help Dad with his problems. Of course they could help arrange something if that was Dad's wish.

The therapists will work hard to keep the sessions safe for everyone involved, making sure that the sessions don't get too hot. We need to count on everyone to take care of himself/herself. If that means staying away from a session, or leaving in the middle, that is perfectly okay.

It is also important to be clear that this new plan does not affect the individual therapy. Mrs. T's individual sessions with Dr. S and Mike's sessions with Mr. D are separate issues.

We are having some difficulty scheduling the first session because of the holidays. It has been tentatively scheduled for Nov. 23rd [about 2 weeks later]. The therapists will call and confirm.

VI. LEAVING THE SYSTEM

OBJECTIVES OF THIS STAGE

The consultant's goal at the close of the session is to achieve maximum impact, yet to leave the system with the therapist in an effective position. To accomplish the first of these aims, the consultant may wish to deliver a final intervention in order to extend the impact of the consultation into the future. To accomplish the second, specific attention should be paid to how the consultant leaves the system and what messages are conveyed about the therapy and the therapist.

TASKS AND OTHER INTERVENTIONS

The consultant may leave the family and therapist with a recommendation, task, or some other specific steps to be accomplished. This may simply consist of specific recommendations concerning the family's involvement in future treatment. If some restructuring has occurred explicitly during the consultation session, it is useful to give specific recommendations of activities that would consolidate those changes. Even when the family will not continue in family therapy, it is still desirable to give tasks that support positive changes that have begun during the consultation.

Paradoxical interventions can also be effective and safe, particularly when they make primary use of restraining (Todd, 1981) and pretending (Madanes, 1981), rather than prescribing. (These techniques are less dependent upon therapist follow-up.) Example: "I think it is good for you to reassure your parents that you will not get better too fast and that you will go as slowly as anyone needs; even if you are feeling better, it is probably good not to show it, or even to pretend to feel good."

MESSAGES TO THE FAMILY

Final messages to the family can be very helpful in increasing the probability of success of non-family treatment. When the primary content of the consultation session has been a straightforward effort to get the family to be more supportive of treatment, such efforts can be underscored with an optimistic pep talk to the family. The consultant can stress the importance of their continued cooperation, give them credit for their willingness to be involved, acknowledge what a sacrifice this represents, and so on.

Final messages can also be helpful in enhancing the role of the therapist. The consultant can express confidence that the therapist will continue the positive direction begun in the consultation session. It is important to portray what has happened in the consultation session as continuous with what has occurred in the previous treatment, rather than a discontinuous event that has come out of the blue. This implies that all the consultant has done has been to speed up the process that was already in motion, rather than that the therapist's previous efforts were incorrect or useless, or that the consultant has done something that would have been impossible for the therapist to accomplish.

Paradoxical predictions can be effective in two situations. At one extreme, the consultant may sense that the consultation session went so well that progress is unlikely to continue at that level. This could be a particular problem for the therapist if any slippage is attributed to the therapist's lack of skill as compared to that of the consultant. In these situations it is important for the consultant to predict a relapse as inevitable and no one's fault. At the other extreme, even the consultant may have been faced with extreme resistance. In such cases, the consultant can "throw down the gauntlet" by offering a pessimistic challenge to the family that they cannot tolerate change. It is definitely better for the consultant to be the one who is pessimistic and challenging than for the therapist to assume such a role; doing so gives the therapist the opportunity to side with the family in affirming the possibility of change.

MESSAGES TO THE THERAPIST

It is usually effective for the consultant to summarize the session by outlining the recommended future course of therapy and relating this to the events in the consultation session. At times, it may be useful to share hypotheses about the case in front of the family. (If interventions have been more strategic, the consultant should usually refrain from sharing such hypotheses with the family.) When the situation is well entrenched and the therapist is clearly stuck, the consultant can follow up with a paradoxical message that includes the therapist, such as positively reframing the lack of progress in therapy and even implying that progress might be dangerous.

Case Example (Continued)

Leaving the System and Follow-Up. The helpers and the family seemed to be enthusiastic about this plan (with the father yet to be heard from). Probably the biggest question mark other than the father was the inpatient therapist, who did not have a major role in this plan. On the other hand, he had been an active participant in the consultation session and had functioned as Mike's advocate, so he felt some ownership of the plan.

Leaving the system proved difficult for me—something that could have been predicted in view of my multiple roles in the system. Everyone, family and helpers alike, felt relieved and grateful that the session had gone so well; my diplomacy was clearly seen as contributing to the lack of warfare between agencies and to the development of a positive plan that had some promise of including the father without threatening him. Everyone expressed hope that I would remain at least indirectly involved in the case; since this wish seemed to be shared by all of the major factions, some continued involvement seemed safe.

One immediate consequence of the consultation was a second meeting of all the helpers in the case (except me). In this meeting, the halfway house program agreed to accept Mike back on one month's probation, on the condition that the family sessions and the day hospital program continue. They also stipulated that I supervise the case. Mike was discharged from the inpatient unit shortly thereafter.

The family sessions continued every 2 weeks for approximately 6 months. The father was surprisingly positive about them; even more remarkable, his sense of propriety led him to stay sober for almost an entire week prior to the sessions. The mother practically adopted the two therapists; at first she served coffee, then gradually progressed to elaborate meals. Both parents seemed to accept Mike's move to the halfway house, with the stable connection provided to the family sessions. Mike seemed to find the sessions reassuring; they kept him connected to the parents and allowed him to check on their welfare, yet provided him with needed distance.

In the long run, the sessions were not sufficient to prevent the father from slipping back into heavy, episodic drinking. The important difference was that Mike and his mother continued their progress. Mike made a smooth transition to the day treatment program and began to work in a vocational rehabilitation program. Despite his father's deteriorating condition, Mike managed to hold onto the gains he had made and stay out of the hospital. Mike's mother was able to let go of Mike and continue to develop a life of her own.

FUTURE DEALINGS WITH FAMILY AND THERAPIST

SUPPORTING STRAIGHTFORWARD CHANGES

If the consultant has any further contact with either the therapist or the family, it is important that he or she make certain that the primary credit for any progress is given to the family and the therapist. It is dangerous, though tempting, to accept accolades for wonders performed in the consultation session.

If the treatment plan has succeeded where previous treatment has failed, it is also important to avoid competition with other agencies or other treatment modalities. Often consultees will attempt to ally with the consultant by touting the superiority of family treatment over the prevailing patterns in the agency. Agreeing enthusiastically with such views would probably involve the consultant in undeclared professional wars and could result in the consultant suddenly being seen as dispensable.

SUPPORTING PARADOXICAL CHANGES

When paradoxical interventions have been made by the consultant, it is important to remain consistent. This includes the consultant remaining skeptical about any reported changes. He should advise the therapist to convey his skepticism to the family; this should help to consolidate such changes. More of a problem is the issue of handling therapist's efforts to undo paradoxical interventions. It is usually a mistake to let the therapist "in" on the thinking behind the interventions, because in most cases the therapist's entrenchment is one of the factors that led the consultant to move in a paradoxical direction. On the few occasions in which I have relented, the therapist has invariably become defensive and attempted to demonstrate all the ways in which change is impossible. (The obvious remedy for such a mistake is to agree quickly with the therapist and de-escalate to a more extreme, pessimistic position.)

CONCLUSION

Obviously no single chapter can hope to convey all of the skills needed by a family therapist who is attempting to provide family consultation to other mental health colleagues. The consultant must already possess solid skills in rapid assessment and intervention with families. More than in other situations, it is important for the field of vision to include the interplay of other helpers and components of the treatment system and other agencies. It is hoped that this chapter has provided a conceptual framework that can be useful to the experienced clinician in organizing the mass of data available and in guiding the decision-making process.

REFERENCES

Madanes, C. *Strategic family therapy*. San Francisco: Jossey-Bass, 1981.

Papp, P. The Greek chorus and other techniques of family therapy. *Family Process*, 1980, *19*, 45–57.

Stanton, M. D. An integrated structural/strategic approach to family therapy. *Journal of Marital and Family Therapy*, 1981, *7*, 427–439. (a)

Stanton, M. D. Marital therapy from a structural/strategic viewpoint. In G. P. Sholevar (Ed.), *The handbook of marriage and marital therapy*. New York: SP Medical & Scientific Books, 1981. (b)

Stanton, M. D., & Todd, T. C. *Integrating structural and strategic therapy*. Workshop presented at the Philadelphia Child Guidance Clinic, December 1982.

Todd, T. C. Paradoxical prescriptions: Applications of consistent paradox using a strategic team. *Journal of Strategic and Systemic Therapy*, 1981, *1*, 28–44.

Todd, T. C. *Structural and strategic therapy: The case of integration*. Paper presented at the Annual Meeting of the American Association for Marriage and Family Therapy, Washington, DC, October 1983.

6

FAMILY THERAPY CONSULTATION AS INVASION

CARL A. WHITAKER
University of Wisconsin Medical School
Madison, Wisconsin

In collaboration with LYMAN C. WYNNE and SUSAN H. McDANIEL

Within the medical community, the use of consultants has been standard practice for many years. Presumably, any physician may need help in understanding and treating the infinite complexities of the human organism. It is mysterious to me that psychotherapists have not availed themselves of the second-opinion phenomenon that now has become legally accepted by such diverse groups as insurance companies and the federal government. Perhaps the difficulty for psychotherapists arises because there is no doubt that the consultant is always an invader into the ongoing process between psychotherapist and patient or family. The consultant's invasion may make the therapist aware that he or she has adopted the family under treatment, or has been adopted by the family, precipitating such painful components of adoption as the imitation of biological parenthood and the presumption that the responsibility goes on forever.

My first experience with consultation came in 1948. Because I had been working with the wife of a psychotic physician and realized that the therapy had gone on for a year and a half and had become more and more boring, I asked a colleague to visit. The colleague's arrival precipitated an immediate free association for me about the patient: "She looks like my mother." The patient did not look like my mother, but she and I had set up an implicit contract: "I will be your make-believe mother if you will be my make-believe mother." This had gone on for a year and a half without either of us being aware of it.

Consultants in family therapy can intrusively disrupt the power that families have to co-opt therapists by making them members of the family or by excluding them, that is, keeping them either inside or outside the impermeable rubber fence around the family system, as described by Wynne, Ryckoff, Day, and Hirsch (1958). However, if the therapist does dare to be vulnerable by inviting the consultant in, he or she models for the family members the idea that they too can be vulnerable without being destroyed.

In my paradigm, the primary therapist automatically takes on the nurturant role of the foster mother, whether it is with a person, a family, or a couple. This is a temporary, surrogate role structured around the imminence of leave taking. Over the years, I have become more and more impressed, at times awed, by the power of the consultant, whom I call a foster father. Even a brief 10 minutes in the second interview, or at the point of diminishing movement or growing impasse, this outsider's perceptions and contributions can create a new force and raise the temperature of the therapeutic group. As primary therapists listen to a consultant's investigations, interaction, or opinion, they expand their experience with the persons who are being treated. In this way, therapists not only get a second view, but also binocular vision (with depth) that makes possible a greatly broadened orientation.

Because the consultant is an outsider and is relating to the total group that includes the therapist as well as the family, there is greater freedom to precipitate a new experience that may have the symbolic power to enable the family to break out of their standard protectionism. For example, the ongoing relationship between a family therapist and a husband, his divorced wife, and their two children was making a therapist feel uncomfortable. The therapist invited me to consult by way of long-distance speaker phone. As an outsider, I was able to be much more invasive, much more directive, and much more supportive of the therapist. This allowed the therapy to get back on track so that the children could have a new freedom to relate to each of their parents without having to defend one of them out of perverted loyalty.

My first use of telephone consultations took place when 10 mental health workers in a rural Minnesota welfare agency asked for a speakerphone conference. These calls took place once a month for two years. Each time, the problems of family stress in one or two cases were presented and discussed within the group while I, as consultant, participated on the other end (by myself), using my telephone.

Unique to the consultation role is the capacity to increase the pressure for including the extended system. One therapist started working with a wife because she was depressed over her husband's affair, and he later went on to develop a working relationship with the couple. After months of hard work, he decided that things were not going well and asked me to consult in a long-distance telephone conference call. I said yes, if the husband included his girlfriend in the consultation. This was agreed. During the telephone consultation, the girlfriend decided that the husband was not "faithful" to her. The consultant suggested that the wife's psychological affair with her therapist was also fading and that really the therapist and the girlfriend were being left with the empty nest syndrome. The dynamics of the extended system were changed dramatically even though the husband did not understand what was going on.

A single consultation with the extended family can be valuable. This allows the therapist to stay loyal to the nuclear family while the consultant does a historical review with the two sets of grandparents or siblings of the parents. This may expose for the therapist and the nuclear family carryovers from past generations, such as family rules and myths, and hidden dynamics of the relationship between the therapist and the nuclear family. The consultant can also expose the bilateral fantasies that have led the family to dream of being adopted by the therapist, and can even tease about sexual attraction between the therapist and a family member, or about the seduction euphoria of one or another member of the family group.

"Back on the ranch," the therapist is free to listen, to transcend developed, ongoing patterns of relating to this family, and to learn bits of a colleague's wisdom from this consultation as well as from the family members as they respond to the consultant's invasion. The consultant may help the therapist individuate from the family within the appointment hour and thereby enable him or her to avoid the usual ploys of allusion, cynicism, intellectual isolation, or vacillation—from overinvolvement to boredom—as revealed by daydreams of golf scores or sailboat racing.

Meanwhile, the consultant also is learning a new role, discovering that it is not always necessary to be the nurturant therapist/mother. There can be a new freedom to act in the foster father role of adviser instead of therapist or supervisor. That discovery could even lead to a decision to escape some standard, expected role functions and to retain the right to be one's self at any moment, with no excuses needed.

One unusual kind of consultation is that in which the mental health professional does not accept the role of being therapist but, rather, acts as a kind of nonparticipant observer/consultant. There are four or five schizophrenics whom I have never treated but who report back every 6 months to a year (or 2 years) to complain about the mental health system, or the world as a place in which to earn a living. The therapist becomes a consultant on the horrors of life, without accepting any role, nurturant or otherwise, except as a kind of "colleague."

Sometimes it is less embarrassing for a therapist to utilize a consultant who is a nonprofessional. For example, an ex-schizophrenic patient can be a beautifully creative consultant for another family in treatment over the problem of their schizophrenic child. Even less embarrassing is the use of extended family members, especially grandparents. The therapist can say to a family, "I feel we are not doing the kind of work we should be doing.

Would you please ask both sets of grandparents to come in and be my consultants for an interview." Once they have arrived, the therapist can complain about the failure to be effective. The hope is that these grandparents can be helpful in telling how it was when they were the age that their children are now or how it was when they were raising these two adults. This kind of request launches the grandparents into an extended description of the good old days, and may lead to further discussion of their own grandparents and parents. The therapist can get a perception of a five-generation family unit while treating the last two generations. This usually turns out to be a successful hour whether or not the content is of any significance. The grandparents are talking about their children to someone else, while their children listen. If the hour is unsuccessful, it should still be seen as symbolically useful. It is best to request that the grandparents, should they have any further interest in visiting, take that up with the parents; they are not parents of the therapist but consultants to him in the effort to be a temporary foster parent to these, their children.

Another reason for consultation is professional isolation and burnout, with loss of creativity. One therapist who has been in practice for 20 years and is known as a therapist to therapists was in tears because she had been entrusted with so many secrets about therapists. "They restrict my professional life." She did not dare reveal these secret patterns to anyone. She felt alone, worn out, overloaded, and that her patients imposed upon her. Such feelings are an indication for using a consultant.

Another example involves a therapist who works with sex offenders. Because of concerns about confidentiality, this therapist does not bring in consultants. He talked about how tired he felt after work and how overloaded he felt. To me that means he is working too much in isolation and needs consultants.

Finally, consultation can help to diagnose an abnormally normal family, and offer an identified patient the choice of declining or postponing therapy, or of expanding from individual to couple, couple to family, nuclear family to extended family. It seems best not to change to a subgroup or to an individual during a consultation process or as a recourse if therapy later on is floundering. (Moving to smaller units may be useful as a deliberate plan in the later phases of *successful* therapy.)

HOW TO DO A CONSULTATION INTERVIEW

I have developed a pattern for doing consultations that I think is effective. In an impasse with any family, I bring in a peer as a consultant, someone who knows me and my style. There are some special situations in which I seek out a consultant for some personal characteristic. When working with a black family, a white therapist may request a black therapist to consult. When working with a divorcing family, a consultant or a cotherapist who is divorced may be valuable. When the family is deeply religious and mistrustful, it can be very helpful to bring in a consultant of similar religious faith.

It is best if the consultant knows nothing of the family before the interview. The introduction can be simple and brief. "This is Dr. Schmaltz. I asked him to come in because I am concerned that we aren't getting anywhere. I feel like the stakes in this family are unusually high, and I need some help." If there is danger in the family, such as the threat of physical violence, it is important to acknowledge this. Where a father has been extruded from the emotional life of the family, I may tell the consultant: "I was afraid that the father would commit suicide, not by conscious decision but by working himself to death or getting involved in a car accident."

It is a mistake to ask the family to agree to the consultation. That would be analogous to a heart surgeon asking the patient for permission to bring in a second surgeon. If the patient or family members do not agree, they are then in the position of deciding how the therapist should practice; the therapist then becomes ineffectual. Although consultation can only be implemented by the therapist as consultee, it may be precipitated by the family members who decide that a consultant is needed because the therapy is not satisfactory to them.

The therapist reviews with the consultant in front of the family their family history as well as the process of the therapy to date. The impasse should then be described. It is helpful for the family to hear how they are perceived. It gives the family an opportunity to transcend their past views of themselves. It is most helpful for the therapist to describe them as a group and work down to the subgroup and individual concerns if necessary.

This report to the consultant also does away with the assumption that the therapist knows all about the family. Families often assume the therapist knows how they should live but is unwilling to tell them because it goes against professional custom. The family also can see that the therapist may be confused. Finally, the review with the family present takes the consultant out of the position of being a voyeur. The whole experience is flavored with uncertainty, which causes it to be much more alive. The task is not just to utilize expert knowledge but also to handle a new experience effectively.

In this report to the consultant, it is best if the therapist describes the family in a third-person narrative. If the therapist's anxiety is high, however, the history may be presented in the second person as a series of questions to the family. The information then is being cleared with them, but the family loses the opportunity to be transcendent and instead acts like a supervisor correcting the therapist. If the initial report is in the third person, the family can restate it in their own way after the therapist has finished.

The therapist should try to present the family history in simple, direct language, not language from psychology or medicine. Also, I tend to amplify deviance so the family can see patterns more clearly. For example, the father's outburst to the mother might be characterized as a rage attack that occurred when the mother turned her back on him and went to visit her mother. The family may never have put those pieces together. The therapist may be able to teach the family members something about systems and circular thinking by the way that their history and current functioning is reviewed.

Loaded words may be used to intensify the family experience symbolically. If the father and son have been fighting, for example, the therapist may describe the son as trying to drive the father away so that he can have his mother to himself. When the father then defeats the son, mother scolds her husband and he goes out and gets drunk. At the Family Institute of Rome, therapists are encouraged to present a fantasy picture of the family, with no effort made to be factually accurate. Sometimes purposeful distortion helps the family think more creatively about themselves and may induce a language change. They may become playfully metaphorical about themselves, a vital component of family health.

After the therapist presents the family, the consultant takes over. He or she may redo the first interview or address particular issues in the family or in the therapeutic relationship, or may even suggest that therapy seems useless and should be ended.

The best time for a family therapy consultation is the second family interview. The data and the dynamic discoveries of the first interview are reported. The discussion between the therapist and the consultant makes it possible for the family to see themselves in a very different perspective, and for the therapist to see the potential for ongoing therapy, including the freedom to belong to and separate from the family. As the consultant evaluates the family in the presence of the therapist, the triangulation taking place enables the family to see the therapist differently, the therapist to see the family differently, and the two of them to perceive their potential for teaming in a much more operational framework. The consultant extends the history of the family and thus highlights dynamics; this leaves both parts of the therapist–family relationship with greater flexibility and greater awareness of their differing responsibilities in the alliance.

Such a second-interview consultation also makes the consultant an available resource for the breakthrough of later impasses or the clarification of the termination process, and it helps keep the therapeutic alliance from becoming frozen. Bringing the consultant in early means that the consultant will be present in the mind of the family and on call for either the family or the therapist when things begin to become ineffective or too uncomfortable.

The recurrent question, "How can patients afford consultation?" is a red herring. The therapist may simply eliminate one of the therapy interviews to help the family understand how important a second opinion is. It is possible to see families once every other week, once every third or fourth week, and still make the same or even better progress. Avoiding the consultant is a way of hiding anxieties.

Calling in a consultant is a step that mental health professionals can or should take in the first contact with clients, whether with an individual patient, couple, family, extended family, or group, before therapy begins. In a strange way, the initial contact is always like a blind date that involves such questions as: Who is the therapist? Who is the patient or family? What do they expect? What do they want? What can they accept? What will benefit them? The ultimate question is: What can the therapist offer? Out of these original questions, the final issue is: Can the therapist and family evolve a concurrent project, or does the family need only information about a further or different referral?

For example, one patient wanted to begin her fourth psychotherapy attempt in a new city with a new therapist. It became clear during the first "consultation" hour about possible therapy that her previous therapists had been effective and that she had developed a good investment in them. Her plan for renewed therapy was to extend her discovery of herself by another symbolic, interpersonal experience. In the role of consultant, the new potential therapist suggested that instead of reentering therapy she should read Anne Morrow Lindbergh's book, *Gift From the Sea*, and set out on a solo discovery of herself. A long series of dyadic relationships does not facilitate the necessarily solitary rite of passage to selfhood. In consultation, options are considered, and therapy is not necessarily the best choice as the next step. A consultant may suggest to a therapist or directly to family members who are seeking therapy that they do not need psychotherapy because it would be most advantageous if they just continued with their own living process without a foster parent.

REFERENCE

Wynne, L. C., Ryckoff, I. M., Day, J., & Hirsch, S. Pseudo-mutuality in the family relations of schizophrenics. *Psychiatry*, 1958, *21*, 205–220.

7

IS THERE THERAPY AFTER CONSULTATION?

A Systemic Map for Family Therapy Consultation

PEGGY PENN

MARCIA SHEINBERG

Ackerman Institute for Family Therapy
New York, New York

As consultants about impasses in family therapy, we often have found that stalemates between therapists and families in treatment are curiously similar; the problematic theme of the family connects to an important problematic theme in the therapist's family or work system, and both are stalemated. In an impasse, it is these concomitant themes that govern the therapy. We have developed a systemic map for consultation with five stages that help break the stalemate between the family and the therapist.

In consultations with therapists, we have formulated the impasse as arising when a thematic resonance has developed between the double contexts of the therapist and the family. For therapists, the context may include their family of origin, current family, team, or any area of their work. Information can be elicited and defined by a consultant even in the first interview with the therapist: "Does the problem in this family have any resonance for you?" Resemblant but unrecognized connections can be found between the participants; a common but unidentified theme flows between the two, resulting in the impasse. Such an impasse appears to be what Gregory Bateson (1972) called a "double description," in which each component is essential to an understanding of the whole therapeutic system. The first task of the consultation, therefore, is to identify these thematic connections and then to design interventions that will unify them in the service of the entire therapeutic process and thus break the impasse.

Earlier, we and others regarded change in the "simple loop" of family dynamics as the sole indicator of treatment progress. With the development of cybernetics, we have learned to look at more complex loops and now look for changes in the system or context of the therapist and the family.

Any therapeutic loop that develops into an impasse has the capacity for reorganization as well as stalemate. The most thorny place in any consultation is not the appreciation of systemic wholeness and potential but, rather, the addition of another observing loop—the consultation—without derailing the ongoing therapeutic system. We wish to conduct that transaction in such a way that the therapy remains superordinate and is able to integrate the perturbations of the consultation. Our continual question is: How can we use this perturbation of the therapeutic system to resolve the impasse while protecting the centrality of the therapist and insuring continuity of the therapy as needed?[1]

We have designed a consultation process that consists of five steps carried out in three interviews with two consultants, the authors.

- *First Interview*
  Step 1: Consultant 2 interviews the therapist about the therapy impasse, while Consultant 1 observes.
- *Second Interview* (1 week later)
  Step 2: Consultant 2 interviews the family, while therapist and Consultant 1 observe.
  Step 3: Consultant 1 interviews the therapist regarding the consultation.
  Step 4: Consultants 1 and 2 break to confer about an intervention, and then deliver the intervention to the therapist.
- *Third Interview* (months later)
  Step 5: Follow-up interview of therapist with both consultants.

There is a week between the first and second interviews and a follow-up some months later. The second interview is in three parts that take place on the same day. During the course of all interviews, the consultant behind the one-way mirror communicates by phone with the consultant in the interview room and periodically suggests a discussion break.

The first interview (Step 1) is usually conducted by one of the consultants with the therapist alone, while the other consultant observes through the mirror. We shall differentiate the consultants by calling the observing consultant behind the mirror Consultant 1, and the interviewing consultant

1. The idea for this form of consultation came from Dr. Tom Andersen's work in Norway (1985). As a supervising psychiatrist, he consults with general practitioners and conceptualizes his work in terms of cybernetic loops designed to protect the general practitioner's relationship to the family.

Consultant 2. In the first interview we identify the double contexts and their isomorphic themes.

One week later, Consultant 2 interviews the family in treatment while the therapist joins Consultant 1 in observing behind the mirror (Step 2).[2] In the next part of this second interview (Step 3), Consultant 1 interviews the therapist regarding his or her responses to the consultation with the family in treatment. The final part of the second interview (Step 4) is the *break*, where the consultants confer together without the therapist, prepare their intervention(s), and then rejoin the therapist to deliver the intervention(s).

Step 5 is a follow-up at a later date agreed upon by the consultants and the therapist. In the follow-up interview, the consultants receive feedback about their consultation and the progress of the therapeutic system.

FIVE PROPOSITIONS

1. It is the intention of the consultation to protect the centrality of the therapist in the event that a decision to continue therapy is made after the consultation. This is achieved by having the therapist either in a position of dominance to the consultants or paired with one of the consultants in each of the five steps.

2. The consultants never investigate only the therapist's dynamics or only the family's dynamics. Instead, they observe and comment on the connection between them that has contributed to the impasse. The intention is to trigger change in the therapist *in relation to the work with the family*. To accomplish this, interventions are made only with the therapist; there are no *direct* interventions with the family.

3. The interventions are often twinned. This means that though they do not resemble each other on the surface, interventions are targeted toward the shared areas of impasse, so that even if the therapist uses only one, the whole therapeutic system will be affected.

4. The interventions are flexible as to their timing. The therapist is encouraged to use them when he or she feels it is the "right time," which could be now, never, in 3 months, next year, and so on. This use of the element of time, in which the therapist decides when to use the suggestions, restores the therapist's place in the therapeutic system.

2. In the example to be described here, Consultant 2 did the first two interviews, but we have alternated interviewers with no noticeable differences. The decision about who goes first reflects our attempt to remain as neutral as possible toward the therapist. Therefore, if one of the consultants knows the therapist, the other will interview first.

5. The consultants have chosen to work in a team of two, alternating between interviewing the therapist or the family, or observing from behind the one-way mirror. We have chosen to work as two consultants rather than one because in that way we are a system observing a system, with the capacity to observe ourselves.

STEP 1

As exemplified by the following case example, in the first stage of the consultation a connection is identified between a theme in the family's dynamics and a theme in the therapist's context that may have resulted in a therapeutic impasse. As noted, the process begins with Consultant 2 interviewing the therapist while Consultant 1 observes from behind the one-way mirror. Though Consultant 2 elicits information about the therapist's professional setting and the family's dynamics, the emphasis remains on the therapist's perception of how her work with the family is progressing. By challenging the therapist's definition of the impasse, the consultant obtains *a problem definition that includes the therapist* and that organizes the therapy and the impasse. Through a question, she elicits the connection to the therapist's personal context. The therapist's response confirms and expands the thematic relevance of both contexts. It is in this manner that the impasse is doubly described.

What follows is a verbatim transcription of the initial consultation interview conducted by Consultant 2 (*C2*) with the therapist (*T*).

THERAPIST–FAMILY RESONANCE: A CASE EXAMPLE

T: I work at an adoption agency in New Jersey. This is a family that adopted a child, Derek, when he was 3 months old. He is interracial and the adoptive parents are interracial. Mother is white, father is black. Derek is now 13. The family has not been back to the agency since the adoption. At one point they did consider adopting a second child, but found that they would have had to take an older child and were not interested. So it's a family with one adopted child who is presenting problems. They came back to the agency saying, "Can you help us?" I'm working structurally with the parents to set limits and work together, but I don't think I understand what is keeping them so involved with the child, what keeps them all in such a tight triangle. Then I wonder how life would be for these parents if Derek was no longer involved in their life.

C2: What was the problem that brought them into therapy?

T: The child was kicked out of school last year. He had been in therapy for 4 years, beginning with a recommendation from his second-grade teacher. He was seen once a week, the father was seen once a week, and the mother was seen twice a week for 4 years. Only mother felt that therapy helped her. She felt less depressed and she lost weight. She felt it was helpful to the marital relationship. They communicated better. I don't think they felt therapy helped Derek at all.

C2: So it helped everyone but Derek.

T: Helped everyone minimally, but not 4 years' worth, according to them. It culminated in Derek behaving violently and being kicked out of a very nice school. He beat up two girls. He is not able to handle any frustration. He's not able to acknowledge that he is responsible for anything. Anything that gets lost, anything that gets broken is always someone else's fault. Also, his parents are totally intimidated by him. He rules the house. He intimidates them with threats of violence, threats of running away, and threats of breaking things.

C2: I see. Now, you've worked with them in a particular way. Do you feel that it's been successful? Are there any improvements?

T: I think there is some change. They reported recently they said no to him for the first time. I asked who that was more difficult for, and it was the mother's fear that he would feel lonely if she ever said no to him. It's important that this is a family where the parents were both older when they adopted. The mother is now 56 and the father is 47. So she was really 40 when she got married. They adopted Derek 4 years later. Also, both parents come from families that avoided confrontations at all cost.

C2: All right. Your basic assumption is that he's having all this difficulty because his parents have not been able to say no to him; they have not been able to set limits.

T: Yes. Absolutely, absolutely.

C2: This is the question I want to ask you. You've been helping them set limits and work together, and there's improvement. So why do you feel at an impasse at this moment?

T: I think that the improvement is minor compared to what they could do.

C2: What is your reason for wanting to find another level, to work in a different way with the family?

T: They're very bright and they've been in treatment a long time, and I think that I'm not saying anything terribly new. I have a sense when I speak to them that they already know what I'm saying. But I'm really not getting at the—maybe the marital struggle. I think that's really a part of the problem; although they didn't come in for that, I think that that's really what's keeping this child so involved. I have hesitated to work with them on their marriage.

C2: I see.

T: This is a couple who has never gone out without him.

C2: If you were to be more disrespectful and say, "Invite me in to talk about your marriage," what do you think would happen?

T: Well, they're very cooperative people. They probably would go along with me. I did try to find out if they would be concerned about each other if Derek was not a problem. I asked the boy what his concerns would be about his parents. Mother feels that the father needs more time alone, but she'd like to have more time with him. However, I didn't get a feeling from the father that he misses time with the mother.

C2: So you feel what might become obvious is that the mother desires the father more than he desires her.

T: Um-hum. He's a kind of quiet, independent person.

C2: If that were to emerge as a result of your working on another level, the marital level, what might happen?

T: The mother might be able to recognize that keeping the child involved is in some way a substitute for her.

C2: And if she were to realize that?

T: I think that could be very helpful. I don't know why I've been so reluctant to work on some of the—to see what's behind keeping this child so involved.

C2: All right. Well, let me ask you something different. Is there any event in your own life that resonates around the theme of "not intruding on the couple?"

T: That's interesting. I was thinking about that question coming over here.

C2: You were?

T: I was. I was just thinking about the case. I realized that I'm in the same position in this family as in my family of origin because my brother was very much like this boy. At a younger age, he really had my parents totally intimidated. He ruled the show. He had tantrums, and really kept them from going out very often by threatening to break something, and I was the one who, as the bigger sister, was coaching my parents—unsuccessfully.

C2: Oh, really. You were handling it?

T: Yes. I remember saying to them, "Even though he threatens to break this or to do that, and I know you're not going to be able to go out and have a good time, go down to the lobby" [we lived in an apartment building] "and sit in the lobby all night 'cause your evening is ruined, I understand. Sit in the lobby just so he knows he didn't win."

C2: How old were you when you did that?

T: I was probably about 10 or 12. I think that's why I became a social worker, so I could struggle with clients.

C2: Did your parents listen to you?

T: They didn't listen to me. Eventually, he had to go away to a school where the structure was imposed, and he really shaped up.

C2: Do you think, had they listened to you, they would have shaped him up?

T: Yes, I do.

The two consultants take a short break to discuss the emerging themes of being "in" the family or "out" of the family. The interview then resumes.

C2: Let me tell you what we think might be going on. Derek seems to be behaving in a way that assures him of having a place in the family. You must have a place or you don't belong. There seems to be a theme in this family around people having a place, not having a place, getting in and getting out of the family. I think that resonates for you in your own family with your brother. Did he have a place? Did he not have a place? And so on. You were the big sister and you tried to keep him in the family, but it's possible that part of the family also welcomed his being extruded so that things would calm down. So he probably got both messages: You're in, but only if you behave; otherwise, you're not.

T: Absolutely. There was a combination. There was a relief when he left because things really did calm down. It was also hard to have friends over—he was always having temper tantrums. But yet I lost because no one listened to me, and he could have been saved. If they had listened and done what I said, maybe he wouldn't have had to leave. I felt terribly guilty that I didn't tell him that he was leaving.

C2: You knew?

T: I knew. It was one of those "I Never Promised You a Rose Garden," where you get driven on a summer day somewhere, and then told you're not coming back. I knew.

C2: Your parents had told you?

T: Yes. And I think I felt very guilty that I didn't tip him off in some way.

C2: The idea of having a place in a family versus being extruded is an important idea in your family, and I think this family you're seeing is struggling with similar issues. Does this boy have a place? Does he belong or is he to be extruded?

T: Right. To extrude him by setting a limit when it's an adoption is doubly hard for people.

C2: So you even see limit setting as an extrusion of the boy?

T: Well, I think these parents do because if they were to say, "We're going out tonight," he would feel rejected.

C2: Do you feel that, or do the parents?

T: They've said that.

C2: And you feel that, too?

T: Well, no, but I've heard that a lot from families with adopted children. After all, he's had the ultimate rejection. How can you do it again?

C2: So you feel there is a tremendous amount of confusion around creating rules and discipline for adopted kids. It's hard to say, "Of course you belong here and of course we go out without you, because you're the kid and we're the grown-ups."

T: Yes.

C2: Those issues get confused and you have a particular sensitivity to them yourself. We would like to suggest you bring in the family next week and that you join [Consultant 1] behind the screen to observe the interview.

T: I would like to do that.

C2: Please inform the family about the arrangements before the session.

STEP 2

At the next session, one week later, Consultant 2 meets with the family while the therapist and Consultant 1 observe from behind the one-way mirror and both are in a meta position to the interview. The interview begins with questions about the progress of the therapy and then moves to a discussion about the family's coalitional patterns before and during the therapy. When the consultant asks an existential question about how the couple would fare without their son to fight over, it removes Derek from the conflict between his parents, and begins to expose the pseudomutuality (Wynne, Ryckoff, Day, & Hirsch, 1958) of the couple. Asking this question allows the son to comment with his ideas on the state of the art of marriage; that is, conflict is needed in marriage to insure its survival.

C2: Let me ask you what might be missing in your therapy. In all good work, there's always something that someone might feel is missing.

Mother: On our therapist's part or on ours?

C2: Either.

Mother: Oh, she still hasn't broken us down as to being firm with Derek.

Father: I think that—

C2: She hasn't broken you down.

Mother: It's a hard job.

Father: Well, I think that—I think that the problem, as far as I'm concerned, the problem is one of consistency.

Mother: Umm. That's what I'm saying.

Father: I'm absolutely certain of that. I know that within myself. I'm not always consistent in my handling of issues. I tend to vacillate.

Mother: We don't like to face the issues.

Father: But, you know, I'm seeing results and I'm making a really concerted effort to be more firm and consistent in the way that I handle things.

C2: Okay. Now your therapist, as you said, has been trying to break you down, to get you to do these things, and it seems you both agree you want to do them, but you're vacillating?

Mother: Fearful.

C2: Fearful in what sense? What would happen?

Mother: Well, we don't like conflicts. We just don't like to face a lot of things. Peace at any cost has been our rule.

C2: Would you agree, the two of you, in recalling these fights with Derek, that generally it ends up with you, Father, and Derek together at the end of the fight?

Son: It always does.

Father: Yeah. More likely than not.

Mother: Is this true?

Son: Yeah. You're just—

Father: Well, I think that—

Mother: Oh yes. I just leave because I see no sense in the arguing back and forth.

C2: You leave. Do you feel that your husband has been strong enough with Derek?

Mother: No.

C2: Has he gotten stronger with Derek?

Mother: Yes. We both have. We've worked together on it a lot lately.

C2: How does it work now?

Mother: Now we do nothing until the two of us can talk privately, and then we get together on it and that's it.

C2: Derek, if your parents had never adopted you, do you think their life would be nice and smooth?

Son: No.

Mother: You don't?

Son: No.

C2: What would it be like?

Son: I don't know.

Mother: We would get bored. We would get bored with each other. Yes.

C2: Do you think they'd have fights? What would they fight over if not over you?

Son: I don't know.

Mother: I've often wondered about that.

C2: You knew right away that it wouldn't be peaches and cream, it wouldn't be totally smooth?

Mother: Nothing is.

Son: If it were, then they wouldn't be married; but I don't know.

C2: Do you mean that marriage needs the expression of some anger?

Son: If you don't vent off anger, then some time when you try to vent it off, it will blow up.

C2: It gets to be too much if you let it all accumulate? Is that what you're saying?

Son: Yes. Yeah.

Mother: You're in no danger of that.

Son: Ha, ha, ha.

C2: You're saying that, even without you in the picture, for them to have a marriage that would last, they would have to find a way to have some conflict because, without it, someone would explode? Or what would happen without it?

Son: I don't know. I'm just saying that there would be a lot of anger.

C2: Would someone leave?

Son: I don't know. I can't predict something that didn't happen.

C2: That's interesting. You really feel that it's important for a marriage to have some anger expressed in it, and your parents are saying that they think it's important for a—

Son: Not just in marriage. Any relationship.

C2: Any relationship.

Son: Sure. I meet friends at camp on the first day. We fight on the second day. And we are better friends on the third.

C2: It's like two opposing philosophies. Hmm?

Son: Yeah.

C2: Their idea is that their relationship needs to be conflict free, but you have this very important idea that a marriage must express some conflict; otherwise, it wouldn't last.

STEP 3

Step 3 takes place on the same day, immediately after the family leaves. Consultant 2 moves to the meta position behind the mirror, observing Consultant 1 and the therapist. In this interview, the therapist discusses her responses to watching Consultant 2 interview her treatment family. She immediately recognizes the "theme"—the difficulty Consultant 2 had getting "in" to the family—as a problem she herself is having, Derek is having, and her brother had in her family of origin. The therapist deals with being "out" of the family by moving toward the mother, and we hypothesize that this move also happened in her family. When the consultant talks about the mother's alliance with the therapist, she is indirectly talking about the therapist's alliance with her own mother, which we see as a response to the hidden coalition between father and son. Toward the end of this interview, direct reference is made to the resolution of the brother's place in the therapist's family of origin and to the pseudounity of her parents. This is confirmed by the therapist's recognition that her mother was more upset about her brother, and that her intervention has mediated this upset. This interviewing process addresses the double contexts by identifying the similarity of dynamics in the families that has contributed to the impasse. The next task of the consultation will be to intervene in such a manner that the entire therapeutic context or loop will shift. Consultant 1 (C1) now interviews the therapist.

C1: Tell me what was different for you.

T: Well, well, let me just say what was the same.

C1: Okay. What was the same?

T: I watched the way they didn't let [C2] in. My experience was of mother's really not answering the question and talking about social issues, using a lot of humor, a lot of sarcasm, et cetera. I think I've gotten to know them over the course of time, and they give the sense of not jumping in, although they really do think about what's being given to them. They really digest it.

C1: That was clear, yes.

T: But they don't always let you know that. You don't always know whether you've got them or not.

C1: How do you deal with that, this feeling from them that they keep you out?

T: Well, one thing I do is I fight my impulse to go to the mother. She's humorous, she's alive, she always has something to say; whereas the father is more ponderous. She fills up the space more. When I force myself to really hear what he has to say, I often get some of the richest material from him. I noticed they were on their best behavior today, so you didn't see Derek challenge them. When Derek feels frustrated, he talks in a shrill voice. He's at the edge of his voice: "What do you mean I'm—" da, da, da, da, about to explode, and they don't hear it. They answer him as though he was speaking very nicely, and I have often said, "Is this how he talks to you at home?"

C1: Do they act like he's not there?

T: They pretend that they don't hear the *way* he's saying things. They just hear what he says.

Cl: That's a way of not really hearing him. It's a real disqualification, isn't it?

T: Yes. He also engages them in content struggles. For instance, could he really get to class in time when, in fact, he has to climb up forty-seven stairs to get to class?

Cl: So he's good at engaging them. He's better than you are or than we are.

T: Oh. (*Laughter.*) Absolutely!

Cl: He's the best, and that's how he gets in rather than being out.

T: That's right. Yes.

Cl: Now, if you had to choose one person in the family who thought that this therapy was most in his or her behalf, who would you choose?

T: Well, I would agree with what the mother said. She's the optimist, and the father is more cautious.

Cl: So she feels more allied with you in the therapy. Is her sense of therapy that you're helping her? If so, what are you helping her to do?

T: Be less intimidated by her son.

Cl: I see. The basic theme of the family is an interesting one: For an adopted child who is an interracial child of a white mother and a black father, the expression of anger, or extreme difference, makes him feel like an outsider. But Derek has indicated that, on the contrary, he will use his difference and anger to become an insider. He will aggressively "stay" in this family. Now you work in a foster-care agency, so you recognize that belonging is an—

T: It's an absolutely crucial issue.

Cl: Crucial issue. I have to assume that these issues around belonging often come up in these families and you deal with them over and over again.

T: Yes. Oh, absolutely.

Cl: Now let me ask you something about your own family. Did your brother ever resolve whether he belonged in your family? I know you tried to get your parents together, just as you try with these two parents. You encourage them to get together, to take charge and et cetera, to listen to you, to save this boy, give him a place, keep him in, et cetera.

T: Well, you know what's so interesting is that I saw today that they were much more together than I had formerly seen them. But I also experienced my parents as very together. They also were a tight unit.

Cl: And possibly hard to get to?

T: Certainly. Clearly, they were a unit. That was very clear in my family.

Cl: Did you have as hard a time as your brother getting into that unit?

T: Yes, and I feel closer and closer to my brother as we get older, and more protective. I still dive in, head first, to protect him against my parents when I feel they are up to something.

C1: That's still necessary?

T: Yes. And he will call on me to do it. I feel—I feel more like a big sister.

C1: What would happen if you didn't do that?

T: I feel he needs it. He can't stand up for himself. They're overwhelming. It needs the two of us.

C1: They're overwhelming.

T: Yeah. They have demands of what nice Jewish children do for their parents.

C1: Well, you certainly know how to handle that. (*Laughter.*) Although your parents are very close, is there one who would be more upset with him?

T: Yeah, my mother.

C1: Your mother would be more upset. And would your father plead his son's case?

T: Yes. He's actually been the one

C1: So you have to intercede in order to make sure that she doesn't get too upset? Is that right?

T: Well, she does threaten to push him out. It's always "the end," but I don't take it all as seriously as I imagine I used to.

STEP 4

INTERVENTION

Although the intervention tasks, one for the family and one for the therapist, appear quite different, they are structured similarly; their intention is to focus on the pseudomutuality of the parental couples through addressing their differences. When the differences are addressed, the coalitions open up, and the systems can no longer maintain the appearance of "unity." Both interventions are targeted toward the whole therapeutic system so that if only one is used, it will still affect both systems.

The element of time is introduced to underscore the therapeutic context as ongoing, with the therapist's centrality remaining intact. This allows the therapist to determine when the consultation will end. Consultant 1 delivers the intervention to the therapist.

C1: I am going to talk to you about your own family. I'll offer a couple of suggestions that you may or may not use at whatever time you think best, tomorrow, next month, next year, never, et cetera. You have a crucial spot in your family, an important place. Our first suggestion would be to say to your brother: "I don't think I should protect you anymore. I think you are able to make your own place in the family." Then you would need to say to your parents: "I cannot decide which one of you is right. I know both your positions about this issue with my brother, and I absolutely cannot decide which of you is right. So I'm not going to intercede because I can't make a decision." Now that means your brother will either have to make a place for himself or he'll have to go to your father to find out how to negotiate with your mother. Your father knows. Or he'll do something we can't anticipate.

T: So he's got to be allowed to make his own place.

C1: This would let him decide how to get into the family, accompanied by you saying to your parents: "I don't know which of you is right. I can't decide."

T: Even if I understand or think I know who's right?

C1: You don't know who is right.

T: (*Laughing.*) Okay. No. I can see two sides.

C2: Now, we do have something for the family. We recommend that for 3 days mother takes total charge of disciplining Derek, handling all the conflicts that may emerge and any misbehavior he drums up. She does it totally on her own for 3 days. Then the next 3 days the father takes charge and she steps back.

T: Three consecutive days.

C2: Yes. He's totally in charge. However he organizes it, it's his domain. And for the last 3 days, they do whatever comes spontaneously. Anyone can take charge. If they fall back, that's fine too. Everything is acceptable.

T: Well, I think that will—could do some interesting—

C2: What I'm concerned about is that both of these suggestions will really change your position, both in your family of origin and in your treatment family. So I think that you ought to think about it and only do it when you feel that there's a *time* you're ready to do it. Otherwise, I think you should hold back until you're ready for some change.

T: Puts me out of a job.

C2: When you're ready for a change, then you'll draw on this. Okay?

T: All right. All right.

STEP 5

FOLLOW-UP INTERVIEW

C2: Do you see this family any differently than you did before you met with us?

T: I saw the parents as people who were in their own kind of trap, and the boy was acting up to bring them together and to bring the father in more. I don't think I saw the hidden coalition between the father and the son. Before, I saw the couple as such a tight unit and the boy was struggling to make a place. So, yes, I do see it a little differently. I feel that I have more of a handle on the level of their marital disagreements, though I still am working very structurally with them.

C1: How did it work in your family? One of the things we had said to you was to take time to decide when you wanted to use our suggestion, if you wanted to use it in 5 years, 2 months, et cetera. How did you—

T: I had one opportunity to use it with my brother and I used it in the smallest way I could at the final moment that I could. (*Laughter.*) But this consultation was very significant. I really started to do a lot of thinking about the family I brought in, my current family, my family of origin, and my first marriage. I just went through many different phases for a long time, thinking about it in different places, thinking about my place in each of those families, and the families' similarities, and my brother, and this boy. It stayed with me a very long time.

C1: So those connections made sense.

T: They made sense. Now, if I jump in to rescue my brother, it will be with a total awareness of what I'm doing and how that really may be blocking him from moving into the family. It's going to be a lot harder to do because I see it in a much different way.

CONCLUDING COMMENTS

This consultation describes a double context: the family system, and the personal system of the therapist. The latter is thematically similar to the situation in the family in treatment. We hypothesize that it is the unrecognized connection between these systems that results in an impasse. We collect information about the coalitional structure and themes in the family system, and this guides us to the information to be collected about the therapist's system. Taken together, they produce a feedback process, with data from one context informing the other until a hypothesis about both contexts is developed. Using two consultants permits the integration of these isomorphs into interventions that are relevant to the impasse but do not usurp the therapist's place. How the interventions are used, whether therapy continues or not, are issues for the therapist and family to decide.

This systemic approach to consultation may be modified if a one-way mirror and two consultants are not available. In such an adaptation, Step 1 remains the same. In Step 2, the therapist tells the family in advance that he or she will stay in the room to observe the consultant and family. The major difficulty occurs in Step 3, where the consultant has to remain objective when the therapist comments on the consultant's interview. The degree to which one is able to maintain the observer position will affect how one uses the therapist's comments to generate a fuller hypothesis. In Step 4, the consultants take a short break to think through translating the information into paired interventions. Step 5, the follow-up interview, remains unchanged.

We have used this form of systemic consultation in a variety of circumstances and with increasing flexibility. In some cases, we have not performed all the steps. In other cases, we have seen only the therapist. We also have adapted the model for use when the referring context includes professionals from different disciplines who have developed a problem among themselves that is isomorphic to the family problem. More commonly, however, we have seen both the family and the therapist, and we have completed all five steps, as illustrated in the case example.

Our title, "Is There Therapy after Consultation?," highlights the differences between the terms "therapy" and "consultation." The term "therapy" has emerged from a medical context, and its essential meaning has remained "the curing of a disease." By extension, in the field of human relations it has come to be regarded as a process that changes or adapts "ill behaviors" to the social norm. The term "consultation" has sometimes been regarded as a higher form of therapy; in a sense, it has become a therapy of therapy. Given that perspective, consultation, like therapy, is cut from the same curative cloth. If there were no "family therapy," and we only *consulted* with family systems, families might come to feel less labeled, less ill, less crazy, and so on. Eventually, family systems could obtain consultations about family matters when needed, just as they consult many other professionals when they need them. Following that idea, families sometimes could have consultations with one consultant and, on occasion, with more than one. Eventually, we could drop our medical-therapeutic characterization and adopt the term "consultation" as a more respectful descriptor of our activities with family systems.

REFERENCES

Andersen, T. Consultation: Would you like co-evolution instead of referral? *Family Systems Medicine*, 1985, *2*, 370–379.

Bateson, G. *Steps to an ecology of mind.* New York: Ballantine Books, 1972.

Wynne, L. C., Ryckoff, I. M., Day, J., & Hirsch, S. Pseudo-mutuality in the family relations of schizophrenics. *Psychiatry*, 1958, *21*, 205–220.

8

CONSULTATION WITH MENTAL HEALTH SYSTEM TEAMS IN ITALY

GIANFRANCO CECCHIN

LAURA FRUGGERI

Centro per lo Studio della Famiglia
Milan, Italy

In collaboration with LYMAN C. WYNNE and SUSAN H. McDANIEL

Since 1978, when mental health services in Italy were deinstitutionalized, Italian mental health centers have worked not only with psychiatric problems but with social problems as well. The concepts underlying deinstitutionalization can be traced from the theoretical formulations of Maxwell Jones (1953). In Italy, Jones's ideas were elaborated in a political–social form by Franco Basaglia (1973) and his collaborators. Inspired by a movement called Democratic Psychiatry, Italian mental health workers introduced attitudes and approaches that were opposed to institutionalization of patients. In 1978, these changes were codified in national law no. 180, which ratified the closure of the psychiatric hospitals and gave responsibility for psychiatric intervention to mental health centers in the community.

Before deinstitutionalization, mental health services functioned in a way that kept the patient a patient. The implicit message to patients was the same whether they were in the hospital or outside, namely: "You are a chronic patient. You have a chronic problem that needs medication and continued care inside or outside of the hospital. If you cannot maintain yourself outside of the hospital, you will need to be rehospitalized." From the patient's standpoint, it was advantageous to be regarded as "chronic" in order to get social services. The mental health worker had to define the patient as chronic in order to get medication, to provide help finding a job, housing, and so on. Thus, both the patient and the mental health worker were reinforced for maintaining the patient's status.

The 1978 law for the deinstitutionalization of patients changed the implicit message to patients; it now became: "We can help you if you are not chronic." Since deinstitutionalization, the services that formerly were provided only for "handicapped" or "chronic" inpatients are provided only for nonchronic, self-supporting patients. Given this state of affairs, patients began to change their behavior. They now had to avoid being labeled chronic in order to receive help. In Italy, deinstitutionalization took place on a more sweeping scale and from a different starting place than, for example, in the United States, and the changes in Italy were greater than in places where deinstitutionalization has been only partial.

SYSTEMIC FAMILY THERAPY WITHIN ITALIAN PUBLIC SERVICES

Nearly all staff members in the Italian mental health programs understood that the public services were keeping patients dependent. Even with deinstitutionalization, the patterns of dependency were recreated when the staff took the same kind of roles that the institution previously had taken. The system of services now was located outside of the hospital but could function in the same way as it had before deinstitutionalization. In some centers, the new custodial hospital is the home. Instead of being in the back ward of the hospital, patients now are in the back room of the home. In these places, members of the mental health staff have tried to continue in the old way: Patients are more or less left to their own devices except that they are given medication, some nursing care, and an occasional home visit in order to monitor whether they have regressed too far—in which case, they are rehospitalized for 2 to 3 weeks at a time before being released. In these settings, the consistent message is: "You have to go back home."

In other centers, there was a furor among the mental health people who wanted to help, wanted to cure, and who perceived their proper function as the provision of broad public services. Staff members of a number of these mental health services began to come to the Centro per lo Studio della Famiglia in Milan with the more or less explicit goal of learning how to counteract dependency dynamics by learning the skills of systemic family therapy in the Milan model. However, when the Milan family therapy model was applied in the context of public services, it became apparent that the cases were being treated ineffectively and many were ending in failures. We concluded that the model was being applied without enough attention to the broader context, that is, with a too narrow or literal application of the family therapy model that did not take into account the specific context of public services.

In this context of public services, many types of interventions take place, including conversation and interviews with clients, home visits, pharmacologic prescriptions, and socioeconomic assistance. Within each catchment area of about 200,000 people, mental health services are now integrated with other types of medical, psychiatric, psychological, and economic intervention. The services are accessible to all persons free of charge, with institutions responsible for intervention when compulsory treatment is necessary after referrals by neighbors, police, families, priests, and so on. Also, staff members have the same salaries regardless of the number of clients seen; they work on the basis of personal motivation rather than on a fee-for-service basis.

This public mental health context differs greatly from that in our private practice and teaching systemic family therapy in Milan. In dealing with the difference, we could have tried to modify the context of public services so that it would fit our techniques of systemic family therapy. Obviously, this would have been very complicated and difficult to accomplish. More realistic was the opposite idea of modifying our family therapy techniques in order to adapt them to the context. However, both of these approaches would have rested on the premise that systemic family therapy is a primary, generalized solution to the problems involved in providing services. This premise would have involved a confusion of levels between family therapy as a specific set of techniques and family therapy as a theoretical model. In our approach, family therapy includes techniques such as meeting with the family in a certain setting and with a structure of interviewing in stages (presession, session, team conference, and intervention). In addition, the model includes theoretical principles for therapeutic intervention that are intended to introduce information about new connections and new maps of the world.[1] Differences between relational patterns can be identified directly, as in reframing or, more indirectly, as in prescription of rituals and the use of circular questioning and neutrality by the therapist (Penn, 1982; Selvini Palazzoli, Boscolo, Cecchin, & Prata, 1980). Regardless of the type of intervention chosen, systemic family therapy is always oriented to stimulating the family to look for new relational patterns.

In applying family therapy principles in the context of public services, we have regarded our role as that of consultants to the service teams who are the primary implementers. We found that family therapy techniques are possible and adequate only in certain cases, while different methods are more appropriate and effective in other cases. If one accepts the idea of doing something other than therapy, it becomes very clear that social assistance (or whatever) is the job that the staff is paid to do and needs to do. There can be a therapeutic effect to such an approach without doing therapy. The staff is introduced to the idea of accepting what the family

1. "Information" was defined by Bateson (1979) as "any difference that makes a difference."

shows them. If the family members show that they are helpless, then a natural kind of caretaking by staff is accepted. Any member of the service team can do useful interventions. That is, each staff member can take care of particular needs, depending on the division of team roles and special training of each person.

When new staff members come to programs with a more systemic approach, they take to the new systems ideas quickly. Often there is an administrative director who leaves the staff members free to do what they want. Administrators usually are political appointees who know nothing about therapy. When a patient has been chronically ill, two or three staff persons are assigned to the case. Perhaps a nurse, a social worker, and a psychiatrist will visit the patient's home together. After the visit, they meet and try to arrive at a hypothesis about what is going on and to decide what kind of intervention can and should be attempted. Very rarely is it in the form of a purely psychological intervention; usually it will involve some action and not just verbal intervention. "Talking" therapy is not important for most of these people; they want and need action. Family therapy may be one of the types of services provided, but only one.

Overcoming dependency: A case example. Marguerita is a 35-year-old, married, depressed woman who had been a "chronic patient." Her husband had left her and was not available when she was to be discharged. She was incapable of doing anything for herself or of caring for her two young children at home. She needed a nurse or social worker to help her on a daily basis. Her mother began to go to the home quite frequently after Marguerita was discharged, but she soon became rather bored with taking care of her daughter, preferring to be with another daughter and son. The more the nurse and social worker visited the home, the more the patient became dependent upon them for giving her medication and care. The mother finally stopped coming to see the patient in order to have more time with the patient's sister and brother, and the patient became increasingly dependent upon the nurse and social worker.

What were the nurse and social worker to do? Our role as consultants to this team came about when the mental health staff (a social worker, psychologist, nurse, and psychiatrist) brought the case to us. When they had tried family therapy in this situation, they found that it did not work very well. At first they brought the family to the consultation, with the idea of continuing family therapy. But the problem was not helped with family therapy. Other approaches were needed: monitoring medication, home visits, finding a job for the patient. We believed that there were far richer possibilities for helping this family than through formal family therapy.

We learned that it was much better to consult with the four service team members, and not directly with the family. Sometimes the team would bring audiotapes for us to hear or would present a report that they had prepared about what was currently going on. Trying to educate the mother in this case had not worked, yet the staff realized that the mother was much more effective in helping the patient than they were. A decision was made not to help the patient directly but to talk to the mother and the daughter together about the problem. The team told the mother and daughter that the nurse would assist the patient only when the mother was present, but would not come if the mother were not there. They said that they respected the patient's decision to be totally helpless and, therefore, the nurse would visit only to help the mother.

When the nurse visited with the mother present, she would help the mother to cook, clean the house, and so on, but she would leave when the mother left. This approach had a tremendous effect upon the mother. She perceived herself as the "best of mothers," better than the nurse who was only there to help her. The daughter/patient then began to do some things for herself when she was alone—a response perhaps to the mother's being more helpful to her.

One day the mother announced that she wanted to go on vacation. The staff suggested that she not go too far away in case Marguerita needed her and wanted to call her. The staff emphasized that they were not going to help Marguerita without the mother being present. The mother did go on vacation, but Marguerita, knowing that she could contact the mother, never called her.

Soon, the mother informed the staff that Marguerita wanted to find a job. With the mother's help, she began looking for a job and found one. Thus, when the staff worked with the mother and refused to help Marguerita directly, Marguerita was mobilized. Thereafter, Marguerita only occasionally came to the clinic to pick up medication, and the mother slowly began to cut back on her visits to her daughter.

At this point, the staff was able to utilize only a nurse for direct contact with the family. The rest of the staff became a team of consultants to the nurse and met with her to discuss the case from time to time. The nurse was very pleased with the way things were going; she felt supported and effective. There did not need to be a sophisticated intervention; the nurse understood exactly what to do and knew she had the support of the team.

Some of our consultations have involved problems in which the staff members were presented with requests that led to conflicting responses. When staff members take sides against one another, the result is likely to be a stalemate that does not yield to nonsystemic directives or confrontations.

A blinding double bind: A case example. Elena, 50 years old, came to a mental hygiene center accompanied by her common-law husband. He said, "For a few months she cries, cannot do anything, moves slowly, and speaks to some voices." For these symptoms she had been previously admitted twice to psychiatric services without any stable improvement. The common-law husband asked openly that

Elena be put in an Old People's Home because he could not tolerate the situation and did not want her with him any longer. The team responded by saying that in order to find an answer adequate to such an important request, it was necessary to have a deeper knowledge of the situation, and to do this, it was necessary that the couple should come for a few meetings. The team did not refuse the request but, rather, redefined it.

At the first meeting the team obtained some information that suggested the possibility of formulating a systemic hypothesis and intervention. Three years earlier, the common-law husband had been left almost blind by a car accident. Because of this handicap, he found himself compelled to close his business. Since then, he lived almost locked up in the house, very depressed, and not working. It was soon after this change in her husband that Elena started to show her first symptoms. She herself observed, during one of the meetings with the team, that everything suddenly had changed: While at first she was the one to take care of the husband, afterward, because of her symptoms, it was the husband who was dedicating his time to taking care of her.

The team then explained their hypothesis and intervention to the couple: Elena was behaving as a sick person while the husband was handicapped and remained without work. Because she felt that his life had collapsed, she had decided to fill his empty life. If Elena felt this way, it was necessary to think more about the situation before sending her away from home; it was necessary to understand the consequences that such a change would have on the husband.

As a response to this intervention, the husband left the home, withdrew to a country hut, and let the wife know that he would not come back until she would agree to go to live somewhere else. This represented a complete reversal of his earlier position. Elena called the mental hygiene center and said that she felt terrible. She did not know what to do without her husband and she "trusted completely" the team to solve her problems. The team asked for a consultation from our Milan group because they beleived that the situation had come back to the starting point. Initially, the therapists had succeeded in redefining the request to admit Elena to a home for the aged as a request involving the couple. Now Elena (and the husband) had reacted by redefining the therapy as assistance with their joint living arrangements.

It became clear that the team was in a double bind. It could not refuse to help Elena find a placement in a home for the aged because this request was consistent with the role and tasks provided by the Italian social services. On the other hand, if the team confirmed the couple's "punctuation" (Bateson, 1972) of the situation, which defined Elena as incapable of taking care of herself, the team would not be helping the couple to move beyond their rigid premises.

According to this analysis, the response of the team had to be twofold: on the one hand, to accept the role of the center staff (to provide assistance) and, on the other hand, to introduce into the family system new information that would help it become less rigid. The following response was worked out in the consultation: "We are very worried about your husband because not only has he no job and has lost his eyesight, but now he also risks losing his family and a home where he can stay. We cannot do anything at the moment directly for him, but we can help you, Elena, to find a new house so that he can at least come back to his own home."

From the follow-up later on, we learned that this intervention appeared to enable them to resolve the situation. Elena now lived in a home where she could take care of herself without the help of anyone, and the husband was back home. They were now seeing each other regularly "as if they were engaged."

When a public mental health service team asks for a consultation, we initially specify that the consultation should take place with all the staff members who are involved in the case. If such a condition is satisfied, one of us meets the team members in our center in Milan or where they work. The consultation consists of a meeting with the team, followed after 6 months by a telephone call from us to obtain information about the development of the case. These consultations are usually paid for by the public service administration.

The consultation consists of a discussion that does not focus so much on the structure of the family as on the effects of therapist interventions on the interaction within the family. In the consultation, we do not formulate hypotheses separately from the team, nor do we suggest interventions. Rather, the hypotheses and the intervention come from the full group of caseworkers and consultants; the consultants only introduce a different level of analysis.

We prefer not to include the patient together with the staff members in the consultation. In those cases in which the patient is present and the patient and the therapist are observed by the consultant, the consultant considers the relation of therapist and patient, formulates hypotheses, and intervenes, remaining always within a perspective that is isomorphic to the therapeutic situation in which the patient is observed by the therapist. Without the patient present, the consultant stimulates the therapists to observe themselves while observing the patient, and in this way introduces a meta perspective of the therapeutic process.

Systemic psychopharmacology: A case example. Maria is 26 years old and was sent to the mental hygiene clinic by a family doctor. She is married and has two daughters. Her presenting symptom was a serious state of anxiety; she would not eat for fear of being poisoned. She talked of having many difficulties with her husband, but she did not want him to come to therapy because "he would not understand." She complained that the bond that the husband had with his mother and his sister is very close, and she felt that they all were in an alliance against her. She said that she could not speak in the family of her problems because everyone answers: "They are all stories." At the end of the conversation, she thanked the therapists very much for the attention that had been given to her and said, "For a long time I have been looking for someone with whom I can bring up my problems. I told this to my husband too."

The team understood the danger of a quick response to the patient. Their conclusions were:

1. Maria seems to look for a therapist in order to use him in her relationship with her husband. She had ruled that the husband should not come into therapy. Individual therapeutic meetings with her would only have confirmed her idea and her relational problem.

2. Yet, undervaluing her problems would have meant accepting the punctuation of the problem by the husband and his family.

Because of these considerations, the team decided to redefine Maria's problems, telling the family that she suffered from a sickness that needed an intensive pharmacological treatment with intravenous injections that would be carried out in the mental hygiene clinic. For this treatment, it was necessary that the husband be present to assist her. The team also added that they would not bring up the problems of the couple. Both Maria and her husband happily accepted this solution. A week later, Maria reported feeling better.

At the time of a pharmacological follow-up a month later, the couple came together and reported that they had been intensively discussing their difficulties as a couple. Also, Maria began to speak of her desire to find a job for herself. For the staff members, the problem appeared to be reaching a positive solution. However, a week after the follow-up meeting, the team received a telephone call from the husband who asked for a home visit because Maria was feeling so badly that she could not come to the clinic by herself.

At this point, the team requested a consultation from the Milan Center. The consultant focused the discussion on the last meeting: What did the therapist do in the interaction between the couple? It was reported that the therapist had not asked any questions about the couple and about their problems, but had accepted what they had spontaneously said about them. By listening to a description of the couple's problems, the therapist had broken the couple's rule, that their problems should not be talked about. This rule had been recognized at the beginning of therapy, and was at the base of the rigidity of the couple's relational problems. By listening, even passively, the therapist had begun to infringe upon this rule.

How was it possible to escape from this impasse? To go back to the definition of sickness would have been redundant, repetitive behavior devoid of "informational" meaning. To propose psychotherapy would have been going against the couple's rule. We decided that the intervention that could avoid these false alternatives would be "not intervening."

The team was given the job of calling Maria and her husband to inform them that they had made a mistake, that they had gone too fast in talking about their problems as a couple, and that it was very dangerous to talk about them at this moment in time. Because the risk of talking about the problems was very high both for the therapist and the couple, and to do so would not be therapeutic at this point, the team had decided to interrupt the meetings for 3 months.

At the follow-up, the therapist informed us that the intervention had been accepted with relief by Maria and with enthusiasm by the husband: "This is really good news!" After 3 months of interruption, the couple did not show up. They did show up, however, 5 months later to inform the therapist that things were going well.

The idea of observing yourself while you observe the family has been a central idea in the training in Milan. Dividing into groups of therapists, supervisors or consultants, and observers has been a concrete way of introducing this idea in teaching. The observation of the relation between family and therapist cannot be the specific or exclusive job of the consultant. It is part of the therapeutic process to introduce analysis of the therapeutic process itself. However, the therapist occupies a position in the therapeutic relationship that often makes it difficult for him or her, in spite of a high level of competence, to adopt this different point of view. The more external position of the consultant in relation to the therapeutic process, by contrast, facilitates adopting a second order, cybernetic, meta perspective.

After the Italian psychiatric hospitals were closed, residential community placements were opened for the purpose of helping the chronic patients return to their earlier social contexts. In order to achieve this result, caseworkers also carry out assistance activities, such as finding homes for the chronic patients of the community.

When a home is not a home: A case example. Rosa, 60 years old, had been in psychiatric hospitals for 20 years and was now living in a community residence. She had a married son who had responsibility for his old, handicapped father, and who was not willing to take care of Rosa. Rosa also had two elderly sisters who came to visit her occasionally. On the basis of their experience in the community, the mental health team believed that there was little possibility that Rosa would go back to her family. For this reason, they had written a letter to the township for Rosa (as had been done in other cases) asking that she be assigned an apartment where she could go to live by herself.

When the news came that a house had been found for her, a meeting was arranged between Rosa and her family members in order to give them the news. They all were very happy about it. This reaction perplexed the clinic team because Rosa used to say that she would leave the community residence only to go to live with her son. Nevertheless, when presented with the happiness shown by Rosa and her family members, the team decided to continue the program and to proceed with moving her to the new home.

A few days later, when Rosa was invited to go to the township office to sign the papers for her home, she answered with anger that she would not sign any paper and asked everyone to let her alone. Her family members now also expressed doubts about the kind of house assigned to Rosa. Everything seemed to be back at the starting point. The caseworkers could not understand the change and asked for a consultation from the Milan Center. The consultant proposed to analyze the meaning of "home" within the larger context of patient–caseworker. What happened in other cases? Usually the assignment of a house produced a deep crisis in older patients, and firm opposition from the family members. The caseworker found that, in response to such reactions, it was useful to say that the house was available, but that for the moment the patient did not have to go to live there. In the face of opposition, they intervened with words and actions to slow down the process and only later would take up the problem of the house again. But in the case of Rosa, in which neither she nor her family members had shown opposition, why was there a change?

We hypothesized that "home" had acquired in time, and in the more general context of the whole community (patients/staff/family members), a different meaning. We hypothesized that in light of the intervention of slowing down the process of assigning the home, the initial announcement about "finding a house" was not significant information and was not very dangerous. For this reason, Rosa and her family did not oppose the news. They reacted to the meaning that "finding a home" had come to have over time, namely, "finding a home" did not mean actually going to live there. However, staff members had responded to the nonopposition of Rosa and her family as if they really had accepted this solution. Understandably, the opposition emerged a few days later when the caseworker actively pursued this program.

In consultation, the following intervention was decided upon: "During that last meeting, we did not understand one thing and we apologize. Luckily, Rosa, with her refusal to sign the papers that would assign her a home, and you, the family, with your doubts, made us understand that you are all very happy that Rosa might have her own home, but not now. At present, it would be very dangerous for all of you. Unfortunately, we do not yet understand for whom it would be more dangerous. For this reason, we ask you to come here for another meeting. In the meantime, it is very important for Rosa not to leave her old place. As for signing the papers for the house, we regard it as a simple, bureaucratic act that has no effect. Even if Rosa were to sign it, we would not ask Rosa to go and live in the house."

At the follow-up, the staff members informed us that Rosa later went to the office and signed the documents; in the meantime, her family members started family therapy meetings with the mental health team.

Compared to the more fragmented mental health services in North America, the Italian services now are more receptive to systemic approaches to problems of psychiatric patients in the community. The national health services in the United Kingdom function somewhat like the Italian system. The U.K. mental health services are unified in such a way that they can more easily cooperate with one another than can those in North America, where there are many competitive services at different levels: private, public, nonprofit, and religious. After their creation in 1968, American community mental health center (CMHC) programs were usually staffed with people who were either part-time workers or who were regarded as less qualified than those in the non-CMHC services. In the newer Italian system, the community services are now primary. As in England, only a very small proportion of people obtain services through expensive, private psychiatrists.

Our consultations with teams in the Italian mental health system are approved by the administrative director of each service unit. However, if *only* the administrative director wants us to meet with a team, we consider it a poor basis for consultation. For example, there was a case in which the administrator said to us, "I want my team to learn your ways. Will you come here to teach them?" If we had done that, the team probably would have found reasons for not being available at the time of our visit. Anything we had to say would be contaminated by their viewing us as working for the director. Staff members come to the Milan Center on their own initiative, though with administrative approval, and they at least partially pay their own expenses.

When somebody from a mental health team wants us to consult or to teach, we ask that everyone in the treatment team attend. We will then wait unitl they can all come. We will not, for instance, meet with only two members of a four-member team. If the whole team cannot meet, for whatever reason, we cancel the meeting. With a family in therapy, we will meet with them and ask why some of the family is missing. With a team, we assume that there must be some disturbance in it if the entire team is not present. They first have to agree with one another.

Our impression is that in Italy there is a quiet revolution going on in the field of mental health services. It has not been announced that systemic approaches are being used. Teams do not report to others that we are the source of their authority, ideas, or techniques. Instead they just start to do things differently.

An interesting phenomenon is that each team feels as if it alone has to discover what to do in specific situations. If students at the Milan Center try to transfer our suggestions literally from one situation to another, they will not be successful. The team may tell us that they understand everything we do, but that they simply cannot do it, and they have to invent their own ways of doing something else. If we ask why they then look so happy about coming to us, they say that the training was very useful because everything we told them did not work and they *had* to do something differently. If we ask why they then come back and why don't they come to us for something that they can use, they reply, "We hope that you will keep proposing something so we can do something totally different. We learn how to learn from your mistakes and from what you do that we don't think is right." We answer, "Perhaps we should copy what you are doing and in this way each of us can learn from the other's mistakes."

REFERENCES

Basaglia, F. *Che cos'e la psichiatria. Einaudi:* Torino, 1973.

Bateson, G. *Mind and nature: A necessary unity.* New York: E. P. Dutton, 1979.

Jones, M. *The therapeutic community: A new treatment method in psychiatry.* New York: Basic Books, 1953.

Penn, P. Circular questioning. *Family Process,* 1982, *21,* 267–280.

Selvini Palazzoli, M., Boscolo, L., Cecchin, G., & Prata, G. Hypothesizing, circularity, neutrality. *Family Process,* 1980, *19,* 3–12.

9

FAMILY CONSULTATION IN PSYCHIATRIC EMERGENCY PROGRAMS

RICHARD A. PERLMUTTER
Sheppard and Enoch Pratt Hospital
Towson, Maryland

JAMES E. JONES
University of Rochester School of Medicine and Dentistry
Rochester, New York

Family systems theory and family therapy techniques have great potential for application in psychiatric emergency programs. In a given year, between one third and one half of all cases presenting to a psychiatric emergency department (ED) come as families. Family issues are salient in at least 70% of these clinical presentations (Perlmutter, 1983). This chapter will describe a consultation project at the University of Rochester Medical Center that had the explicit goal of learning in what way family theory is applicable in emergency rooms and how the theory and relevant techniques can be taught in that setting. An unintended side effect of the project was that staff and residents of the ED gradually assimilated a family point of view into their general clinical thinking. The process of this consultation and subsequent teaching will be considered here.

THE SETTING

The Psychiatric Emergency Service of the University of Rochester's teaching hospital is a physically separate section within the general hospital emergency department. Approximately 4500 visits are made per year. It is staffed 24 hours a day, 7 days a week by psychiatric nurses and either psychiatric residents (usually in their first year of psychiatric training) or a faculty psychiatrist. In addition, numerous trainees rotate through the service.

There are four interview rooms, one large enough to see families, one smaller office, and two rooms equipped with restraints for emergency care of violent patients.

THE PROBLEM AND THE QUESTIONS

The anxiety and fear evoked in the staff by angry, distressed families can be overwhelming. Staff members may experience families as oppositional to their attempts to treat the identified patient. As power struggles emerge, the families can become angrier and more rigid and threatening, and staff members can become more fearful of being devoured or at least thwarted.

One of the authors (R.A.P.), who was at that time Director of the Psychiatric Emergency Service, observed that the ED staff was being asked to deal with the most highly charged and difficult family cases daily, and yet, overall, they had had minimal experience in formal family therapy or training in family interviewing. Psychiatric residents in this hospital are assigned to work with the staff of the emergency department at the beginning of their training. Emergency psychiatric nurses expressed an interest in acquiring family-related skills but had little opportunity for formal training. While the nurses and other staff members were highly skilled and experienced in emergency psychiatry, they were not family therapists. Families were handled routinely, usually with good clinical judgment and common sense. Nevertheless, the staff constantly had the sense of being abused, defeated, and overwhelmed by the families.

Repeatedly (and after a while predictably), we experienced and observed the "family dance" that ended with the interviewer feeling trapped, de-skilled, and helpless. It was not unusual to watch a carefully designed intervention with an individual, often taking several hours of work to carry out, destroyed in seconds by family members who had been outside in the waiting room and ignored. Neglect of the family's need for information about, and some shared perception of, the problem, agendas, and dynamics seemed to lead to a doomed outcome to the ED visit. The staff was being asked to deal with a wide range of clinical problems, all of them challenging and many of them replete with the potential for chaos, violence, immature defenses, desperation, and defiance. What seemed unfortunate was the mismatch between what was needed in the way of a wide range of possible modalities and what was actually being used.

A number of questions began to emerge:

• Were therapeutic opportunities being lost? Or, at least, would the staff be more comfortable if they had better skills with which to approach families?

• In a situation in which the proper use of words and voice tone contribute to staff members' survival and integrity of bodily parts (verbal and physical abuse is a hazard), would greater awareness of principles of communication and language be helpful?

• In a situation in which staff members are frequently in difficult situations with rigid, frightened families, could knowledge and skill in the positive reframings of the presenting problem be useful?

• Given the urgency "to do something immediately," which easily leads to self-destructive or unwise decisions by families, is it possible for staff members to channel this energy toward more helpful options?

• When it becomes clear early in an evaluation that a family wishes both to be helped and to thwart any change, how can this conflict be addressed?

• As it becomes clear that a family has a need to project years of pent-up rage onto whoever is working in the emergency room, how can the staff prepare for and use this awareness in designing an intervention?

• Often it becomes painfully clear that a family will leave enraged at the staff no matter what is done. How can staff learn to see beyond the inevitable dysphoria of such a scene, and to observe that some families are able to leave with the splits that precipitated the crisis realigned or temporarily healed?

These questions suggested to us that the fields of family and systems approaches might have something to offer to emergency staff workers if they could be taught in a relevant way. We needed an approach and a way of thinking that was flexible and did not require special understanding of dynamic principles to be effective, yet could be used in dealing with resistance and defiance. A conceptual model for emergency interviews with families and the tasks of the assessment phase of these interviews has been presented by Perlmutter and Jones (1985).

THE NATURE OF THE CONSULTATION

As awareness of these issues grew, the director of the Psychiatric Emergency Services (R.A.P.) decided that there was a need for family-oriented consultation, and at first sought this in a relatively informal and unformulated way. In 1979, family therapists were invited to conduct rounds in the ED and to interview any families that were present. At quiet times they began to consult with staff members about specific problem cases. In 1980, one of us presented to the Family and Marriage Clinic study group the preliminary results of a questionnaire study assessing family involvement in psychiatric emergencies (Perlmutter, 1983). The Director of the Family and Marriage

Clinic (J.E.J.) and the Director of Psychiatric Emergency Services (R.A.P.) began to discuss the feasibility of a joint project to study the implications for emergency psychiatric practice of such family involvement. Two specific project goals emerged: (1) to see if the principles of family systems theory and therapy could be applied to the practice of emergency psychiatry in a way that would help develop staff members' skills and competence in dealing with desperate and distressed families, and (2) to develop a way to teach these skills to incoming psychiatric residents and staff. (An additional, longer range goal emerged later.) Gradually, we conceptualized the project as a *consultation* to the ED as a system, with the authors serving as collaborative consultants—one from inside the system and one from the outside.

The consultation was viewed as long-term, with the goal of indirectly modifying the ED system as a result of the clinical teaching project. In the process of developing and teaching a systems approach to interviewing families in emergencies, it was hoped that staff attitudes about working with families would gradually change. Ideally, a flexible interview style would be developed that would enable staff to address some family issues more effectively. Part of the long-range strategy of the consultation was the hope that some staff members and residents would become interested in further learning and begin to experiment with a systems approach to these difficult problems. Since the consultation was on-site, it was hoped that this might happen as staff and residents observed us in our attempts to help families in slightly different ways, as they engaged with us in dialogues and were exposed to systems thinking, and as they watched us experiment and learned to profit from our mistakes. Hence, we were primarily clinicians and teachers who, in the process of developing a new teaching model, were allowed to become consultants. The system itself was influenced and began to change as the focus was maintained on clinical observation and teaching. However, the staff was not directly requesting consultation about their problems in dealing with difficult families. Staff involvement was voluntary and free of administrative demand for participation. Thus, the consultation that resulted was as indirect as the request.

The first step was to assess what kinds of problems were typically encountered and what most staff members wanted to learn (Perlmutter & Jones, 1985). The authors scheduled a block of time the same afternoon each week to spend in the ED. We interviewed various people who happened to be there—individual patients, families, and friends—and used a system perspective as our conceptual framework. If no patients were present at this scheduled time, we would discuss difficult family cases of the past week with interested staff. Over a period of 1½ years we interviewed 24 families and discussed these cases in depth. In the last 6 months of that period, eight interviews were videotaped in order to have tapes available for use in teaching psychiatric residents. We thus had the opportunity to examine a small number of families in detail, and were able to focus on the interview, the relationship of the family with the ED, and systems aspects of the crisis presentation.

Concurrently, we worked together to set up a system of referrals from the ED to the Family and Marriage Clinic without the usual clinic waiting lists and delays. This was very useful for some families and very much appreciated by ED staff who wanted rapid follow-up on emergency family referrals. However, it became evident over time that the number of families who followed through with the referrals was less than expected and much less than those identified as needing family meetings. Many factors contributed to this noncompliance with "direct referral for family therapy." Although staff members would try to help the family see the problem as a family problem and directly encourage the whole family to go for therapy, this approach was rarely successful with emergency service families. A common result of such referrals was an angry family that reacted as if they as a family were being blamed. They certainly did not intend to comply with "family therapy" or, for that matter, with anything else that had been suggested.

Hence, we experimented with other interventions to help staff become more effective in making family referrals. Strategies included suggesting to the family that while the focus would be on the identified patient as the "sick one," their participation and information would be absolutely essential to the new therapist for the work to succeed. Such an approach was consistent with the fact that the hospital emergency system insists that a billing and clinical chart be made out for one person, who is identified as the patient. To expect the family not to see that person as the patient would be unrealistic and incongruent with administrative procedure.

FRAMING THE PROBLEM

Choosing a frame for the central presenting problem became one of our more useful and teachable practices. Typically, after about 30 minutes of the family interview, we would recess to meet with staff and trainees who had been observing, and discuss the most helpful way to frame the problem for the family. Then we would return to the family and present the frame and discuss the painful binds that both they and we were in. In many cases the frame served as an example of a new way in which staff could change or defuse the intense power struggles that often characterize emergency work with families.

GRANDPARENTS AND EXTENDED FAMILY

Another technique involved routinely taking an extended-family and multigenerational history, with an emphasis on grandparents or other important and often-ignored people in the extended family. This allowed anxiety to be lowered and valuable information about the family to be gathered. In this way we quickly came to know the family better and could be more empathic with their plight.

The effects on some families of an empathic systems approach were immediately noticeable. Belated awareness of striking multigenerational patterns intrigued and deeply moved some members. For instance, a mother, who became aware that her cold control of her daughter was exactly like her mother's treatment of her, became more nurturing of her daughter by the end of the session. As long as the family could tell their story without feeling blamed by us, covertly or overtly, then problem solving and a new way of looking at the world was at least possible with some, though certainly not all, families.

SYSTEMS THINKING

One central aspect of the consultation was the introduction of systems thinking. As we discussed cases, the emphasis was on interactive rather than simple lineal, causal effects. The role of each family member in the family, at work, at school, and in society, was considered. As the relationships of the family to agencies and other groups became known, the context of their crises became more understandable.

When a health professional had been previously involved with family members (as in over 50% of the cases), the visit to the ED was framed as "a consultation to an ongoing therapy relationship," with the ED staff member as the consultant, and the staff was encouraged to think of themselves as consultants. The following is an example of the problems that developed when we paid insufficient attention to an ongoing therapeutic relationship.

A case example. A chronic schizophrenic man presented with his wife and 1-year-old son. Their chief complaint was the identified patient's violent ideation. They had shared this concern with a new therapist, who had sent them to the ED. The couple seemed to be in a family crisis and were amenable to being helped. We chose a problem-solving mode and reframed the patient's symptoms in the larger context of the family and multigenerational factors. The couple became more aware of their interactive patterns and miscommunications. The wife became aware of her tendency to distance from and provoke her husband because of her anger at him for not being "as good a man" as her dad. The problem-solving phase of the interview by itself was quite powerful and immediately useful. An admission to the hospital was avoided, and the family felt more interested in working as a unit with their therapist.

Our "creative" intervention at the first ED visit looked wonderful but then failed miserably. The couple returned the following week to the therapist, who sent them again to the ED. This time it was necessary to arrange an admission. During an argument, the husband had slapped his wife, and their therapist was scared and anxious. By focusing on the "family issues" and moving for family systems change, we had deemphasized the context of their coming to the ED in a crisis, not to a family therapy clinic. We did not attend sufficiently to the medical–psychiatric assessment of violence and, most important, we did not attend sufficiently to the task of consultation with the ongoing therapeutic system.

Working from this vantage point under time constraints, we did not see that the moving force behind both visits was the therapist. Had we understood this "hidden agenda," the problem might have been resolved in an entirely different and much more satisfactory way. It turned out that the wife had spoken to the therapist privately after their final session and revealed that she had decided to leave her husband. She and the therapist were in collusion to postpone delivery of this devastating message to him until *after* he was in the hospital. The wife could then leave while he was safely in the hands of the hospital staff.

A THREE-PHASE EMERGENCY INTERVIEW

The conceptual model for a three-phase interview process (see Figure 9-1) includes a consideration of the relevant social systems in each phase. Social system assessment is a task of Phase I (see Perlmutter & Jones, 1985); social system brokering and therapy consultation are tasks of phase II; and consideration of the family's alternative resources is the task in phase III.

Another dimension of systems thinking that we stressed is the concept of multilevel and "circular" causality. In emergencies it is essential not to assign equal importance to all levels. For example, physical illness must be considered early in all evaluations; a "stable biologic base" (Abroms, 1983) is essential before addressing levels such as family interactions. It was essential that we continually remind ourselves that we too were a system, a cotherapy team operating within an ED system that, in turn, was part of a hospital and social system. Because these systemic interactions are complex, during an evaluation we would focus, for efficiency and clarity, on one or two system interactions but remain aware that other forces also were operating. Discussions often focused on whether enough attention had been paid to the school principal, to the medical doctor, to the therapist, and so on.

It is useful to examine the effects that the interviewers had on the family

Phase	Tasks needing attention
I. Assessment	Opening of the assessment Engaging Reducing anxiety Identifying the request
	Traditional assessment of the identified patient Organic differential diagnosis Bizarre behavior and ability to care for self Suicide/homicide potential
	Social context assessment Social systems Family system
II. Crisis intervention	Social systems brokering Therapy consultation
III. Negotiation of disposition	Preparing a frame for "the problem" Decision to admit Enhancing compliance with referrals Taking leave

FIGURE 9-1. Conceptual model of the emergency interview of the family.

and hypothesize how they may have induced or encouraged a family response. This could range from an observation that we had made a family more defensive by allying with an adolescent member to the observation that our restructuring had helped them become more caring of one another. If a family member became angry, we would first consider whether we had missed a point or failed to be empathic before we attributed the anger to patient psychopathology. Also, we had to consider the effect on families of our team of two male interviewers and a male cameraman. When a wife was discussing her marriage and commented that "all men are animals," we had to be prepared for her resistance to any direct intervention from this team. Therefore, we preceded our intervention with a comment on how difficult it would be for her to follow our advice because we were men and she might distrust any of our suggestions.

THE USE OF MISTAKES

We repeatedly drew attention to our errors of omission and commission. When discussing the cases and interventions, and teaching with videotapes, we shared with staff members and trainees what we did not understand about the family and what opportunities for clarification we had missed. For instance, if we had only observed a patient's nonverbal behavior in the first minutes of the interview, we could have predicted behaviors and sometimes prevented blunders or wrong tactics in later phases of the interview. But, because no interview is ever perfect, we were able to use and focus on our errors even in reasonably successful interviews. Since the ability to be self-critical is quite natural for us, our contribution as "experts" seems to have been made palatable and allowed us, as consultants, to enter the system in a way that did not seem to provoke undue defensiveness or defiance. Staff members' fear of having their deficiencies and mistakes exposed by judgmental, observing experts was mitigated in an atmosphere that valued self-examination and a critical, though not harsh, evaluation of one's work.

The openness to admitting possible errors seemed to have a salutary effect on psychiatric residents and other trainees. If two faculty members can view their work in this way, then perfectionism and performance anxiety of residents and trainees about seeing their first families in crisis may be reduced. The teaching goal was to effect a change in attitude—from expecting the interview to go perfectly to doing the best one can and learning from whatever happens. Our hope was to provide models for staff and trainees by asking questions about their own behavior and in recognizing what they can learn from patients and families.

The following case illustrates how, in our urge to help, we made the mistake of not attending to risks involved in a hospital intervention.

A case example. A 16-year-old boy, who had been adopted at age 9, was brought to the ED by his parents at the request of the police and school principal, who wanted an evaluation of his running away, school truancy, and past firesetting. The boy's natural mother and two sisters had been killed in a fire when he was 4. Family relations in the adoptive family had never been good, but conflicts had been more severe since the boy became an adolescent. Numerous psychiatric and counseling contacts were seen as unhelpful. There had been a question of possible seizure disorder.

An interview with the boy revealed a desperate, depressed, angry adolescent with fantasies of killing his adoptive parents. The interview with the family showed a disengaged, angry father and a mother who left us repeatedly confused. She probably exhibited the highest level of communication deviance (Singer, Wynne, & Toohey, 1978; Jones, 1977) of any family member in our series. One of her requests was that we write a letter to help her son get into a special education class. Another request was for hospitalization, which for the parents represented expulsion and for the son represented escape.

Yielding to the family pressure, we reluctantly agreed to hospitalization. We justified this decision in our own minds on the grounds of a need for a neurological examination, the high level of family tension, and the possibility of violence if respite was not achieved. Our reluctance involved a fear of the family closing ranks so that the boy would have nowhere to go, of hospitalization becoming a way of solving life problems, and of family tension being reduced so far that motivation to solve problems would evaporate. Our fears proved justified. After a long hospitalization, there were no options other than for the boy to return home, with minimal change, against the parents' vigorous objections.

For months afterwards, the family repeatedly sought rehospitalization by "upping the ante," that is, the boy behaved in more and more destructive ways in a circular pattern with his parents, who provocatively engaged in open marital hostilities.

In retrospect, an attempt to prevent the initial hospitalization by more active social system brokering (for example, calling the school principal, returning the family to a prior therapist) might have avoided the pattern of destructive help-seeking behaviors. In subsequent ED visits, the family confronted some of the residents whom we were teaching. The residents were able to stand firm in their resolve not to admit the boy. The family responded with increased anger and threats of lawsuits. When forced to go away angry and dissatisfied, they also were forced to problem solve in a more mature way than by expelling the patient. Surprisingly, after months of effort, they engaged in outpatient family therapy and even requested help with underlying marital issues. This case allowed us to praise beginning residents for doing better than we had done in holding to the very principles that we espoused.

SPECIAL FEATURES OF CONSULTING WITH EMERGENCY PROGRAMS

INTEGRATION OF THE CONSULTATION WITH THE SYSTEM

For any consultation to be effective, the unique features of the consultee organization must be carefully considered. For us, the special features of a busy university hospital ED had to be respected in designing our project. Mathews (1980) has described in more detail the subculture and values of emergency departments. In our consultation to the psychiatric ED at the University of Rochester Medical Center, it is important to note two points: (1) the request for consultation came from the leadership inside the system (R.A.P.) and (2) the consultation was a collaborative project of that member with an outside "expert" (J.E.J.). Together, as inside and outside team members, we were viewed as consultants to the ED around an identified problem. The expertise of someone in the system (in this case the director's knowledge of emergency psychiatry) was blended with the expertise of a family therapist, then the Director of the Family and Marriage

Clinic in the Department of Psychiatry. In this way, much of the resistance and ambivalence toward an outside expert trying to enter a system was mitigated.

The contract with the system was carefully designed to respect the specific needs and beliefs of the system. The time and space boundaries of the system were a priority. The schedule of time blocks when we would be in the ED were specified months in advance and were adhered to. We incorporated the emergency concept of time in another way—by constant attention to how long our interviews ran, to keeping them brief, and to noting whether our intervention took more or less time than a more conventional one.

We worked to minimize disruption of other ED functions, recognizing its intense task orientation and its need to maintain a rapid flow of all patients through the system. We defined and maintained our roles as clearly as possible, designating ahead of time who would be responsible for follow-up, disposition, or continuity. In fact, we were often viewed more as front-line help who could facilitate the work of the ED because of our willingness to handle the family, whenever possible, from the beginning to the end of their visit and, thus, leaving one less case for the rest of the staff.

Staff members and trainees were free to join us as they wished—observing through the one-way screen, participating in discussions, debriefings, and critiques. We explicitly did not try to encourage staff to join the project. We anticipated that there would have been resistance if we had interfered with the routines of the ED staff. Therefore, we were very careful to structure our work so that it did not add any burden to the staff's often heavy caseload. This open invitation recognized the unpredictability and variability of ED clinical duties and staffing patterns. We believed it was important to allow staff participation but without pressure or coercion. Generally, we were joined by all available staff on days when clinical demand of other cases was not intense. Some staff members even joined us on their days off or came in a few hours early before their evening shift began.

DISPOSITION

Another aspect of crisis programs that must be respected by consultants is the necessary and central concern for rapid decision making and disposition. This became the focus of much of our discussions of individual cases and, later, of our conceptual model of intervention. Clarification of the request, followed by problem solving, led to framing the problem in a way that would facilitate more healthy and mature solutions. Failure of family therapist consultants to recognize disposition factors will prevent acceptance of their ideas and principles into the pragmatic and pressured world of frontline emergency work. In that system, patients must be evaluated and sent somewhere as quickly as possible, preferably before the shift ends, in order to make room for the next emergency.

There is pressure not to admit to the hospital for several reasons—most prominent is the shortage of beds and the awareness that if a bed is filled, it will not be available later when an even sicker person may need it. A majority of visits do involve a request for admission. ED workers become expert in assessing certain chronic conditions. They are aware that, for a subgroup of patients, repeated hospitalizations have been repeated failures and might aggravate, more than alleviate, the person's problems in living. Here again, the field of family therapy has much to offer. For instance, there is literature on hazards of inpatient treatment that can jeopardize future functioning and other social supports (Mendel & Rapport, 1969), on alternatives to hospitalization (Langsley & Kaplan, 1968; Rubinstein, 1972), and on specific approaches to suicide, violence, psychosis, and other emergencies in family contexts (Everstine & Everstine, 1983; Richman, 1979). We found ourselves strongly drawn to approaches that emphasized strategic reframings that would increase our leverage and help us to help families avoid potentially harmful extrusions of one family member into the hospital.

Literature on how the decision is made to admit from an ED suggests that it is often dependent on variables other than the level of symptomatology (Bartolucci, Goodman, & Streiner, 1975; Gerson & Bassuk, 1980). Family pressures for admission, characteristics and preferences of the interviewer, and bed availability may be more salient factors (Tischler, 1966; Mendel & Rapport, 1969). To admit or not to admit is most clearly an interactional and multidetermined issue.

THE ED AS A DUMPING GROUND

The word "dumping" is omnipresent in the ED. Staff members frequently perceive (often with good reason) that patients are deposited in their area for poor reasons and often leave without any follow-up support. Because of 24-hour availability and acceptance of all comers, emergency programs are arenas for group projection processes. Families may wish to extrude an adolescent member or a demented parent; an agency may have internal troubles or become fed up with long-term, difficult clients. Such referrals to an ED for definitive treatment and disposition often occur on Friday afternoons or before a holiday. Medical services refer patients who need a place to live, who are aggravating, who are drug or alcohol abusers, or who have no interesting, demonstrable disease. The vagaries of defining what is a "psychiatric problem" are immensely compounded in medical emergency settings.

The ED becomes the court of last resort. Consultants would do well to be aware of the sense of vulnerability, lack of control, and anger that are then inevitable. This also contributes to ED staff members' attitudes about families, because families are among the most frequent "dumpers." Families, in turn, can apply the energy of their desperation to angry confrontations of ED workers who are not willing to accept total responsibility for the "sick" family member.

THE ED AS PROJECTIVE SCREEN

One of the most common phenomena is the use of the ED and its staff as receptacles for years of accumulated distress and anger. Patients and their families, as well as therapists and agencies, are all capable of displacing intense blame or anger onto whoever is working in the ED at that hour. This is a general phenomenon of mental health work and not unique to the emergency room. But it is more intense there, as a result of factors such as time pressures, bed shortages, more severe levels of psychopathology, crisis issues of violence and suicide, desperation of families to find immediate relief, and so on. We emphasize to staff members that they should think of themselves as blank screens onto which families will project pictures of their past experiences, often involving abuse and rejection.

In a videotape we made of one of these families, a disturbed alcoholic woman never raised her eyes to look at us and kept referring to us as "Mr." and "you social workers." It became clear as the interview proceeded that she had identified us as being like other people and agencies that had not been helpful years earlier in her frightening encounters with her brutally violent daughter. She seemingly became enraged with us because we had not offered a solution to that dilemma many years ago. For our emergency family teaching, that tape is labeled "The Case of Mistaken Identity," and is a dramatic example of the projective process.

SOME EFFECTS OF THE CONSULTATION ON STAFF THINKING

It is our impression that systems thinking is not easily introduced into a medical setting where staff members are under considerable pressure to work quickly and get patients out of their area. Our project did change some aspects of staff thinking and practice, but in some areas it was not effective. The project, for instance, seems to have had minimal effect in encouraging conjoint family interviews. Even staff members who were influenced by our approach tell us they still prefer to interview family members separately. There also seems to be little use of strategic interventions with families.

Our hypothesis is that there are three factors that contribute to resistance to systemic approaches in the ED:

1. Practice of emergency psychiatry incorporates a wide range of modalities but focuses on medical–biological interventions and on the problem of violence and how not to get hurt.

2. It was not the staff as a whole that contracted initially for the consultation (although they were eager participants); the original request was from their director. Perhaps formal, prior involvement of nursing and frontline staff could have increased the overall effects of the project.

3. There appears to be particularly strong resistance to those nonintervention techniques and approaches that superficially seem to be counter to the stereotyped view that health professionals should give nurturance, expert advice, and "help."

In the following example our nonintervention was structurally useful for the family and yet it seemed to do little more than amuse or shock the system.

A case example. A 45-year-old chronic alcoholic man presented to the ED with his 80-year-old father and 70-year-old mother. He asked to be admitted to the state hospital. He had visited our ED 4 times in 4 weeks and had had 38 prior state hospital admissions. He evoked a moderate revulsion in ED staff to whom he was known as the "nose-picking drunk." At the time we saw him, the chief complaint was that he was driving his parents crazy. Indeed, his parents were fed up and wished to extrude him because he was so disruptive and disrespectful of their retirement life. Interestingly, his life had been more stable in the weeks before the ED visit, that is, he had not been drinking or getting into legal trouble.

We supported the family in their decision to have him leave the home and, much to the surprise of other staff members, we did not ask the social worker to arrange a place for him to stay. This had been done dozens of times in the past with multiple agencies, after which he would act in a way that made him *persona non grata*. We refused to arrange or suggest a disposition because we had repeated evidence that it would be sabotaged. Instead, we confessed helplessness in knowing where the best place for him to go would be. We stated that he knew best what to do and knew community resources better than anyone. The family left saying, "At least those guys tried." The patient seemed to appreciate our faith in his survival skills and competence. The staff seemed both intrigued and puzzled and asked, "How could you do that?"

The proclamation of helplessness is an indirect approach that would not be regularly appealing to staff members in psychiatric emergency rooms. Hence, it is incumbent upon those of us who teach family therapy principles to find alternative ways of helping psychiatric professionals deal with defiant, disturbed people who do not benefit in any long-term way from the usual direct approaches.

The project did have a noticeable impact in several ways. Psychiatry residents showed an attitudinal change and seemed to take for granted that "of course, evaluating the family is part of the workup." Some of them identified with us in a way that helped them to be comfortable with skills that were still being learned. One resident who had to work with a very difficult family in the middle of the night later told us that he tried to imagine what "Rich and Jim Edd" would have done. Months after the project had formally ended, one staff nurse had a similar experience when confronted by a regressed, angry, borderline woman who was demanding to be back in the hospital after a recent discharge. The nurse tried a maneuver similar to one she had seen us use. She told the patient that she blamed herself for participating in an earlier admission because the hospitalization seemed to have left the woman worse off. She said she was sorry for giving in to the patient the last time she demanded hospitalization. Of course, the patient had then seen it as a helpful option but, the nurse said, it was her responsibility to help the patient with a more long-sighted arrangement. The patient left without a fight and even without the usual raising-the-ante: "If you don't admit me, I'll kill myself."

There has been a shift away from the staff's practice of trying to redefine to the family that the psychiatric illness of one member is really a family problem for which the family should go for "therapy." We emphasized the futility of this approach with an emergency population (Perlmutter, 1983). More often, alternate approaches are now being tried. Also noticeable since the project in ED ended is the increase in family and systems thinking by staff members. Nurses are taking family courses and proposing research projects about family problems during emergencies. At least one doctoral dissertation is being written about family influences on the decision to admit a patient to the hospital. After attending our teaching sessions, one resident designed a two-month, intensive, elective experience in interviewing families in crisis and ways to teach these skills. There is also an increased demand for teaching sessions utilizing the videotapes of family interviews.

CONCLUSION

The change resulting from the consultation was made possible by our knowledge of frontline, psychiatric emergency work. This knowledge enabled us to respect the emphasis on time, disposition of cases, rapid decision making, and differential diagnosis, that constitute the value system of emergency rooms. Incorporating these principles, we could begin to design an adaptation of systems thinking for an emergency system.

In the planning stages, this consultation was narrowly conceived as a project to develop teaching principles to staff members who deal with families in ED. However, some of the unintended side effects on the ED system were similar to those that result from a more traditional organizational development consultation. We believe that some features of this project can be used intentionally in explicit organizational development consultations. It has often been remarked that research projects will change the thinking and behavior of those involved in them. This occurred here. The work had similarities to a research project: We were trying to learn how to apply family therapy ideas in an ED and then how to teach what we had learned. Some projects in organizations generate antipathy toward the content and members of the project. How did this project avoid that and end up with generally positive, unintended effects?

We can only speculate about answers to this question, but we have had occasion to test our hypotheses in other organizations with whom we consult. Both the outside consultant and the director of the ED were careful to assert repeatedly that neither were experts in how to achieve the goals of the project; one was competent in ED work and one was competent in work with outpatient and inpatient families. Neither had firm, empirical knowledge about interviewing families in an ED. We were repeatedly clarifying what we knew and did not know; what we were doing was based both on conventional ED practice and on conventional family practice outside the ED. This emphasis was important in establishing for all who came in contact with the project that we were not coming to show them the true or only way to do their jobs. We were also careful to structure the boundaries of the project so that it did not interfere with the jobs of staff members, residents, and trainees. When an ED is busy, it takes the staff's full resources to do this difficult work. If there is any explicit or implicit demand to attend to something else as well, then the source of the demand will inevitably be resented. Therefore, we made it clear that personnel were free to join with us as their work or desire allowed. We continued to interview families and to think through the issues, regardless of whether staff members and trainees joined us. The project was conceived as a collaboration between two persons who wished to evaluate principles for working in an area where a hybrid of their two areas of expertise could be developed.

In summary, in our description of a consultation model for family therapists as consultants with crisis programs we suggest three central precepts: (1) to know and respect the generic, unique features of emergency work, (2) to minimize disruptions of the ED tasks, and (3) to be aware of the nuances of the particular program requesting the consultation. Because there is wide variation in any system's pressures and politics, it is essential to tailor the consultation to the system with minimal a priori assumptions.

REFERENCES

Abroms, E. M. Beyond eclecticism. *American Journal of Psychiatry*, 1983, *140*, 740–745.

Bartolucci, G., Goodman, J. T., & Streiner, D. L. Emergency psychiatric admission to the general hospital. *Canadian Psychiatric Association Journal*, 1975, *20*, 567–575.

Everstine, D. S., & Everstine, L. *People in crisis*. New York: Brunner/Mazel, 1983.

Gerson, S., & Bassuk, E. Psychiatric emergencies: An overview. *American Journal of Psychiatry*, 1980, *137*, 1–11.

Jones, J. E. Patterns of transactional style deviance in the TAT's of parents of schizophrenics. *Family Process*, 1977, *16*, 327–337.

Langsley, D. G., & Kaplan, D. M. *The treatment of families in crisis*. New York: Grune & Stratton, 1968.

Mathews, D. B. *Disposable patients*. Lexington, MA: D. C. Heath, 1980.

Mendel, W., & Rapport, S. Determinants of the decision of psychiatric admission. *Archives of General Psychiatry*, 1969, *20*, 321–328.

Perlmutter, R. A. Family involvement in psychiatric emergencies. *Hospital and Community Psychiatry*, 1983, *34*, 255–257.

Perlmutter, R. A., & Jones, J. E. Assessment of families in psychiatric emergencies. *American Journal of Orthopsychiatry*, 1985, *55*, 130–139.

Richman, J. The family therapy of attempted suicide. *Family Process*, 1979, *18*, 131–142.

Rubinstein, D. Rehospitalization versus family crisis intervention. *American Journal of Psychiatry*, 1972, *129*, 715–720.

Singer, M. T., Wynne, L. C., & Toohey, M. L. Communication disorders and the families of schizophrenics. In L. C. Wynne, R. Cromwell, & S. Matthysse (Eds.), *The nature of schizophrenia: New approaches to research and treatment*. New York: John Wiley & Sons, 1978.

Tischler, G. Decision making processes in the emergency room. *Archives of General Psychiatry*, 1966, *14*, 69–78.

Editors' Commentary on Consultation in Mental Health Systems

The chapters in this section on consultation in mental health systems can be considered from the standpoint of how the different authors define the consultee in their work, and how this consultee relates to others in the particular setting. The case example presented by Todd illustrates a common situation in which the consultee is a junior family therapist who requests the help of a senior family therapist colleague. However, because both the consultant and the primary family therapist are part of a broader mental health program, they need to define their roles not only with each other but also with other members of the treatment team. Therefore, in order to avoid competition that would be confusing and counterproductive, the consultant must clarify the roles of each participant. Todd makes clear that his goal is to "leave the system with the therapist in an effective position," that is, with the family therapist having received recommendations for specific steps that he or she can thereafter carry out. Many pitfalls as well as opportunities for consultation in such a setting are richly illustrated in Todd's case example.

The work of Perlmutter and Jones also occurs in a hospital setting, but calls for crisis intervention and triage rather than longer-term treatment. In the emergency service in which Perlmutter and Jones have worked, the staff members are not experienced family therapists. Their consultation requires role modeling and the teaching of principles of family functioning and intervention with families. Whereas Todd's consultation is oriented to resolving a therapeutic impasse, Perlmutter and Jones are consulting about highly fluid problems in which crisis provides the opportunity for rapid change.

Whitaker's work is, characteristically, difficult to describe in terms of traditional categories. He describes being both a consultant to a family therapist colleague and a consultee who requests consultation from colleagues. Furthermore, he views therapy, as we do, as most appropriately preceded by a consultative phase in which the family, as consultee, requests help in considering their options and their need for therapy. The fact that Whitaker's role as a consultant differs from that of a therapist/consultee is used with great effectiveness by him to help unlock a therapeutic stalemate. This complementarity frees the consultant and the primary therapist to move in and out of engagement with the family members. Whitaker's active and fluid style helps both therapist and family to gain a new perspective. He regards the consultant as usefully invasive and enlivening for a boring or stuck therapeutic process.

In another method of using consultation to resolve impasses in family therapy, Penn and Sheinberg work as a team of consultants who take interchangeable but differentiated roles. They have developed a format for applying systemic principles in which one consultant is an observer and the other is a participant/interviewer. A special strategy in the Penn and Sheinberg approach is to identify isomorphic problems in the therapist–family system and in the therapist's own family system. The Penn–Sheinberg hypothesis is that unrecognized connections between these two contexts have resulted in the impasse. The consultant team can take a meta perspective partially outside both of these systems and free the therapist to facilitate change when he or she is ready, beginning either in his or her own family or in the family in treatment. The concept that the consultant takes a meta position is fundamental to systems consultation, but the systematic method with which Penn and Sheinberg implement and dramatize this principle of consultation is an innovative contribution.

Max van Trommel (1984)) has recently described another way that a consultation team can help a therapist–family system become unstuck. While Penn and Sheinberg emphasize the importance of maintaining the centrality of the family therapist as consultee, van Trommel hypothesizes that the impasse has arisen because the therapist has lost this position. The consultant interviews the therapist and the family together in order to examine their relationship. With the help of a consultation team of observers, an intervention is then proposed that will help the therapist and family to become better differentiated. The therapist can thereby regain a functional position and the consultation team's task is completed. Van Trommel's approach exemplifies how the therapist–family system can be regarded as a unit that has systemic properties of its own and that, in turn, the consultation team plus therapist–family system is a temporary suprasystem.

With the deinstitutionalization of psychiatric services in Italy, the Milan family therapy teams have turned to consultation programs in the community. Cecchin and Fruggeri describe their version of systemic consultation in which they work with staff teams of psychiatrists, psychologists, social workers, and nurses, most of whom are not trained in family therapy.

More often than not, the systemic approach used by Cecchin and Fruggeri leads to the recommendation of services other than family therapy, such as social welfare services that utilize the special skills of a team member. This approach to systems involves the clear recognition that the treatment team involves persons with differentiated roles and skills. In considering what kind of services are most appropriate for a specific problem at a specific time, a consultant can provide an invaluable overview. In the model described by Cecchin and Fruggeri, the consultants do not interview the family directly but assist the team members in identifying interventions that will reduce chronic dependence of patients and families on mental health services.

Parallel work in community services in Italy that more recently has come to our attention is carried out by Mara Selvini Palazzoli (1983). Her consultations, like those of Cecchin, Fruggeri, and Boscolo, are carried out in a district, or catchment area, that provides services. With her guidance, the staff members initially respond to requests from families by becoming consultants to them. In these consultations, the nurses and other staff members meet with each family to help them identify and clarify the nature of their problem and to consider their choices and resources for what to do about the problem. These "direct" consultations with the families may or may not produce a plan for the provision of some form of social service or, more rarely, family therapy. Selvini Palazzoli is a supervisor or, in effect, a meta consultant to the staff members who are functioning as consultants with the families.

Selvini Palazzoli's approach is very similar to the one that we have proposed for working with patients and families: to define the initial direct contacts as consultation rather than as the beginning of therapy. The consultation phase, usually one to three meetings, consists of problem identification and selection of a method for resolving the problem, if resolution is still wanted or needed. Family therapy, or therapy of any kind, is a possible option, but the consultation may lead to the conclusion, after the situation has been assessed systemically, that some other approach is preferable or that *any* change would bring more losses and dangers than gains.

Rather than imposing and teaching the systemic model in an abstract fashion, Selvini Palazzoli helps the staff teams construct pragmatic strategies for service delivery to their clients. Selvini Palazzoli now believes that a consultation model in a primary service setting is preferable to the routine provision of services such as family therapy. If a clinical service or professional has the reputation of *only* providing "family therapy," even professionals trained in systems theory are apt to become isolated in private practice or within an institution, where they "carve . . . a niche to practice family therapy," but do not have contact with primary services where clients come with diverse needs (Selvini Palazzoli, 1983). As in our model, the Milan approaches of Cecchin and Fruggeri and of Selvini Palazzoli may evolve into family therapy, but requests for therapy may also be refused. What seems especially encouraging and exciting about the seemingly diverse approaches to mental health systems that have been described in this section is that a newly defined consultation component in these services seems agreed upon. A consultation model induces us to pause before plunging into therapy and increases the likelihood that further services, family therapy or whatever else, will be thoughtfully, not automatically, offered and accepted.

REFERENCES

Selvini Palazzoli, M. The emergence of a comprehensive systems approach. *Journal of Family Therapy*, 1983, *5*, 165–177.

Trommel, M. J. v. A consultation method addressing the therapist–family system. *Family Process*, 1984, *23*, 469–480.

III

CONSULTATION IN MEDICAL CONTEXTS

The biopsychosocial medical model, first discussed by Engel (1977, 1980), emphasizes the many different levels of a system that may benefit from intervention. This new medical model is controversial in its conceptualizations, its usefulness, and its implementation. (See "The Risks of Change" by McDaniel & Amos, 1983, and other articles in the new journal, *Family Systems Medicine*, for a survey of current efforts and problems in implementing a systems approach to medicine.) The biopsychosocial model of medicine is, however, quite consistent and compatible with a systems approach to consultation. The chapters in this section reflect work in this area.

Bloch has surveyed the opportunities available to the systems consultant in working with health care organizations. McDaniel and Weber describe the implementation of systems theory in a family medicine residency program, particularly the teaching and consultation that were a part of this exchange between family therapists and family physicians. Sluzki on hypertension, Wellisch and Cohen on cancer, and Munson on pediatric problems each have described a biopsychosocial systems approach to medical case consultations. These consultants take a focused but flexible view, assessing the illness, the individual, the family system, and the treatment system as they work toward specific consultation goals. The McDaniel, Bank, Campbell, Mancini, and Shore chapter describes using a larger system, a group of peers, to provide case-oriented consultation to a physician or other provider.

REFERENCES

Engel, G. L. The need for a new medical model: A challenge for biomedicine. *Science*, 1977, *196*, 129–136.

Engel, G. L. The clinical application of the biopsychosocial model. *American Journal of Psychiatry*, 1980, *137*, 535–544.

McDaniel, S., & Amos, S. The risks of change: Teaching the family as the unit of care. *Family Systems Medicine*, 1983, *1*, 25–30.

10

THE FAMILY THERAPIST AS CONSULTANT TO HEALTH CARE ORGANIZATIONS

DONALD A. BLOCH
Ackerman Instítue for Family Therapy
New York, New York

This chapter focuses on the special contributions the family therapist can make to health care organizations. The phrase "health care organization," as I will use it, is a generic term referring to all members of that class of social institutions that are charged with preventing or treating disease. In this chapter, I will limit myself to physical disease while recognizing that such a definition violates the primary holistic perspectives of the family systems paradigm. The social organizations under consideration may be of many kinds; consulation may be to any level or component unit. Thus, the family therapist, as consultant, may be addressing a legislature in its funding capacity, a health commissioner as planner, a medical director of a hospital, a chief of medicine, the staff of a cardiac-care unit, an organization of dialysis nurses, a diabetes self-help group. In all of these and analogous instances, the focus of the consultation is on the gains to be made from including family systems perspectives in the ongoing work of the social unit at hand. In many instances the family is the sole "health care organization." Consultation is either to the family or about the characteristics of the family that apply to health care.

Consultation in family systems medicine is a personally and professionally exciting venture, with rich and complex possibilites and challenges. Recent changes in medicine speak more insistently of the need for intelligent and active inclusion of family therapy perspectives in the health care process. Of particular interest is a new set of iatrogenic risks and stresses to which modern family systems are exposed in the course of lengthy, painful, and costly care for diseases that only recently have come within the therapeutic capabilities of medicine. The simple prolongation of life heads the list of biomedical successes that, as they unfold, generate hitherto unknown problems for families; we must include on this list such well-known medical advances as treatment of malignancy with radiation and chemotherapy, and of end-stage renal failure with dialysis. The recent interest of medicine in developmental epochs inevitably requires attention to family processes, as well as to individual life stages. Pediatrics, adolescent medicine, and geriatrics all involve the family; nor can we forget that sexual medicine is a family affair.

Despite these and many other apparently persuasive reasons, the inclusion of family systems perspectives in the operations and planning of health care organizations has been considerably less common than one might expect. The family therapist proposing to consult with these institutions must acknowledge that this is so, understand the reasons for it, and develop collaborative ways of working that respect the different traditions, tasks, and perspectives associated with biomedicine, on the one hand, and family therapy, on the other. The two disciplines are profoundly different in their epistemologies (Auerswald, 1968), theories of knowledge and action, social organizations, economic rewards, assigned tasks, and technologies (Auerswald, 1983). To the degree that they overlap in their concern with solving human problems, they have both competitive and collaborative aspects.

Perhaps the most appropriate way to summarize this issue is to speak of the difference in paradigms. As professionals with a family systems persuasion become involved more and more with programs that take biomedicine as their orienting paradigm, the problems and possibilities associated with this collaboration will become more evident. The consultant is well-advised to think through carefully his or her epistemological stance and to consider the impact of that stance in the specific settings in which such work takes place. The failure to recognize this issue can result in efforts that have no chance of success, or that may provoke unnecessary and destructive confrontations.

Thus, let it simply be noted that at the beginning of each consultation one should undertake as best one can an epistemological and paradigmatic diagnosis. Such a diagnosis should consist of a detailed description of the cybernetic characteristics of the work unit with which the consultation is taking place; what events are defined as data and how they are collected, organized, and transmitted. Information overload may rapidly overwhelm care providers for whom incoming data should be screened to eliminate all but essentials. Contextual information may burden the care provider with the obligation to solve insoluble problems. Pain, misery, despair, may need to be denied so that daily functioning can go on. Lineal causal paradigms are more useful than systemic paradigms in highly instrumental situations such as emergency rooms, surgeries, and even busy medical and pediatric practices. In work situations, people acquire the information necessary to complete the task while minimizing their own personal discomfort. Thus, prevailing patterns of data acquisition and processing are essential data for the work of the consultant. It is essential to have as clear a grasp as possible of the "reality" that guides the program's actual operations. Events that otherwise would be inexplicable will be less baffling as they are seen to express and support this orientation.

The general rules governing consultation with an ongoing, functioning, social system must always be kept in mind. In relation to the paradigmatic issue just touched on, it is well to remember that the decision to invite consultation is related to some systemic disequilibrium that has taken place in the inviting organization. This may be associated with political shifts or institutional malfunction; it is also possible that the invitation reflects increased strength and growth: "Now that we have successfully established our adolescent inpatient program, we are ready to add the perspectives of family therapy." In any event, the request for a consultation is always related to a prior disequilibration, and consultation is expected to be problem solving in nature.

The kind of solution associated with a family therapy perspective, however, may be more wide-ranging than anticipated because of paradigmatic differences between family therapists and other professionals who serve as consultants. The initial contract may not extend at all to including changes, let us say, in intake procedures or billing. Such changes have political and economic consequences that may not have been contemplated in the original contract. This requires continued clarification and renegotiation before proceeding further. Organizational-development or management-consultant skills may need to be part of the process to the degree that the consultation is, among other things, a political act that is associated with the possibility of power redistributions in the organization.

CONSULTATION PARAMETERS

Here we will consider the major types of issues in health care provision with which the family therapy consultant is likely to be involved.

THE FAMILY AS A HEALTH CARE AGENCY

Increasingly, clinicians have become aware that the family, however defined, is an intrinsic part of the health care delivery system. Its ability to function in health care is of great importance for the ill. Indeed, the family is always the health care agency of last resort; it may be the only social unit providing this function, and, together with the individual, it provides the early warning system for recognition of health care problems. Thus an orientation to those aspects of family functioning that permit this system to function well or poorly generates vital information for the consultant.

Indeed, this perspective in itself is a major orientation that can be brought to health care systems.

Some of the factors that affect the competence of the family as health care provider are the ability to:

- shift roles flexibly,
- process painful affect,
- communicate freely and appropriately with other health care providers,
- observe the physical functioning of its own members,
- tolerate disability,
- deal with body products or surgical wounds,
- adequately mourn its losses.

The creation of family-sensitive health care systems requires considerable revision in current modes of practice. For example, home visits are highly desirable but often hard to arrange, although there are considerable data to indicate their usefulness, particularly in chronic illness or when patients are undergoing physical rehabilitation. Office hours that are arranged conveniently for families may not fit with other scheduling needs. Convening the family for a diagnostic management conference requires the availability of appropriate physical space, as well as knowledge of the techniques for getting a family history and a genogram. These simple, practical arrangements can be beneficial to families and actively engage them as partners in the health care enterprise. However, instituting them in ongoing operations that are differently oriented may not be at all easy.

The costly triad—overutilization, underutilization, and noncompliance—are often symptomatic of a poor fit between the goals and paradigms of the family, and those of the health care professionals, although they are presumably engaged in the same tasks. Caution requires modesty at this juncture as to the ability of family systems approaches to make a contribution to the solution of these problems. Some gains have been made, however; relevant research is accumulating, and there is good reason to believe that the future will provide better concepts and intervention techniques in these areas.

DIRECT TREATMENT: THE DIRECT APPLICATION OF FAMILY THERAPY SKILLS TO THE TREATMENT OF MEDICAL AND PSYCHIATRIC CONDITIONS

In many instances, a mixed treatment approach is most appropriate and the family therapist as consultant or direct purveyor of treatment must hone those skills and attitudes necessary to working with other disciplines. The combined psychoeducational, psychopharmacological, and family treatment of schizophrenia (Anderson, Hogarty, & Reiss, 1980) or the combined pediatric and family therapy approach to the abdominal pain syndrome in children are cases in point.

Direct treatment skills are called for under those conditions in which family factors are significant in the etiology or maintenance of physical disease. The list of these conditions is lengthening as the immunological link between levels of physical and psychological organization is explored. The list includes what used to be known as the psychosomatic conditions, as well as the neoplastic diseases, the autoimmune diseases, and certain infections (Schmidt, 1983).

The consultant here is a clinical case consultant and needs to be able to reach into family therapy techniques for those treatment skills appropriate to the clinical material at hand. This area is rapidly expanding; it is essential that knowledge of the available family therapy techniques and their applicability to medical situations be kept up to date by the consultant.

THE FAMILY AT RISK

Our focus in treating the family at risk is on the public health aspects of physical disease: the consequences of severe illness for the psychosocial functioning of the family. This concerns those shifts (usually unnoticed and unattended to) in individual and family funtioning—specifically, psychosocial breakdown—that are associated with severe, acute, physical illness, and/or protracted treatment regimens. The family therapist, as a clinician, has long been aware that problems seen in the consulting room are connected with the failure of the family to cope successfully with such biomedical stresses. There is increasing awareness in the medical and surgical community that lack of attention to this dimension of care is costly, both clinically and economically. Many specialists wish to mitigate the adverse impact of their procedures on families. Much research is needed in order to define those elements of disease–treatment–family systems interaction that significantly affect families. It is desirable to be able to triage families in these high-risk situations so as to use scarce therapy resources efficiently; however, sound knowledge as to how to do this has yet to be achieved. Most often family therapy consultants are brought into such high-risk situations as consultants to renal dialysis units, oncology programs, gerontology units, and hospices, to assist with pressing management problems, because it is in this area that the most visible instances of breakdown occur.

It is often difficult for health care providers to know what impact their procedures have on families. Much useful information along this line can be routinely obtained from appropriately organized self-help groups. The consultant working with a major disease program such as diabetes or cancer care can secure much relevant information from appropriate patient, parent, or family self-help groups. (Such groups have their own systemic properties, including preferred explanations of the meaning of the disease, its etiology, and the direction research should take.) They can be valuable sources of information about the impact of disease–treatment configurations on families.

DEVELOPING TRAINING PROGRAMS IN FAMILY SYSTEMS THEORY AND TECHNIQUES FOR HEALTH CARE PERSONNEL

Developing training programs in family systems theory and techniques for health care personnel is frequently defined as a consultative task. Illustrative of this kind of activity is the collaboration of family therapists in training family practice residents; primary care medicine also draws upon family perspectives in its teaching programs.

An example of an important but more limited teaching consultation is a current effort (Simon, in press) to prepare teaching materials for ostomy nurses so as to enhance their ability to add a family dimension to their work. Teaching family therapy skills in this fashion will become widespread, as the recognition of the importance of the family perspective infiltrates the specialty subdivisions of health care, the generic disease-oriented professional, and the self-help organizations. Demand will increase for the preparation of appropriate teaching materials, as well as for active participation in teaching programs; consultants need to familiarize themselves with both appropriate content and presentation methods.

GENERAL HEALTH POLICY DEVELOPMENT

The development of public health policy by governmental, third-party, consumer, and provider organizations rarely includes family systems perspectives. This is unfortunate. Admittedly, this is an area in which the family therapy community has yet to develop much expertness or experience. The proper starting point for making the appropriate contribution to public policy on health care should occur in the family therapy community itself. The organization of task forces, the preparation of white papers, and consultative expertness at this level of decision making develop together.

To illustrate, we consider briefly the problem of current clinical and cost-accounting procedures, which are inadequate from the family systems point of view. The clinical record-keeping procedures ordinarily used reflect this deficiency. Specially, there is the absense of information that relates the functioning of the family and its individual members to the disease–treatment of one of its members. Consider the sequence that begins with the birth of a child with a severe neurological or orthopedic deformity. Large amounts of money are expended in the care and rehabilitation of this infant. For some families, these steps are attended by improved functioning: The child is treasured; a proper balance of attention to his or her needs and those of other family members is attained; other functions are protected. For other families, such an event is an unmitigated calamity, initiating a stream of consequences leading to family breakup, psychosis, addiction, and so on, with all kinds of costs to society for further malfunction and treatment.

This issue has both clinical and public policy consequences. It is highlighted here because of recent controversies over public policy in regard to such instances as the "Baby Doe" case. Rational public policy decision making depends *inter alia* on there being an empirical base of information on the consequences of such events for families. There are of course other dimensions for public policy considerations: the sanctity of life and the right of self-determination, for example. The family therapist, as public policy health consultant, has a contribution to make to these debates. Substantial changes in both the family therapy and health policy communities must take place for these possibilities to be actualized. Not least of these is the development of record-keeping and accounting systems that more adequately reflect the systemic consequences of disease and treatment (Huygen, 1982).

RESEARCH

A brief note about the family therapist as a research consultant in health care settings should be added here. As is true in the public policy area, the family therapist rarely serves as a consultant to biomedical research enterprises. This is unfortunate because a substantial contribution ought to be forthcoming in this direction, particularly in regard to the inclusion of family systems level variables. It appears likely that many ambiguous or inexplicable findings—particularly the inability to discriminate significant subgroups of patient populations—are related to sampling difficulties associated with such variables. Specifically, it has been traditional to look at the meaning of disease, or treatment events, or risk reduction procedures, as they are perceived by the individual targeted for the procedures. It is appropriate as well to consider the meaning of these events for the family system. Such a perspective is particularly important in regard to understanding compliance and noncompliance, chronicity, excessive somatization, and certain kinds of unexpected failure-to-thrive-in-treatment configurations. In all of these instances, it is well to recognize that the disease, or the treatment, or the relationship with the health care providers is significantly meaningful to the family system.

Reciprocally, a second research area of interest has to do with the contribution that can be made to family systems theory and therapy by work in biomedical settings. It is easy to see that natural experiments occur here that could not be duplicated elsewhere. An example is the tragedy in which an accident cripples a young adult parent, forcing major role revisions in a family. Perhaps the surgical trauma team of the future will include a family therapist able to take speedy action to limit the damage to vital social organs. Sad as such situations are, they also provide a chance to understand better how families function, where a malfunction originates, and how intervention can ameliorate these defects. Family therapists are uncomfortable in biomedical environments and unfamiliar with how they work and with their possibilities for research. The establishment of good consultative, collaborative relationships can reverse this trend with considerable profit to all concerned.

FEATURES OF HEALTH CARE ORGANIZATIONS

Health care systems are not unique; in many respects, the principles that inform their organization, structure, and function are similar to those of other operating social institutions. However, health care systems are distinctive in important ways; this section will indicate some of the issues to which the family therapy consultant should be sensitive. The list is by no means exhaustive; to some extent we are talking about differences of emphasis. I will describe them under two headings: Economic Realities, and Workplace and Psychological Realities. Together, they make up the overall reality, the constraints, facilitations, tasks, and information of the environment within which the health care provider functions. It will help the consultant to pay attention to these parameters, whether he or she is dealing with a solo practitioner, a small group practice, a large health maintenance organization, a department within a hospital, or an entire hospital.

ECONOMIC REALITIES

The most important single question to be asked when consulting for any program is: How is this program paid for? Although it may appear on the surface that the economic issue is tangential to the clinical concerns of the family therapist, it is, instead, central. The constraints that are embodied in current economic relationships must be known and respected; and economic consequences of a shift in the patterns of services must be attended to. As an example, consider the introduction of a part-time family therapist into a small fee-for-service group practice. The fee-for-service arrangement requires that each procedure fit into a prevailing reimbursement structure, a structure established for most patients by third-party payers, usually government and insurance companies. Though the appropriate use of family therapy might cut overall health care costs, the fee-for-service practitioner may see this as economically threatening. Moreover, the usual accounting systems do not reflect these savings, nor do reimbursement schedules easily permit the addition of new procedures, especially in the psychotherapy domain. Thus, the economic consequences of a procedure that may be clinically desirable must be recognized if the commitment to generating change is serious.

Similar examples proliferate in all kinds of health care settings. The heart of the situation is that severe cost-containment requirements at all levels limit the total available funding. Health care providers are keenly aware of this and recognize that any reallocation of resources away from their area of competence is a threat. One can see this happening between such major divisions of health care as medicine and psychiatry. The process is played out from the national level down to the most minute clinical setting.

If we broadly dichotomize health care provision into fee-for-service and health maintenance organization (HMO) structures, family therapy is likely to fare better in the latter configuration insofar as economic considerations are concerned. The health maintenance organization, in principal, is tailored to reducing overall costs and substituting less expensive procedures (although one may often question how it achieves this). If a single family interview at the outset of the management of a difficult and protracted treatment can improve compliance and reduce overutilization, it will have been cost-effective. The HMO may be in a better position to realize these benefits both conceptually and economically.

The principal economic problems of the HMO arise from difficulty in maintaining productivity and quality control. The health care provider in the HMO is not motivated by competitive materialistic goals to work long hours but seeks instead improved professional and personal life. As a European colleague put it to me, the HMO does not completely solve the problem of the lazy doctor. One might hope at least that the activation of the family as a consumer–partner in the health care enterprise would go a long way toward remedying these liabilities.

At the very least, the consultant should have a broad understanding of these economic issues, including the importance of consumer groups, generic disease associations, and self-help groups in maintaining focus on patient- and family-oriented definitions of adequate service. The maternity center movement, for example, emphasized natural birthing, preservation of family values, and lower overall costs. It has had a twin impact on hospital-based obstetrics: more inclusion of families and a higher cesarean-section rate. Systemic effects of an action are rarely unidirectional.

WORKPLACE AND PSYCHOLOGICAL REALITIES

The consultant must look at every workplace with great care and ask in the most sensitive way possible what arrangements and attitudes are necessary in order for workers to survive and function in that particular setting. This does not mean that current arrangements cannot be changed, but it is essential to respect them as reasonable efforts to adapt to the exigencies of the situation rather than as signs that somebody has been foolish, self-aggrandizing, or worse. The scope of such an inquiry can only be indicated here. Consider, for example, the radiologist and other personnel who must subject their cancer patients to disfiguring and debilitating doses of radiation, knowing that while some will be saved, most will languish and die. Consider the primary-care physician who needs to see at least six patients an hour in order to earn a competitive income. Consider the young internist in solo practice who needs to develop a referral network and guard against frivolous malpractice suits. The list could go on and on; indeed, it would ultimately cover everyone, including the consultant. The consultant is obliged to understand and respect the solutions as they operate at any given point in time, keeping clearly in mind that any change must provide better answers to the same questions.

At the psychological level, two themes that diverge in regard to the orientation of the family therapist and the biomedical practitioner should be noted here. The biomedical practitioner needs to limit the information available about any particular subject to precisely those items that bear on a focused, clinical, usually *tissue* event. In addition, greater emotional distance must be maintained because the practitioner is exposed to much, often overwhelming, human misery and pain for which little amelioration is possible, particularly under the conditions of medical practice. The family therapist on the other hand is oriented to defining *treatable* social situations (Glenn, Atkins, & Singer, 1984).

Finally, let us add certain personal factors: First, there is the self-selection of those people who are comfortable working in such an environment. Second, we must note the possible invalidation and de-skilling that may be associated with major changes in paradigms for work roles. For the health care worker to be de-skilled by the consultative process is enormously threatening, and this is particularly true where high levels of skill acquisition have enabled her or him to achieve important work status. The dimensions of the consultant's dilemma, as noted earlier, become more clear as we consider this mix of factors.

In order to offset the disadvantages of a shift to a family therapy perspective, the consultant must provide benefits that outweigh the negative factors. Improved clinical functioning is certainly one of these benefits: Clinicians greatly appreciate solutions to their patient's problems. Substantial improvement in work satisfaction and in the overall interest level can be brought to the work place by virtue of this transformation. For the health care provider, there are the possibilities of an easing of stress, of a greater sense of satisfying his or her idealistic values, and of a general improvement in personal and professional functioning that may offset some of the economic losses and discomfiture associated with a changed work definition.

REFERENCES

Anderson, C., Hogarty, G., & Reiss, D. Family treatment of adult schizophrenic patients: A psychoeducational approach. *Schizophrenia Bulletin,* 1980, *6,* 490–505.

Auerswald, E. H. Interdisciplinary versus ecological approach. *Family Process*, 1968, *7,* 202–215.

Auerswald, E. H. The Gouverneur Health Services Program: An experiment in ecosystemic community health care delivery. *Family Systems Medicine*, 1983, *1,* 5–24.

Glenn, M. L., Atkins, L., & Singer, R. Integrating a family therapist into a family medical practice. *Family Systems Medicine*, 1984, *2,* 137–145.

Huygen, F. J. *Family medicine: The medical life history of families.* New York: Brunner/Mazel, 1982.

Schmidt, D. Family determinants of disease: Depressed lymphocyte function following the loss of a spouse. *Family Systems Medicine,* 1983, *1,* 33–39.

Simon, R. *The family of the ostomy patient.* Princeton, NJ: Convatec Corp., in press.

11

FAMILY SYSTEMS CONSULTATION IN A FAMILY MEDICINE TRAINING PROGRAM
Opportunities and Realities

SUSAN H. McDANIEL
University of Rochester School of Medicine and Dentistry
Rochester, New York

TIMOTHY T. WEBER
Colorado Center for Psychology
Colorado Springs, Colorado

Recently, professionals in family therapy and family medicine have opened numerous channels of communication to explore the areas of interest common to the two fields. The literature at the interface of these two disciplines is growing, as exemplified by publication of the journal *Family Systems Medicine*, edited by Donald Bloch (1983), and the book *Family Medicine: The Medical Life History of Families,* by a Dutch family physician, F. J. A. Huygen (1982). Also notable are contributions by people trained in both disciplines, such as Doherty and Baird's *Family Therapy and Family Medicine* (1983) and publications by Christie-Seely, including *Working with the Family in Primary Care* (1984) and earlier papers (1981, 1983). Recent conferences held by both disciplines offer possibilities for sharing and exploring common concerns.

Opportunities for consultation now exist as a result of this growing interest in the application of systems theory to medicine. Family physicians may seek consultation with family therapists about patients and families they see in their medical practices. Family therapists may seek consultation with family physicians about chronic illness, medication, and other medical issues in families they treat. Profitable exchanges of mutual benefit may occur about any number of theoretical, clinical, professional, and research topics. Family medicine and family therapy have much to offer each other.

FAMILY THERAPY AND FAMILY MEDICINE: HISTORICAL ISSUES

In this chapter, we will consider in detail one particular consultative relationship, that of the family therapist consulting in a residency training program in family medicine. We shall also review the broader context of family medicine, noting the many parallels between the historical development of family medicine and family therapy. The formal disciplines of both fields have developed in the last 30 years. Family medicine began in reaction to the trend toward costly, reductionistic, biotechnical approaches of specialized medicine. Likewise, family therapy began in part as a reaction to the costly, lengthy, reductionistic approach of psychoanalysis. Within the mental health community, many family therapists see themselves as generalists, much as family physicians are the generalists of the medical community. Both disciplines focus on families and early intervention, and both are characterized by innovations and enthusiasm common to relatively new ventures. Family therapy had its beginnings in the 1950s, while family medicine began its transformation from general practice in the 1960s. Both fields have established some credibility and longevity; they are now in the process of integrating with the rest of the mental health and medical communities while at the same time responding to the general public's concerns and needs.

During the period of inception and growth, some pioneers were already working on issues at the interface of the two fields. Richardson's 1945 classic, *Patients Have Families,* foreshadowed many of the issues regarding health and families now deemed important. In the 1970s, Engel (1977) proposed the biopsychosocial approach to medicine, and Ransom and Vandervoort (1973), Sluzki (1974), and Weakland (1977) called for the new disciplines to apply family systems theory to medicine. For the most part, however, the two fields developed in parallel without much exchange, perhaps because of their own struggles to become established and because of the difficulties inherent in this communication (McDaniel & Amos, 1983). Current attempts to apply a systems model to medicine generate many challenges, which include coping with competing assumptions and language barriers (Bursztajn, Feinbloom, Harum, & Brodsky, 1981).

In addition to understanding the development of the relationship between family therapy and family medicine, it is also important to know something of the development of family medicine itself. Is there truly a difference between the practice of the physician recently trained in family medicine and the practice of the more traditional general practitioner? This debate continues in the journals of family medicine; while controversial, one proposed distinction is that family medicine now has a theoretical underpinning consistent with its practice of treating all members of a family and its belief in continuity of care, that of systems theory with a primary focus on the family (Taplin, 1983).

Since the beginnings of family medicine in 1968, residency training programs have had a strong emphasis in the behavioral sciences. ("Behavioral sciences" is the term used in family medicine to refer to the psychosocial curriculum.) The founding fathers, such as Carmichael, Geyman, Stephens, and McWhinney, saw the humanizing of medicine and the integration of emotional and physical problems as central to the new discipline. However, as Ransom (1982) has noted, most of the past emphasis has been on individually oriented psychoanalytic or behavioral approaches. In its early days, family medicine advertised that it treated the "whole person" and emphasized a caring approach. Today, the discipline continues to attract talented faculty and residents with strong interests in psychosocial issues, some of whom might have entered psychiatry but for a desire to treat patients in a more comprehensive way. The question of whether systems theory will be seen as relevant, pragmatic, and effective by family practitioners remains to be answered.

An ongoing issue in family medicine is its status in the medical and academic community. Clearly, the strength of family medicine is its generalist approach to practice. The potential for comprehensive treatment, in which the biomedical is no longer split off from the psychosocial, seems an attainable reality. While the generalist approach of family medicine is clearly a strength, this approach is not universally valued in the traditional community of medicine where subspecialists are revered. It is important for the consultant to understand that family physicians still fight this prejudice against nonspecialists and that family medicine residents will struggle with their identity and question their own competence as they interact with specialists, including the family therapist. In spite of these difficulties, family medicine is a flexible and innovative discipline, ripe for collaboration with family therapists around a common interest in the family.

ROLES OF THE CONSULTANT

A variety of roles may be requested of a family therapist in a family medicine residency training program. A person who has family therapy expertise may be asked to function as teacher, supervisor, administrator, research consultant, and case consultant for patients of faculty and residents. The family therapist may be asked to teach family systems theory to faculty and residents, precept residents, consult on the behavioral science curriculum, or consult with the organization as a whole. In this kind of situation, it is useful to conceptualize one's overall role as that of systems consultant, in this case a systems consultant functioning within an educational system. Regardless of how one may be officially perceived and labeled, taking the superordinate position of systems consultant helps one to clarify the specific roles needed for each given task.

A consultant generally is someone whose primary professional identity is either more specialized than or lies outside the context of the consultee. Most often, a single consultative relationship does not provide the individual with a primary source of income. A continuum of possible involvement exists for the family systems consultant to family medicine, ranging from that of complete outsider to complete insider. All positions have their advantages. At the outsider end of the continuum, a family systems consultant may have no faculty appointment, a position that diminishes the consultant's investment in departmental political struggles, but often reduces that person's status or perceived power. At this position on the continuum, the consultant may be better able to see "the forest" or the system as a whole, better able to make novel suggestions, and less likely to react quickly to the suction of the system. At midrange, a family systems consultant may have adjunct status or a primary appointment in psychiatry and a secondary appointment in family medicine. In this position, the advantage is having freedom of movement that comes with being an outsider, while still having the investment of a relative insider in getting programs accepted and carried out. Finally, a family systems consultant may have a primary appointment in family medicine and become a full-fledged insider. This is most likely to happen only in the still rare instances when an academic family physician is also a trained family therapist. On the insider end of the continuum, the consultant may be less easy to discount; he or she may have more power and leverage for change, more awareness of the overt and covert rules of the organization, and more accessibility. In general, the more roles the consultant assumes, the more possibilities exist for impact upon the system.

Our own experiences are at the midrange of the continuum because we have had roles in both the Department of Psychiatry and the Division of Family Medicine of the University of Rochester School of Medicine. Early in its history, the Division of Family Medicine had a more limited program for the behavioral sciences, with a series of consultants all headquartered in the Department of Psychiatry. More recently, the Division has expanded its program with one half-time, on-site consultant who has a variety of tasks and roles (the first author); another consultant from the Department of Psychiatry participates in a more limited way (the second author). This team approach to consultation, with each of us occupying somewhat different places on the insider–outsider continuum, offers some of the same advantages to consultation as do family therapy sessions viewed through a one-way mirror. One consultant can join with the system, do an assessment from the interior, and carry out many programs; the other consultant remains relatively "meta" to the system, assessing it from the exterior, and consulting about programs more from an outsider's perspective.

As with any consultation to a training program, it is important for family systems consultants in a family medicine program to clarify the difference between their roles as "consultants" and as "teachers." Consultation is a relationship of colleagues, in which one professional imparts specialized knowledge to another. This needs to be distinguished from teaching or training, a hierarchical relationship in which a senior person teaches and evaluates a junior person. In a residency training program, the family therapist may play many roles, including those of consultant and teacher. The family therapist as consultant may share and develop ideas with the faculty about general family systems issues, consult with the faculty on specific cases, and consult with program directors about the place of family systems theory in the residency's behavioral science curriculum. The family therapist as teacher may instruct residents about family systems theory and family interviewing technique and assessment skills. Within this context of teaching, the family therapist also may consult on specific resident cases as a vehicle for teaching about family systems theory and the process of consultation.

The family therapist may find that the initial consultation request asks for a sharing of expertise about families in which the roles of consultant and teacher are blended during preliminary discussions. However, we have found it useful to conceptualize the relationship to faculty colleagues as that of consultant, while conceptualizing the relationship to residents, involving evaluation, as primarily that of teacher. Mixing the roles of consultant and teacher can be problematic.

Mistaken identity: A case example. A family therapist who was hired to consult and teach about family systems to faculty and residents offered to teach the faculty through live interviews with families. While the faculty showed some interest in using this format to learn about family systems, many logistical factors (scheduling, and so on) kept the plan from being implemented. Only later, when the faculty more specifically requested case consultations, individually and in a faculty development group (see Chapter 10), did it become clear that the initiative needed to be theirs. At that time, the relationship was clarified as consultation among colleagues and not teaching or evaluation.

In the medical system, a similar problem can develop in other relationships. Residents frequently ask for formal consultations from specialists in connection with their patients. Though the residents are learning *in vivo* how to consult with specialists, they frequently need more supervision and guidance than is typical of a consultation. In this context, both consultative and educational functions are needed because of the simultaneous service and educational demands of the residency. Again, clarification of roles is essential.

A pregnant case example. An example of such mixing of roles occurred when a resident requested a consultation from a family therapist about a pregnant teenager who had made two suicide attempts during the pregnancy. The family therapist, assuming a consultant role, assessed the individual and family and recommended some general guidelines for primary care in conjunction with an immediate referral to the Family and Marriage Clinic in Psychiatry. In the consultation model, the resident could take or leave this recommendation.

As the situation developed, it became clear that a nurse practitioner involved in the case had also asked for a consultation from a pediatrician. After hearing about the case, the pediatrician recommended to the nurse and the resident that they do the counseling themselves, in-house, as he believed any referral probably would not be followed up and, furthermore, that the teenager's behavior might be within the range of normal adolescence. The family therapist subsequently found that the nurse and the resident were struggling between using her and the pediatrician as consultants (much as the identified patient was struggling between family members). After some reflection, she realized she could better serve in the role of teacher, not consultant, with the resident. Allowing the resident to function as a colleague during the consultation, without appropriate teaching and supervision, had led to conflict and a stalemate in the treatment of the case.

The family systems consultant then discussed with the pediatrician their different perspectives of the case. She and the pediatrician arranged a conference with the nurse and the resident for the purpose of developing a treatment plan and coordinating roles. Once the faculty members took supervisory responsibility in this conference, roles were clarified, and an effective, comprehensive treatment plan was developed by the resident and the nurse practitioner for this teenager and her family. Because the family therapist had a responsibility in this situation to guide and evaluate the resident, the consultation occurred in the context of a teaching relationship with the teaching function being primary. For the family therapist, clarifying the roles and boundaries in each situation allows a rewarding and useful blend of consultation and teaching, with consultation primarily occurring with faculty members and teaching primarily occurring with residents.

JOINING THE SYSTEM

The contract and roles negotiated by the family therapist and the subsequent place of the consultant on the continuum of possible involvement will markedly affect the nature of the joining process. In our experiences, the joining process is somewhat easier the more the consultant is on-site and available to the system, as opposed to residing in an office off-site. This geographic issue may be especially relevant in family medicine, where residents rotate through many other departments; the model outpatient clinic that houses family medicine becomes highly valued home turf.

In any consultation, the joining process involves much listening and only occasional comment. The consultant needs to take time to learn the system, support competence in the system, demonstrate one's own competence, and, in general, earn the right to be a consultant. The formation of mutually satisfying relationships, in which colleagues respect each other's areas of expertise, provides the foundation for successful joining. The relationship between family medicine and family therapy is now in a courtship phase; the strength of the alliance is yet to be determined. Recognizing this, we have found it important to demonstrate competence as well as to understand the daily concerns of the family physician, without overselling family systems medicine. Acknowledging the experimental and innovative nature of the approach allows the consultation to become a collaborative exploration.

Moreover, theoretical misunderstandings can lead to competition and rivalry between the biomedical approach and a family systems approach, making a collaborative consultation extremely difficult. We have found it useful to emphasize what Engel (1980) terms the "biopsychosocial model." Using this medical systems model throughout consultation, we can support other training that residents need to deal with the biomedical levels of a system and then teach residents to conceptualize beyond this level to other systems levels. Finally, they may learn to develop interventions at a single level or to dovetail interventions at multiple levels. The biopsychosocial model allows for an integration of biomedical and psychosocial approaches to health and illness. Accommodating to the dominant models in any system is an essential task in joining.

Joining of the consultant with a family medicine system requires negotiation with the departmental hierarchy. Most important are the chairman or director of family medicine, the director of the residency training program, and the faculty most interested in the family therapist's consultation and education. These initial relationships are essential because they provide the foundation and support for the consultation program as a whole. Much of the joining with the director may occur around early contract negotiations and role clarification and then expand to ongoing dialogues about common interests. Introductory meetings with each faculty member may also uncover similarities and common concerns that allow the consultant to emphasize similarities in the philosophy of family medicine and family therapy that will pave the way for future associations. Next in the hierarchy are the fellows and the chief resident. These senior trainees can often impart useful information about how the faculty and the department work and provide useful liaison with the residents. Joining with the residents often occurs naturally as the teaching and precepting begin. Specific activities, such as being on call with first-year residents, can demonstrate commitment and interest and offer valuable opportunities for teaching.

Using differences and commonalities to best advantage is important to the success of the joining process. If the consultant is a physician, he or she can draw on shared training and a common language. However, many of the consultants we informally polled thought that a PhD, or other degree, allows a consultation to occur without tapping the competition inherent in family medicine's relationships to other specialities. Regardless of training (unless one is a family physician), an important part of joining is acknowledging the family therapist's status as an outsider who is not a family physician, is not regularly on call, and has limited involvement in this context, but who is sympathetic and committed to a generalist approach to medical care.

Setting limits to the consultation and defining what one will *not* do (e.g., be a therapist or process leader) is important for a clear role definition for the consultant and the consultees. Because family medicine is a field of generalists who must be competent with a wide range of skills, being useful in one area of expertise and steering clear of other areas can define one as a specialist within this context. Demonstrating a clear sense of strengths and limitations helps establish reliability and credibility with other professionals.

During the joining process, one advantage of frequently being on-site is that one is available for important meetings. Given the limited time for the consultation, one might question making a faculty meeting a priority. In our own experiences, we have found these meetings to be informative, interesting, and important for successful joining.

Attending national meetings provides a knowledge of family medicine training at other medical schools and offers important access to other resources. The Society of Teachers of Family Medicine (STFM) is a counterpart to the American Family Therapy Association in its focus on training. While there is a Task Force on the Family in Family Medicine and a strong behavioral science group, no official organization exists for family therapists within the STFM. Even so, the organization offers opportunities for academic and clinical stimulation and exchange.

In our own experiences, the joining process has been both interesting and stressful. Being initiated into the system naturally involves many tests of the consultant's competence and commitment. In a situation early in a consultation, one of us was challenged about her effectiveness and style of participation in a faculty development group. Although working through these issues was difficult, the process of doing so began to solidify relationships in the group and facilitate resolution of issues about the group's focus. It was tempting to overreact and view these tests purely as power struggles or rejection, instead of also recognizing that healthy confrontations test the usefulness of the consultant to a new system. Support of colleagues, especially with two consultants working together, can help the consultation to stay on track during this period.

ASSESSING THE FAMILY MEDICINE CONTEXT

WHAT ARE THE CHARACTERISTICS OF THE DEPARTMENT?

The consultation contract may not include a request for systemswide consultation; it is more likely to be focused on teaching or case consultation. However, an understanding of the context as a whole is always useful in knowing how best to implement consultative goals. Family medicine residency training programs vary widely. Of structural importance are whether the department is based in a medical school or in a community hospital and how much the residents rotate through different clinics and hospitals. When family medicine programs staff their own hospitals, residents learn to provide comprehensive care from a family medicine model; rotating through other departments allows trainees to learn in-depth skills from specialists as well as learning to tolerate a competitive atmosphere.

The composition of the faculty by degree, gender, and specialty determines much of the nature of the residency. In the program based at the University of Rochester School of Medicine, all faculty members are physicians except the family therapist and all faculty members are males except the family therapist; about half of the residents are female. Four of the nine faculty members, including the family therapist, are specialists who are not family physicians.

Another important variable is how family medicine is accepted by the other departments. Rivalries and scapegoating frequently exist between traditional medical specialties and this new discipline. A faculty member in the Department of Internal Medicine warned one consultant against joining the Family Medicine faculty, calling Family Medicine the "stepchild" of the medical school and saying that such an association could have negative effects on one's career.

HOW STRONGLY DOES THE DEPARTMENT SUPPORT A BEHAVIORAL SCIENCES CURRICULUM AND APPROACH?

For a consultation to be successful, it must have the support of the director and elicit the interest of some of the family physicians on the faculty. Residents naturally model themselves after the family physician. If they see that faculty members have consultative relationships with the family therapist, they are more likely to be open to family-oriented training. If, on the other hand, the family therapist appears to be isolated and more of a symbol of a systems approach than an effective participant in health care, the residents are more likely to tune out this perspective and avoid any precepting that is offered.

One indication of departmental support for the behavioral sciences is the number of faculty members with an interest and training in this area. Programs range from less than one full-time faculty member to six or eight behavioral scientists. Generally, the more behavioral science faculty, the more widespread is the support for the behavioral sciences program. In the past, the University of Rochester had several part-time behavioral science consultants to family medicine, primarily psychiatrists and social workers. Behavioral science faculty now includes a full-time internist with medical–psychiatric liaison training, one half-time clinical psychologist with family therapy training, several psychiatrists and a psychologist who teach and consult several hours a week, one full-time family physician with medical–psychiatric liaison training, and other family physicians who have interests and skills in the area. With this growth in faculty resources, the behavioral sciences program has become more active, organized, and visible. Other family medicine departments may employ consultants with backgrounds in education, anthropology, sociology, and other social science fields.

Nationally, controversy exists over whether behavioral sciences are best taught by family physicians or by other specialists. Most programs do hire mental health specialists. However, the involvement of the family physician faculty members in the behavioral science consultation and training program is essential if this approach is to stay relevant to primary care concerns and remain credible with the residents.[1]

Another important dimension that should be assessed by the family therapy consultant is the potential support for a family systems approach to family medicine. The approach has generated both enthusiasm and controversy, as reflected in journals like the *Journal of Family Practice* (e.g.,

1. After Dr. Weber left his position in Rochester to move to Colorado in 1983, a family physician whom he helped train in family systems assumed his role at Family Medicine.

Christie-Seeley, 1983) and *Family Systems Medicine* (e.g., Carmichael, 1983; Ransom, 1983). Most faculties have representatives on both sides of this controversy, although only a small percentage of programs actually have family therapists on their staffs. An early assessment of faculty members' beliefs and concerns, especially their attitudes about systems theory and treatment of the family as the unit of care, will help to guide and formulate the nature of family systems consultation.

In our experiences, the faculty seemed to break down into three subgroups: a majority who were receptive and interested, a small, biomedically oriented subgroup whose interests were elsewhere, and a small subgroup who were somewhat interested but were either individually oriented or felt that they needed no more consultation in this area. Residents, having not yet established their own identities or areas of expertise, are usually open and enthusiastic about a family approach.

Our consultations came at a time when the department had had a smorgasborg of other mental health consultants: a few psychiatrists generally thought to be too nondirective, irrelevant, or inaccessible; several other consultants who provided well-received programs but stayed for very short periods of time; and two family therapists who had a few positive reviews but were more generally not well received. The last two consultants had many difficulties, especially because they were headquartered in the Department of Psychiatry and perhaps because they were a little ahead of their time in bringing family systems theory to family medicine. Knowledge of previous consultations can make one both realistic and humble. The year before our consultations began, a family therapist did some limited, successful consultation with the faculty that paved the way for more extensive consultative roles.

WHAT IS THE STRUCTURE OF THE DEPARTMENT?

An assessment of both the official and the unofficial hierarchy, the overt and covert channels of communication and power, is important. The more the unofficial hierarchy matches the official hierarchy, the more healthy the system is likely to be. Assessing the philosophy regarding hierarchy is important in a family medicine department. Much of the strength of family medicine lies in its emphasis on patient education and patient involvement in health care. This emphasis can be distorted when residents with a strong need to be liked confuse an "authoritative" approach with an "authoritarian" approach. In these instances, residents may abandon their own responsibilities as physicians and give mixed messages about who is in charge in a well-intentioned attempt to empower patients to draw upon their own resources. Denying the reality of a hierarchy or refusing a role that is relevant (like that of physician and patient) can lead to dysfunctional communication patterns in the professional system.

An analysis of the subsystem boundaries between faculty and residents, and between residents and patients, can be useful to the consultant in learning about the new system. The nature of the boundary between health care providers and patients can be troublesome; being too disengaged or too enmeshed can be equally problematic. Whereas many of the high-tech specialties may tend to be impersonal and disengaged from patients, family practitioners with their emphasis on caring as well as curing tend toward becoming overinvolved or enmeshed. Like many ministers, family medicine residents often believe that a good doctor should be available to patients at all times.

Marcus Welby, MD: A case example A need for the creation of a more firm boundary occurred when a family physician on the faculty requested a consultation from a family therapist about a family with several members who had multiple somatic symptoms. The physician involved was a friendly, caring, and effective physician who at some level realized that he was being drawn into this enmeshed, extended family. Members of this family were calling him at home with a sense of urgency about nonemergency matters. He was talking to them at length as well as making weekly home visits. Further exploration of the case revealed multiple, intergenerational boundary violations and much ambiguity and hostility that fueled the somatic complaints. Basically a likeable family, they had a history of socializing and even becoming close friends with previous doctors and other professionals involved with them. The consultation centered on delineating the boundaries this physician wished to draw and developing strategies to carry this out (e.g., no more phone calls to his home, other calls to be limited to 5 minutes, increased office visits to replace some home visits). As the physician began to feel some relief from his overresponsible position, family members took more initiative and began to draw more appropriate boundaries among themselves. Somatic complaints were reduced, emotional dynamics came to the surface, and one subgroup of the family entered psychotherapy and successfully resolved some of their problems.

The family medicine philosophy can be misunderstood by young residents who unconsciously may feel paternalistic caretaking is the most appropriate strategy for many patient problems. While some residents do need help in improving social skills and learning to join with patients, much case-oriented teaching and consultation involves reframing idealistic, humanitarian attitudes within practical boundaries. At times, discussion of what is involved in being "caring" and "helpful" and of what distinguishes these concepts from "overfunctioning" can actually help to broaden the resident's humanitarian philosophy. Issues of control between doctor and patient may surface during this discussion, making clear how the resident may preempt the patient's initiative by overstepping boundaries and taking too much responsibility. At other times, reframing is not enough, and a more active approach is needed. Here the family therapist may help the resident to create more appropriate boundaries by suggesting that the resident become more task-focused. Inviting other family members to participate may create a natural boundary because it makes clear that the physician is not part of this natural family group. Encouraging frequent case consultations with other residents and with faculty members also helps to form an appropriate boundary and allows the resident to be less involved and to formulate a workable plan.

Assessing the faculty and residents' responses to physicians who socialize with their patients, date their patients, or encourage other kinds of personal relationships, will help establish the attitudes about boundaries within the system. At times, we have observed that the excessive closeness between physician and patient may compensate for excessive distance between colleagues or between residents and faculty members. Should this be the case, supporting relationships among faculty and between faculty and residents may help to correct overinvolvement of residents with their patients.

HOW FLEXIBLE IS THE SYSTEM?

How well does the system tolerate diverse ideas or ideas that run counter to the beliefs of the organization? Family medicine tends to be very tolerant and flexible, both philosophically and behaviorally. A high premium is placed on new ideas and the pursuit of new approaches. This tendency makes family medicine an innovative and exciting field in which to work. Too much flexibility and tolerance with a low level of communication may result in individuals becoming isolated as each pursues his or her own interests without much exchange.

AT WHAT STAGE OF THE "LIFE CYCLE" IS THE ORGANIZATION?

Is the program at the point of expansion and growth or of decline? Are new ideas welcomed and encouraged, or is the program interested in stabilizing and solidifying its current operations? Are faculty members leaving or joining the program? How stable or fluid is the administrative or fiscal base of the organization?

The University of Rochester program is one of the oldest family medicine programs in the country, having been established in the late 1960s. This particular program has survived and accomplished the early tasks of establishing a new training program. It now is more concerned with developing a distinct identity based upon strong programs in areas of interest to the faculty and residents. As in the assessment of a family, this "life cycle" assessment of tasks can sometimes clarify the covert issues underlying the request for consultation.

WHAT PHYSICAL FACILITIES ARE AVAILABLE?

As Ransom (1982) noted, many medical facilities are not equipped to see families. Most outpatient clinics contain small examining rooms that are just large enough for a physician and one patient. In addition to noting whether there are adequate teaching facilities, one basic assessment question is whether there are rooms large enough for family interviews. One-way mirrors and videotape equipment are now often available in residency training programs.

SPECIAL ISSUES IN FAMILY MEDICINE CONSULTATION

We have found it useful to emphasize several different aspects of the family approach in our teaching and consultation with family physicians and residents.

THE FAMILY IN FAMILY IN MEDICINE

First, we try to expand the use of the word "family," whether in reference to "family medicine" or "family therapy." This effort involves education about the "typical" family constellation as well as about single-parent families, single people, and gay couples. Discussing the variety of family constellations generally tends to discourage idealization or reification of the family (nuclear or otherwise).

ANALYZING THE TREATMENT SYSTEM

In addition to expanding the concept of "family," we have also found it useful to expand the use of interactional analysis beyond the family to include a more ecosystemic view (Mannino & Shore, 1982). From this viewpoint, the family physician is a systems broker working on the front-lines. Residents learn to analyze their professional systems and to see themselves as part of the treatment system. Interactional analysis can help them to communicate and negotiate with their colleagues as well as to deal with interactional problems such as resistance and noncompliance in their cases. It may assist them to define an effective role for themselves when coordinating health care teams around complex cases.

PRIMARY CARE FAMILY COUNSELING

Once the residents' attention is captured and focused, we have found it useful to lower their expectations of themselves by teaching interactional theory and assessment, but clearly differentiating family therapy from primary care family counseling (Doherty & Baird, 1983). We focus on normal family processes, family life cycle tasks, and general education and prevention with families. We emphasize that the family systems model is relevant regardless of the number of family members present at the interview, and regardless of whether the presenting problem is biomedical or psychosocial. We also encourage live supervision in order to increase the residents' family assessment skills. Any resident who undertakes primary care family counseling is expected to request live consultation from a family therapist or another trained faculty member.

"MORE OF THE SAME"

Another common issue in any case-oriented teaching or consultation occurs at the behavioral level: When a case is going poorly, the physician or resident is likely to do "more of the same." In medicine, this will frequently mean gathering more biomedical information or running more tests in order to pinpoint the cause of the symptoms. While entirely appropriate in some instances, somatic fixation can make some problems worse. Introducing a systems view that bypasses issues of cause and effect can be anxiety-provoking to the physician whose scientific identity rests on diagnosis and cure.

Problems with uncertainty: A case example. A family physician on the faculty requested a consultation about a family. He realized that he had done more than enough tests on a woman with back pain, but he could not stop worrying that he was missing some terrible organic cause of the pain. The physician's somatic orientation was identical to that of the family except that he suspected the woman's symptoms might be better treated at the emotional and family systems level. An extended consultation ensued in which the consultant used medical terminology to introduce a new systems-oriented view. The consultant promised nothing, suggested a trial period for a new treatment format, focused on results rather than etiology, and introduced some new diagnoses (unresolved grief reaction and family life cycle issues around bearing children) to reframe the problem and potential solutions. The consultant saw the family with the family physician for five sessions, exploring the symptoms and the family dynamics, and gradually reframing the meaning of the pain. The symptoms remitted and the physician maintained a good relationship with the family, though he continued to have some difficulty accepting the fact that he had never discovered "the cause" of the problems.

THE CROSSFIRE BETWEEN CONSULTANTS

One final example illustrates two difficulties that can occur at the systems level during an extended consultation—getting caught in the crossfire between consultants and being a specialist consulting to a generalist.

Crossfire: A case example. In the context of learning to request consultations on patients, a family medicine resident requested input from several faculty members, including the family therapist, about a difficult patient. The family therapist, not knowing the resident was also consulting with other faculty members, saw the index patient and her son with the resident. She made recommendations for treatment that included setting limits with this woman and referring her to a specialist for psychotherapy. A week or so later, the index patient responded to a crisis by taking an overdose, which she survived after a stay in the intensive care unit. Follow-up after the crisis revealed that the resident had not followed through on the family therapist's recommendations, in part because of her desire to maintain her "special" relationship with this woman and in part because a family physician consulting on the case had recommended against an outside referral. The family physician told the resident that she could handle this sort of "chronic patient" in-house. The splitting, the loyalty issues, and the scarce resources in the professional system mirrored the patient's problems in her family system. This case taught the consultant to always ask, "Has anyone else consulted on this case?" In a residency training program, residents are learning to consult *in vivo*, but still need guidance in difficult situations. At these times, it can be important to coordinate the consultations so that continuity of supervision would be comparable to continuity of care at the patient level.

REFERRALS

Finally, educating about and facilitating referral when appropriate is central to learning to be effective, competent generalists. While some residents refer too soon, feeling overwhelmed and inadequate, other residents refer too late because they feel overresponsible and fear that specialists may not return their patient. Each physician has his or her own degree of comfort and level of skill; we support areas of competence and help the residents to define their limits. We also encourage good communication with the professionals to whom they refer.

Another important aspect of referral is learning to conceptualize the treatment system and negotiate appropriate boundaries when patients are in ongoing psychotherapy.

The right hand and the left hand: A case example. A second-year resident asked for consultation about a couple he was treating. This couple had multiple medical problems but consistently focused on their marital difficulties. The resident felt he should listen, support, and advise, especially the wife, in spite of the fact that the couple were in ongoing marital treatment. During the consultation, it became obvious that these people were stuck and were perpetuating their own problems by splitting the two professionals involved. The consultation allowed the family therapist to suggest that the resident call the family therapist treating this couple. The goal of this call was to develop a coordinated treatment plan in which the physician would deal with X problems and the family therapist would deal with Y problems. Once a plan was developed, the resident was encouraged to have regular phone contacts to discuss the case with the therapist.

CONCLUSION

Many exciting opportunities now exist for collaboration between professionals in family medicine and family therapy. Particularly in family medicine training programs, family therapists may be asked to function as teachers, supervisors, and case consultants because of their knowledge of family systems principles and techniques. Whatever roles the family therapist takes, it is best to conceptualize one's overall role as that of a systems consultant. This conceptualization reminds one, when assuming a multiplicity of roles, to assess each situation and clarify which roles are most appropriate, when, and in what context. This model of consultation is likely to lead to a more successful experience.

ACKNOWLEDGMENTS

The authors would like to acknowledge our family physician and other medical colleagues who reviewed and responded to this chapter: Thomas Campbell, MD; Peter Franks, MD; Drew Kovach, MD; Carmel Perry, MD; Bernard Shore, MD; Stephen Taplin, MD; and Donald Treat, MD. We appreciate their consultations.

REFERENCES

Bloch, D. Family systems medicine: The field and the journal. *Family Systems Medicine,* 1983, *1,* 3–11.

Bursztajn, H., Feinbloom, R., Harum, R., & Brodsky, A. *Medical choices, medical changes.* New York: Delta/Seymour Lawrence, 1981.

Carmichael, L. 40 families—A search for the family in family medicine. *Family Systems Medicine,* 1983, *1,* 12–16.

Christie-Seely, J. Preventive medicine and the family. *Canadian Family Physician,* 1981, *27,* 449–455.

Christie-Seely, J. Teaching the family system concept in family medicine. *Journal of Family Practice,* 1983, *13,* 391–401.

Christie-Seely, J. *Working with the family in primary care.* New York: Praeger, 1984.

Doherty, W. J., & Baird, M. A. *Family therapy and family medicine.* New York: Guilford, 1983.

Engel, G. L. The need for a new medical model: A challenge for biomedicine. *Science,* 1977, *196:* 129–136.

Engel, G. L. The clinical application of the biopsychosocial model. *American Journal of Psychiatry,* 1980, *137,* 535–544.

Huygen, F. J. A. *Family medicine: The medical life history of families.* New York: Brunner/Mazel, 1982.

McDaniel, S. H., & Amos, S. The risk of change: Teaching the family as the unit of medical care. *Family Systems Medicine,* 1983, *1,* 25–30.

Mannino, F., & Shore, M. The wider contexts of family interventions. *Family Therapy Networker,* 1982, *6,* 59–63.

Ransom, D. *The development of a family perspective in health care.* Paper presented at the Conference on Family Systems Medicine: Therapy of Families with Physical Illness, sponsored by The Ackerman Institute for Family Therapy, New York City, October 22,1982.

Ransom, D. On why it is useful to say that "The family is a unit of care" in family medicine. *Family Systems Medicine*, 1983, *1,* 17–22.

Ransom, D., & Vandervoort, H. The development of family medicine: Problematic trends. *Journal of the American Medical Association,* 1973, *225,* 1098–1102.

Richardson, H. B. *Patients have families.* New York: Commonwealth Fund, 1945.

Sluzki, C. E. On training to "think interactionally." *Social Sciences and Medicine,* 1974, *8,* 483–485.

Taplin, S. *Evolution of family principles in family practice.* Extended Grand Rounds–Public Health Service presentation, Division of Family Medicine, University of Rochester School of Medicine, Rochester, New York, April 7, 1983.

Weakland, J. H. Family somatics—The neglected edge. In P. Watzlawick & J. Weakland (Eds.), *The interactional view.* New York: Norton, 1977.

12

FAMILY CONSULTATION IN FAMILY MEDICINE
A Case Example

CARLOS E. SLUZKI
Berkshire Medical Center
Pittsfield, Massachusetts

This chapter describes a consultation that took place in a family-oriented, primary-care center in an inner-city general hospital, site of a family practice residency program. The encounter was prompted by a family-oriented, third-year family practice resident who was the primary physician for the members of the P family, which included the mother (Mrs. P), a 56-year-old woman who had severe hypertension and multiple somatic problems. Until 6 months before the interview, Mrs. P's hypertension had been controllable with appropriate regimen and medications. More recently, it had become refractory to treatment. The resident did not know whether this was due to noncompliance (the patient not taking the prescribed medication properly) or to other factors. The hypertension developed during a period in which Mrs. P was particularly upset and displeased with her husband, who, she alleged, had misused a good part of the family money on trips back and forth between the United States and Jerusalem.

The family members, of Palestinian origin, had migrated to the United States at different times during the last decade. The family is composed of Mr. and Mrs. P, their son and their three daughters, and their respective spouses and children. They live together in the same house or very nearby and constitute a rather closely knit group. The resident, who has treated members of this family for the past 3 years and is extremely fond of them, was worried about the refractory nature of the patient's hypertension and the escalation of her complaints about her husband. She discussed the matter with the author—a behavioral sciences consultant and faculty member in this university-affiliated general hospital—with whom she met weekly to discuss problem patients. He suggested inviting the family for an exploratory interview, which she did. At her request, he joins her for the interview, rather than observing behind the one-way mirror and discussing the session (an alternative in that program). Present in the family interview are Mr. P; his son, S; the son's wife; two of the P's daughters, D1 and D2; and D1's daughter. As may be noticed, the identified patient (Mrs. P) is absent.

Their seating arrangement (see Figure 12-1) shows a clear configuration: The main territory belongs to the women. This probably reflects the fact that the interview is centered on a theme that their culture defines as a female domain, namely, health issues and, perhaps, family issues in general. The men, marginal to the theme, sit against the wall by the door. The boundary between the two sets is occupied by the newcomers: on one side, the consultant and the resident, and on the other, Mrs. P's daughter-in-law (who has been a member of this family for "only" 6 years!). Where would the identified patient, Mrs. P, be seated, had she attended the interview? Perhaps where the granddaughter is, central among women and flanked by the daughters; perhaps by her husband, intermediary between the two sets. The seating position of the son shields his father from the consultant, and their actions throughout the session are quite consistent with this protective role relationship. During the introduction of the family members to the consultant (C), he asks who speaks English in the family. Father looks at the floor and the other family members simultaneously agree that he speaks no English.

With everyone now seated, C begins by asking whether Mrs. P or any other family member is to be expected. The family says that Mrs. P has stayed home, resting. C invites the resident (R) to explain the reason for this consultation. Needless to say, C has already discussed issues about this family with R. However, C first asks R to define the reason for the consultation, in order to have a starting point that is shared by all participants. Starting with a family member who has not requested the consultation and who has been *brought* to it would risk confusion, if not mistrust. It is the consultant's conviction that the initiator of a consultation, be it patient or provider, must bear the responsibility for defining the problem for which consultation has been sought.

R: Well, the main reason why we felt it would be useful to have the family come in is mainly because of Mrs. P—who is not here today—who, I guess, was one of the first people I saw at the Health Center, who has been having lots of trouble with her blood pressure, has been upset a lot lately. I wanted to find out from other people in the family about any problems in the family that may be affecting Mrs. P's health and any solutions. Just, simply, what were the problems in the family.

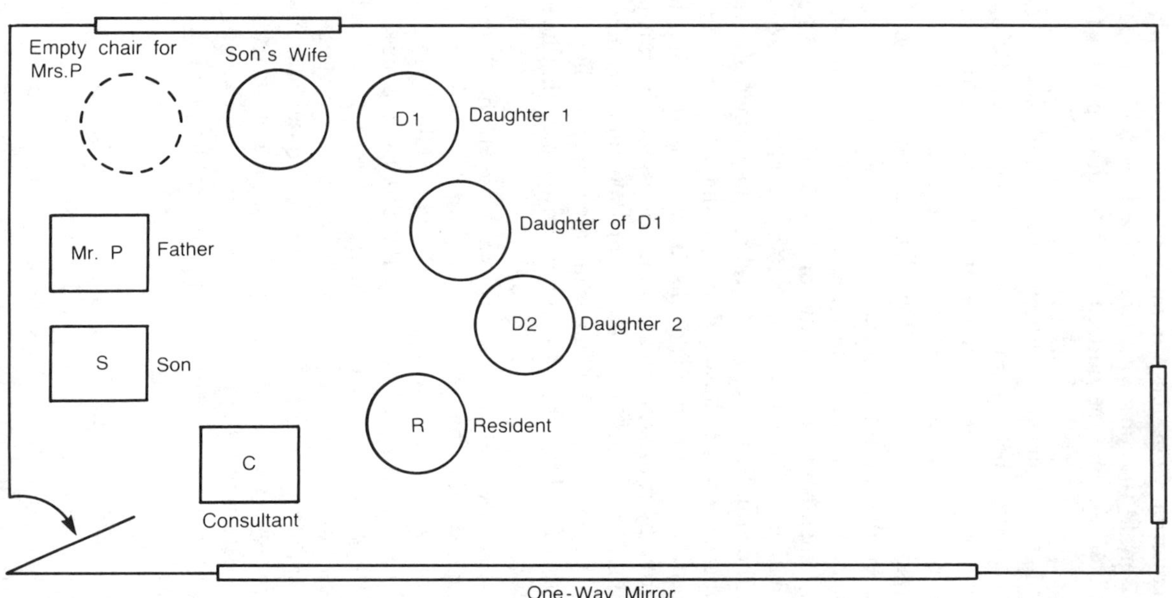

FIGURE 12-1. Seating arrangement in interview with P family.

C comments that there seems to be no place for Mrs. P and pulls up, between Mr. P and the son's wife, a chair. The empty chair will have the function throughout the session of signaling the present-but-absent member, Mrs. P. The interview continues.

C (*to Mr. P*): So in the meanwhile, who is going to translate for you?

First daughter (*D1*): He can understand but he cannot speak English.

C (*to Mr. P*): Do you understand what I say? (*Mr. P nods.*) If you don't understand something, who is going to be your main interpreter?

(*Second daughter, D2, translates into Arabic and an animated dialogue ensues that ends with both daughters saying that they will translate when needed.*)

C (*to Mr. P*): Okay, if you don't understand something that Dr. R or I say, please request help from some members of your family.

As can be seen, Mr. P is addressed at all times by the therapist as if he knows English. This policy of "talk to, not about" (Sluzki, 1978) will be maintained throughout the interview, in spite of the fact that during the first 10 minutes, Mr. P does not even look at C or R and the offspring translate whatever the consultant says to him. The main rationale for this policy is to neutralize the family's attempt to shield Mr. P. By steadily refusing to accept the proposal of the family to exclude Mr. P "because he doesn't understand English," C will progressively incorporate Mr. P into the interview and later in the session will allow open discussion and restructuring of the family's argument around the father. The dialogue continues in an amiable vein.

C (*to all*): What in your view is the health situation in the family? How is the health in the family, in general?

Son (*S*): Perfect, beautiful.

D1: She's [resident R] our doctor.

C: Well, if she's your doctor, then you are healthy for sure. (*Everybody laughs.*) The only person who is not healthy is your mother, your wife. What is your own impression of what is going on with her?

S: Well, you know, mother gets upset so easily. Everything big and small upsets her. That's what troubles her. We try to tell her that she should not be upset for every little thing, but that is her nature. I guess she can't help it.

C: So, in your impression, that is her own way of being. Has she been all her life this way? (*to Mr. P*) You have known her for longer than them. Has she been always easy to get upset, for major or minor things? (*Mr. P makes a statement in Arabic, as do the daughters, and they all agree.*) When did this problem of hers start?

S: You see, she had high blood pressure for many years, 20 perhaps, but these last several years have been very bad. And I'll tell you one more thing. Wives and husbands always have problems. But these sisters of mine, everything that affects them, that happens to them, they come and tell mama. (*Everybody laughs.*) Then my mother gets everything on her head. I tell them, "Keep things away from mama." But this one fights with her husband, or the other one fights with her husband, they have to go and tell mama.

D2: You see, we have another sister. She doesn't get along with her husband.

S: And my mother always likes to see everybody happy. And she gets very upset when they tell her. She doesn't tell anything but she gets very upset. She keeps it all *inside*.

R (*to S*): How do *you* deal with that when you quarrel with your wife.

D1: He never does.

S: I never quarrel with my wife.

C: Never ever?

S: Never.

It should be noted that the style of communication of this family is one in which one person very frequently speaks for another and more than one person speaks at the same time. However, they are not "fighting for the channel" but rather complementing each other's statements with additional statements. Even when they converse among themselves, they tend to talk with extended overlapping. Thus, throughout the interview, the family has to be viewed more as a collective than as a collection of individuals (a statement that goes beyond the family therapy creed and becomes the pragmatic, clinical reality in this case). It should be added that this style, which would be totally anomalous if the family were of Anglo origin, fits their cultural cradle and requires careful calibration by the interviewer: Were he or she to attempt to "correct" this collective-oriented style by trying to enforce a rule of "each person speaks for self only," the result would have been immobilization of the family process (because they literally think collectively).

Another point merits some comment. Why did the son take such an active role in the dialogue, even in affairs that are culturally defined as the domain of women? He probably did so for the same reason that he chose to sit where he did, that is, he assumed that the therapist and consultant would side with his mother in defining father as the culprit, and he wanted to establish a position of power from which he could protect his father from their potential aggression. The interview continues:

D1: They have a perfect marriage. I envy them.

C: I envy them too. (*to S*) And this is a good way of not bringing problems to your mother. But when you have problems of any other kind, what then?

S: I keep it to myself.

C: So, you have learned from your mother to be that way?

D1: He has the same style and character of my mother.

C: So, you are going to have high blood pressure! (*Everybody laughs.*)

S: My problems are minor. They are all minor problems in my life.

C: Do other people come and tell you their problems?

S: Sure.

C (to R): See, there you have another client for you. In a few years he will appear with high blood pressure. (*Everybody laughs.*)

In this last sequence, a semantic equivalence has been established between the presenting complaint (hypertension) and the behavior ("the tendency to become tense and, in addition, to have difficulty in releasing tension"). From now on when we talk about this interpersonal style, we also will be talking about hypertension.

S: You see, it is different when a daughter or son tells something to their mother and when a sister tells it to a brother because, for me, my sister she's married. She has her husband, and I don't care too much. But my mother, she loves her sons better than herself, and better than the love of brothers and sisters. That's why it is so much of a problem.

(*D1 and D2 simultaneously*): *D1*: She loves us too much! *D2*: Poor mother!

C: Let's follow your theory, a very sound one. What would happen if nobody would tell your mother any troubles or any of their problems and everybody would appear to be happy and with smiling faces?

D2: You know, my younger sister is not happy with her husband, so my mother, she *knows*. And we may keep on telling her from the morning to the night that my sister is in good shape, she will not believe it because she *knows* and knows that the situation is never going to change.

D1: She knows the problems *exists*.

S: She knows. (*They chat animatedly in Arabic about this issue.*)

At this point, the exploration confirms the consultant's hypothesis: The family is locked in a tight pattern in which mother's worries generate placating behavior on the part of the rest of the family, mainly her offspring, and that behavior reconfirms her worries, which, when expressed, in turn generate more placating behavior. It is, in fact, a perfect example of the situation described by Watzlawick, Weakland, and Fisch (1974) in which ineffective responses to a symptomatic behavior lead, rather than to a new behavior, to more of the same behavior, despite its having proved to be ineffective. A situation develops in which the attempted solution perpetuates the problem. The stereotyped response, it should be noted, is perceived by all the participants as the only reasonable behavior.

Despite the confirmation of this hypothesis, the consultant decides that it is premature to go beyond this "trial balloon." Mr. P is still an outsider/scapegoat in this interview, and any intervention is likely to be rejected by family members because their view of Mr. P is not being taken into consideration. The consultant thus maintains an exploratory mode while realigning himself with the family and the resident. He will later pursue his hypothesis and develop it into a form of intervention.

D1(to C): Let me tell you something. If I have a problem, I cannot keep it to myself. If I keep it in myself, I'd burst. I have to tell somebody.

C: Okay, so your way of not getting high blood pressure is that, when you are loaded, you somehow unload.

D1: This is the way I am. I cannot do anything about it.

C: No, I am not saying that you have to change. On the contrary, it is reasonable that, when you perceive that you increase your tension, you decrease it by unloading. (*to Mr. P*) How is your style? Do you get loaded or do you open up?

S: Are you asking my father?

C: Yes.

S: He has the same blood pressure I have. (*Everybody laughs.*)

C (*to Mr. P*): How do you unload when you feel loaded?

D1: You know something, he's very, very nervous. He bursts like that (*snaps fingers*) and then he just calms like that (*snaps fingers*).

C: Okay. So you two [Mr. P and D1] have a good method. You get loaded and then you unload. Does your mother, your wife, have any way or anybody with whom to unload?

D1: She talks about it, but still it is *inside* her. She cannot unload and give up and be happy. (*They break into overlapping dialogues, some in Arabic, some in English.*)

Mr. P (*emphatically*): Yes, something happen years ago, and now she remembers it as if 13 years ago were today.

C (*to Mr. P emphatically*): Ah, she keeps it inside and then brings old stuff as if it was new?

D1: That's it. She cannot live with the right-now.

C: When did you all move to the States?

D1: My brother and sister have been here for 6 years. My parents have been here for 2 years. I have been here for 1 year or so.

C: Ten years ago was your mother the same as she is now, unable to forget, keeping things inside? (*Everybody agrees.*)

S: She used to work, you know, and when she was working, she was able to forget. But now she hasn't been working for quite a while. Things have changed. She's at home all the time. She can't work anymore.

C: She cannot? (*to R*) Why? Has she a health problem?

D1: She cannot work.

D2: She would love to work if she could.

C (*to R*): She can't?

D1: She gets tired easily. She does a bit of cooking and her hands feel weighed. This morning she was saying, "I'm feeling so tired." She cannot work much, only do some work in the house in the morning. And in the morning she has to take a rest, or she won't sleep all night.

C: How old is your mother?

D1: She is 56.

C: So, she is a young lady.

Mr. P (*laughing*): Young lady, 56. (*He adds something in Arabic.*)

C: What I mean by that is that at 56 people do not cease working for reasons of age but for other reasons.

R: That was my impression also, that she was responding to some losses with a body depression. In Jerusalem she was a highly skilled worker, translator between Arabic, French, and English, and she lost all that in her move.

C: And everybody suffers with a move. How did *you* do with the move?

D1: We are young and we can deal with problems, but mother is the same as she has been for the last 20 years.

C: She has lost a lot with the move. (*The family members all mutter disagreement.*)

D1: You see, what affects her is us. In our country, the family is, I am sorry to say, the family is more related. We have concern for each other more than here. Whatever happens to me, my brother gets worried, my sister gets involved, my mother gets involved. So, you see, the problem is our relationship. (*Family breaks into conversation in Arabic.*) It is not the move. When mother was in Jerusalem, she hadn't been working already for several years. You see, my sister was here, my brother was on the East Coast, I was in Jordan. So we were far away. Whenever she had a problem we were not around and she would go to the hospital and she would cry saying that she was going to die without seeing us. So having us here, all together, and being here, is very good for her. She has all of us here, and that is what she wanted, and I am 100% sure. (*Short silence.*)

The fact that the onset of the presenting complaint preceded the migration leads to the assumption that some old and ongoing family pattern anchors the symptom, and that the stress of migration may be considered a contributory but not central force in its present configuration. Thus, the consultant chose, after this exploration, to center his interventions on issues other than the specific process of relocation.

It should be noted, however, that an alternative strategy could have been to highlight the stresses of migration and define everybody as equal victims of it. This would acknowledge everybody's increased needs, define Mr. P as competent in his way of handling those stresses by means of his traveling, define Mrs. P as less competent, and then develop from these approaches another way of reframing the problem.

S: You see, in these 3 years, my father went to Jerusalem 6 or 7 times and lost a lot of money in that way.

D1: And she keeps thinking about all that. She cannot *accept* it.

C: Oh, she hasn't gone herself in these 2 or 3 years?

D1: No, it isn't that. It is that my father can't help it. It is his nature. He went 4 or 5 times to Jerusalem.

C: What does it mean that "it is his nature"?

S: He cannot find a job here and he gets bored easily. So he goes back home. He sometimes goes for a couple of months.

C (to Mr. P): So you have traveled a lot all these years?

Mr. P: Yes.

C: Good for you!

D1: So that is the problem, mother cannot forget.

C: What does she have to forget?

D1: That he lost a lot of money during those trips.

C (to Mr. P): But do *you* have any complaints for those trips that you have made? (*Mr. P laughs and everyone laughs.*)

D1: It is *she*, that she can't forget the money he lost in all those trips. That's it, forget it!

C: Has she gone any of these times?

D1 and D2: No, she cannot travel.

C: Why?

D1: The first time she came, after the trip she had to stay in bed 2 or 3 days. I don't know what happened to her.

D2 (to D1): But she recovered, so she could do it.

D1: I have known mother. She hasn't even traveled in our country. She always got dizzy.

C: So she doesn't like to travel. (*Both daughters and daughter-in-law agree with that.*)

This whole section is crucial to the process of realigning with Mr. P and of changing the family's pervasive logic that anchors them in defining Mr. P as the culprit. The consultant carries on his inquiry from a "one-down" position of not understanding or of misunderstanding what seems obvious to the family. He is thus able to challenge those assumptions without being experienced as threatening. By asking what it is to accept and is it that she hasn't gone herself, he challenges the family's seeming assumption that what Mrs. P has to accept is Mr. P's behavior. To suggest that it isn't that Mr. P has traveled excessively, but that Mrs. P has traveled insufficiently, will switch the emphasis from Mr. P's selfishness to Mrs. P's difficulties. This way of shaking basic assumptions about "the way things are" within the family further prepares the way for the following interventions:

D1: But that is the way mother *is*. If she could forget, I would think that she would be okay.

C: What is it that she has to forget?

D: Everything. Something happened wrong yesterday, well, forget it! She doesn't have to remember today! Something that happened 10 years ago, she keeps it. She keeps the same and the same and the same. That is her trouble.

C: I don't know any way to make her forget. In fact, if she has a good memory, that can become an important virtue. She is like the memory of the family. (*Everybody laughs and engages in an animated discussion in Arabic.*)

Mr. P: She has a very good memory.

D1: That is her problem, not forgetting even the sorrows of her life. (*They engage in another discussion in Arabic.*) We are saying that she had a very hard life since childhood, and my father says that we all have difficult lives, and we said that it didn't affect us the same way that it affected her.

C: My impression is that your mother, your wife, is like a specialist, a person who chooses to remember and to worry. My picture in my mind is that when you are together, if anything happens, she will start to worry and you will start to calm her and tell her, "Don't worry, mother." And she is going to wind herself up with worries, and you are going to calm her and calm her. Is that the way it works, all of you calming her all of the time?

S: We don't have really serious problems.

C: But when she brings up whatever is for her a problem . . .

S: All the things at home are minor, an occasional quarrel, but nothing serious. But everything sticks into her mind.

C: The effect of that way of functioning of your mother is to make all of you calming her a lot.

D1 and D2: Yes, we do that.

C: I would like to recommend you to do an interesting experiment. It is a pity that your mother isn't here, because it would be very necessary that she hears what I am going to say too. It is something that will be very difficult for you to do, I am sure. And it is, rather than calm her, instead of saying, "Don't worry Ma," say, "You are right." (*They all shake their heads.*)

D1 (holding her head): Oh, no! She would have a heart attack, I am quite convinced of it! You know, my mother is a very sensitive person. Sometimes, I talk to her in a way that is not very careful, and I can see that she gets sad. So we have to be very careful.

C (*to R*): As you see, even mentioning this generates that action of placating mother, even when mother isn't even here.

D1: Really, I treat her like a baby. My brother comes and caresses her and kisses her. It is something *inside* of her. We try and do our best for her.

C: That's why I said that what I was going to suggest was going to be very difficult and hard, because it sounds like being harsh and cruel. If she comes and says, "I am worried about this or that," you, instead of saying, "Don't worry Mama," say, "Oh, yes, it worries me too."

D1: Oh yes, she will think you are telling her the truth and it will stick into her mind. That is the problem.

C: That is why it would be so important for her to hear all this. And that is the main problem of not having her here. What I would suggest you to do, when you go home, is to tell your mother that we suggested something that was going to be very difficult for all of you. And it is that for the next few weeks you should try, rather than telling her that it is nothing, to step her worries up. You have to *tell* her that, so when you do it, she may not know whether you are doing it because I told you to do it, or because you mean it. You look scared of doing all that. (*D1 nods in agreement and smiles.*) Maybe it is too difficult for you to do. It isn't dangerous, otherwise I wouldn't suggest it to you, but it may be too difficult. And, indeed, it is difficult for her as well as for you to change what has been for years a way of functioning. Apparently she doesn't hear "Don't worry" when you say, "Don't worry." She hears "Worry." Therefore, if you want her to hear "Don't worry," you have to tell her, "Worry." (*They all smile and nod.*)

D1: My daughter would accept that because she generally does the opposite of what we say. (*to R*) Sometimes my daughter wants to eat something and I don't want her to eat, so I tell her, "Come on, eat it," and she won't.

C: We can all learn from the wisdom of your child. So I would recommend to you, first, tell your mother what was our suggestion, and then to do it as seriously as you can, of course. Let her doubt. You don't have to clarify anything. Whenever you are going to say, "Don't worry, Mama," catch yourself and say instead, "You are right, Mother, it is worrisome." (*to S*) Do you think you can do it? I know it is hard. (*Son nods in agreement.*) (*to Mr. P*) For you it's going to be even harder because you have been trained by your wife for many, many years. (*Father agrees. C then requests and obtains one by one the agreement of the rest of the family members.*)

Mr. P (*after a dialogue in Arabic with the rest of the family*): Sometimes I say like that. I say, "You are too nervous."

C: The slight change that I am suggesting is that instead of saying exactly that, you say, "You are right. It is very worrisome." (*The interview ends with expressions of appreciation to the family for having attended the consultation, and other pleasantries.*)

The delivery of this intervention is slightly atypical in the sense that it required C to show considerable skill at persuasion, beginning with a meek suggestion and ending with a strong "selling pitch." The logic of this intervention is based on the consultant's realization of the family's "damned if you do, damned if you don't" dilemma, namely, regardless of what other family members do, Mrs. P will worry. The trap of this situation consists, as already mentioned above, in the fact that any solution they attempt will accentuate the problem. This realization is confirmed by the family members when the assumed pattern is described to them. The consultant then poses the alternative, seemingly nonsensical suggestion, which is followed by an expected initial rejection by Mrs. P's family. The consultant, aware of the family's style, which requires consensus-seeking exchanges between the members before any new idea is accepted, chooses to stick to his proposal, which is totally paradoxical in terms of the family's views.

Contrary to the usual practice with paradoxical interventions, the consultant *explains* the rationale for this intervention to the family. This, in the author's view, does not jeopardize its potential effectiveness. In and by itself, this action goes against the assumption, not infrequent in the field of family therapy, that the effect of a so-called paradoxical intervention (i.e., a type of intervention that is contrary to the family's view of a fragment of reality) is contingent upon its being delivered without explanation of its intended effect. The family finally accepts the proposal. The prescription is then repeated in all its components and the consultant engages each member in an agreement. The chances of compliance are increased by predicting difficulties in compliance, especially for Mr. P who, it is assumed, is firmly locked in the old pattern.

After the family leaves, the consultation ends with a discussion with the resident about the session and her reactions to it. She is astonished at the consultant's closing intervention, and confesses relief that the family accepted it. Other than that, she has felt comfortable with the whole process, which has allowed her to gain some distance from the strong allegiance she felt to the women in the family. The consultant recommends that the resident follow up the family as usual in her clinic, with the only difference being that she herself should also follow the recommendation made by the consultant to the family and she should play along with the mother's worries rather than appeasing her. If Mrs. P comments on the recommendation, the resident is advised to tell her that she, like the members of the family, is following the consultant's recommendation. Further, the resident is to consult with him again if there are any unexpected health problems in the family.

In addition, the resident is to keep the videotape of the interview and is invited to review and discuss it within a month at one of the weekly group supervision/workshops in which she participates regularly with the consultant. At that workshop, the complexity of the interpersonal/psychosomatic package that contained the "hypertension" symptom is discussed with her and the other residents. The didactic emphasis focuses on the viewpoint that symptoms, both in the psychosomatic and psychosocial domains, are interactively powerful behaviors that are part of larger, ongoing, recursive patterns that include both symptomatic and nonsymptomatic behaviors. The therapeutic intervention is aimed at disrupting the interactive pattern of which the symptom is a part, with the hope that the symptom will be dislodged and perhaps disappear.

No other consultation is needed about this family. A follow-up, 18 months later, corroborated by examination of the P family's chart, shows that 2 weeks after the interview, Mrs. P's blood pressure has returned to within-normal limits, without any substantial variation in the type or dose of antihypertensive medication prescribed. Since then, no other major health problems have appeared in Mrs. P or in any other family member.

REFERENCES

Sluzki, C. E. Marital therapy from a systems theory perspective. In T. J. Paolino, Jr., & B. S. McCrady (Eds.), *Marriage and marital therapy: Psychoanalytic, behavioral and systems theory perspectives.* New York: Brunner/Mazel, 1978.

Watzlawick, P., Weakland, J. H., & Fisch, R. *Change: Principles of problem formation and problem resolution.* New York: Norton, 1974.

13

USING A GROUP AS A CONSULTANT
A Systems Approach to Medical Care

SUSAN H. McDANIEL

JOHN BANK

THOMAS CAMPBELL

JOSEPH MANCINI

BERNARD SHORE

University of Rochester School of Medicine and Dentistry
Rochester, New York

Physicians and other health service providers have a long history of consulting with colleagues to obtain advice, support, and information in their efforts to improve patient care. This chapter reports on the use of a group as a consultant, with each member of the group presenting cases in rotation, or as the need arises. This process evolved among the faculty of a family medicine training program. The chapter will begin with a brief description of the group followed by a series of vignettes written by the group member who originally presented each case. These vignettes describe experientially the process and functioning of the group.

A multidisciplinary faculty development group began in early 1982 when some members of the Family Medicine faculty at the University of Rochester became interested in the application of family systems theory to the practice of medicine. Over time this faculty group came to focus on case consultation from a systems perspective. The group now performs many functions. It offers a forum for theoretical arguments about the biopsychosocial model (Engel, 1977, 1980) and its application in practice, and provides support and consultation for its members.

Physicians often are not very explicit in their requests for consultation. It is not uncommon for medical consultations to address content issues only, without considering the underlying reasons for the request. At times, face-to-face interactions between the consultant and the consultee do not occur and, as a result, crucial aspects of a request may be left unaddressed (Rudd, 1981). These ambiguities in the consultation request can result in misunderstanding and frustration for physicians during the contracting and feedback phases of consultation and can ultimately evoke dissatisfaction from patients and their families. One reason for the group's inception and continued vigor may be the members' interest in developing a more effective and less ambiguous consultative process than is now available in the usual medical consulting network.

Membership in the group is open to all Family Medicine faculty members, the chief resident, and fellows. Because of the annual turnover in the residency, composition of the group changes each July, but remains relatively stable in the interim. Most recently, for example, the group consisted of six regular members: three (of six) family physician faculty members, one internist with medical–psychiatric liaison training, one clinical psychologist with family therapy training, and the chief resident. The group's multidisciplinary nature allows the member who takes the role of consultee the opportunity to hear a range of opinions and have the problem discussed among colleagues. This kind of group, in which some faculty members participate and some do not, does have the potential to facilitate splits among different factions in a department. Networking and participation in other groups lessen the potential for the consultation group to become a divisive force in the larger system.

The consultation group has now met weekly in 60-minute sessions for 4 years. The long-term nature of the group has allowed for the development of trust and familiarity with each other's work, counteracting some of the fear of failure described by Krakowski (1971) that can inhibit physicians from requesting help or advice from colleagues. Consultant roles within the group shift with each case, depending on group members' areas of expertise and interest. In any one case, one or two members may provide the main thrust of systems explication, others may provide support, empathy, or interest, and still others may contribute specific ideas for interventions. This use of the group process in sharing the consultant responsibilities allows the expression of many different perspectives, clearly leaving the consultee to decide on the final treatment plan.

The recommendations for the consultee arise out of the group process; sometimes a consensus develops and sometimes diverse views remain diverse. This process contrasts with the simple one-to-one experience of a consultee using an individual as a consultant, with only one opinion likely to be expressed. Theoretically, multiple views could result in confusion; instead, the diversity seems to provide more views of the problem and more potential solutions. The group functions primarily for its members and recommendations are always directed to the consultee rather than to the patients. Even on the occasions when a family is interviewed in front of the group, the group members share their thoughts and advice with the consultee after the session. This structure emphasizes the consultee's primary responsibility for the case.

Topics for consultation in the group are far-ranging. Most common are case consultations approached from a biopsychosocial perspective. In these consultations, interactions among different levels of the system, from the organic to the psychological, from the interpersonal to the social, are usually examined. The format is relatively unstructured. Some consultations are short, one-shot sessions; others are ongoing. The consultee begins by reviewing the case and presenting the group with a question or questions regarding diagnosis or treatment. Assessment and problem solving usually characterize the first half of the consultation. The latter part of the consultation often involves an exploration of how this patient family "triggers" the consultee and makes it difficult for the consultee to treat the family at this particular time. Each member has spent at least one entire session presenting his or her own family. These sessions then provide valuable information for the group's understanding of "stuck" points in future case consultations presented by that group member.

Each consultation includes genograms drawn on large chart paper. The genograms provide a central reference point for all data gathering (Guerin & Pendagast, 1976). For each consultation, the group works with at least two genograms, one of the patient's family and one of the consultee's family (Guerin & Fogarty, 1972). Some consultations also focus on the treatment system as a whole, that is, on the professional systems that are involved in providing care for a family. In these consultations, the group has the patient family's genogram, the consultee family's genogram, and a diagram of the professional treatment system hanging on the wall for review as the consultee's questions are addressed. If the patient's medical problems are complex and many consultants are involved in the case, the group consultation often focuses at the level of understanding and management of the treatment system. These discussions explore what Friedman (1985) has described as the "interlocking triangles" between the patient system, the professional's family system, and the work system.

When the group discusses cases, it functions in many ways like a Balint group (1957), a case-oriented group of primary care physicians that focuses on the doctor–patient relationship. Important differences between this group and a Balint group are that this group has no single leader and it has a family systems rather than individual orientation.

Besides the doctor–patient relationship explored in the case orientation, other interactional topics covered in the group have included personal boundary issues, such as the problems that can occur when a physician is dealing with medical issues found in his or her own family. The group also has consulted on problems between a faculty group member and a resident. Here, the role of preceptor in the training context can mirror that of consultant in the treatment context. Teaching problems can also involve struggle similar to those that are problematic in the doctor–patient relationship.

Theoretical discussions naturally emerge from questions about patient care or other interactional problems. Lively discussions have taken place in the group about such issues as the pragmatic applications of systems theory to medicine, the effectiveness of family systems theory, group process and leadership, the history of theoretical underpinnings of family medicine, and the process of medical consultation. As in the case consultation, members provide information and leadership in these discussions depending on areas of expertise and interest. These discussions have pushed each of us to look beyond our own points of view in a more comprehensive and systemic way.

Describing the group defines its structure, but it does not give the flavor of the experience or the process of using a group as a consultant. For this reason, we offer the following series of vignettes. Each case is written by the person who was in the role of consultee on the case and includes some editorial comment by the consultee about the meaning and usefulness of the consultation to him or her. The second vignette includes a set of genograms to illustrate how such diagrams help to clarify and focus the consultation.

SECRETS OF THE HEART: A CASE EXAMPLE FROM DR. A

I first presented the family of Mrs. C to the group at a time when the family was in crisis. As a family physician, I was contacted by this family a year previously when Mrs. C was hospitalized with a myocardial infarction. During that hospitalization, the family impressed me, in my informal contacts with them, as being very angry. Over the subsequent year, Mrs. C experienced progressive debilitation from her inoperable coronary artery disease. On several occasions she alluded to her view that her family was having difficulties accepting her illness. However, offers to meet formally with the family were always declined with the response, "They won't come." She also frequently expressed concern about her husband's heavy alcohol use and "inability to care for himself."

Mrs. C, an obese, soft-spoken woman, presented herself first and foremost in the role of mother. During the course of her regular visits with me, it became clear that she perceived herself as central to her family, taking care of and being relied upon by everyone in the family. With her progressive illness, she could no longer fulfill that role. In August, Mrs. C was admitted to the hospital again for congestive heart failure. After her medications were adjusted, she was ready for discharge within several days. On the morning she was to be discharged, I received an urgent call from the energency department, where her husband was being treated for an overdose of sedatives and alcohol. This allegedly was precipitated by Mr. C's discovery the day before that his youngest son (Kerry) was gay. The urgent call was from another son (Steve) and a close family friend (Mrs. T). The major concerns of Steve and Mrs. T were to get help for Mr. C with his alcohol problem, and to "protect" Mrs. C by keeping her in the hospital and not letting her know about Mr. C's overdose or Kerry's homosexuality. This encounter served to clarify for me the secretive manner in which this family had dealt with crises. However, I was at a loss for an appropriate intervention plan at that point and so I brought the case to the group.

Initially, the group served to allay my anxieties by allowing me to express my frustration. It then provided a forum for discussion of how best to deal with the situation. This was tremendously helpful in dealing with the crisis. Subsequently, I was able to shift responsibility for solving the problem back to the family by calling for a family meeting. In the hospital, the first family meeting consisted only of the original patient (Mrs. C) and one son (Steve). The husband (Mr. C) had been discharged from the Psychiatry Department and was recuperating at home. I then arranged a second family meeting, which included the husband, for later that week in the office. The focus of that meeting was on how the family could best adjust to Mrs. C's progressive illness and debility. We deliberately did not address Mr. C's alcohol problem nor Kerry's homosexuality at that time. Agreement was tentatively reached that further family meetings would be held.

No further family meetings occurred. There were various reasons offered for this, most of which involved "impossible" scheduling conflicts for the youngest son, Kerry. However, over the next few months, the family did seem to stabilize. I continued to see Mrs. C on a regular basis. During these meetings, she indicated that her family was more supportive and understanding and, in fact, that she seemed to be coping better with her illness. During this period of time, I also had some individual contacts with other family members that corroborated the impression of improved family functioning. Kerry had come to my office once to ask my advice on how best to tell his mother that he was gay. Mr. C did not follow through on alcohol rehabilitation, but did decrease his alcohol consumption, which seemed to decrease Mrs. C's anxiety about this problem. Thus, the issues that had precipitated a crisis in August apparently were being dealt with by this family in some fashion.

However, another potential crisis was developing that involved the role of the medical consultant. Because of the severity and complications of Mrs. C's coronary artery disease, a cardiologist had been serving as consultant. On his recommendation, Mrs. C was given several medications to control her angina. Yet, despite increased dosages, she continued to get worse. She believed these medicines had not helped and considered stopping them. When she mentioned this to the cardiologist, she was scolded for even considering this. She then came to me for support of her decision. However, she did not want the cardiologist to know of her plan and, in fact, it was unclear if she had discussed this decision with her family.

I again brought the case to the group for further guidance. After discussion, it became clear that I was again dealing with another secret in a family that maintains many secrets. The resulting plan was for me to be supportive of Mrs. C's autonomy but to keep communication lines open by discussing her plan with the cardiologist consultant, and by encouraging her to do the same with her family and the consultant.

The pull to become entangled in this family's secrecy and dysfunctional coping mechanisms were great. Part of this may have been due to parallels with my own family, in which my mother (of a similar age and demeanor) is central to family functioning. The group helped me to maintain some therapeutic distance and objectivity and has provided very helpful consultation in my treatment of Mrs. C and her family.

This first vignette exemplifies several functions of the group as consultant. First and foremost, the case clearly demonstrated the importance of treating the individual patient in the context of the family system. Group consultation helped the family physician take advantage of a family crisis to help the family to begin to adjust to the painful reality of the mother's illness. This approach then fostered a more direct, less secretive communication among family members. Second, the group's recognition of parallels between the families of origin of physician and patient enabled the physician to put his relationship to the patient and the family in proper perspective. The use of genograms further helped to organize the personal data relevant to this kind of consultation. Third, the group emphasized the importance of considering other "players" (in this case, the cardiologist) within the medical system, lest care providers find themselves working against one another.

ENMESHMENT AND MORE: A CASE EXAMPLE FROM DR. B

Family T (see Figure 13-1) is a multigenerational family that is cared for at our Family Medicine Center. Over the last several years, two major lengthy episodes of doctor–family interaction have occurred, each of which pre-

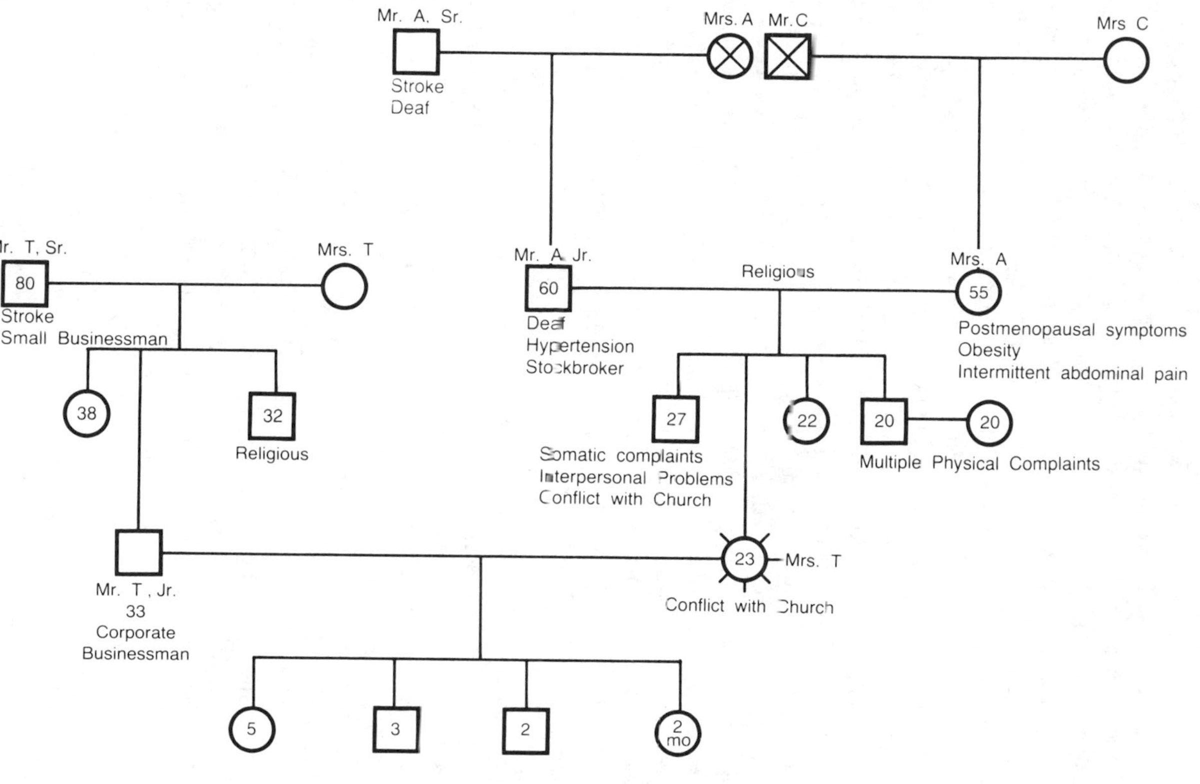

FIGURE 13-1 T family genogram.

sented a strong pull on me, the family physician, to be drawn into the enmeshed behavior of this family.

In the first episode, several years ago, the focal person in the family was Mr. A, Sr., who was living in the home of Mr. and Mrs. A, Jr. He had undergone a series of strokes and falls that had left him essentially dependent and bedridden. Mr. A, Sr.'s deteriorating health and the conflict and triangulation that occurred around Mr. A, Jr.'s loyalty to his father versus his loyalty to his wife gradually made it apparent that Mr A, Sr. might not be best cared for at home. In spite of this inadequate care for his father and his own severe marital problems, Mr. A, Jr.'s feeling of guilt and responsibility prevented him from moving his father out of the home into an appropriate nursing setting. At this point, I was drawn into the dynamics by the family's request to make the decision for them, that is, whether or not Mr. A, Sr. should be placed in a long-term-care facility.

During several months of interaction around this issue, I was under pressure to be drawn into the family dynamics and to overfunction in solving their problem. Upon presenting the situation to the group, I was encouraged to set boundaries with the family by structuring my availability for phone calls and visits. I also redefined my role from adviser to facilitator; by pushing the family members to make decisions they all could live with, I encouraged them to set their boundaries. I then was able to free myself from enmeshment with the family and they were able to work out their own resolution to the problem. The ultimate solution came after Mrs. A announced that either Mr. A, Sr. or herself would have to leave the home. This forced the issue, clearly set the ground rules, and Mr. A, Sr. was successfully admitted to a nursing home.

For several months, the situation remained stabilized; Mr. and Mrs. A, Jr.'s marriage improved and Mr. A, Sr. made a good adjustment to his new home. Family problems then surfaced in the next generation when Mr. and Mrs. A, Jr.'s daughter, Mrs. T, presented with a multitude of somatic complaints around her pregnancy. She eventually required hospitalization for nausea and vomiting. As her pregnancy progressed, she told me of a close male friend of hers whom she had met at church. They began having an affair, but she denied that this friend was the father of her baby. Triangulation occurred among herself, the friend, and her husband, with the husband refusing to believe that the third party was anything more than a friend. The church friend was present at the delivery and ultimately became the godfather of the newborn baby. Tensions mounted when the husband realized that the friend had been intimately involved with his wife. I was drawn into the situation much in the way that I had been drawn into the nursing-home scenario. Once more I presented the family to the group, which again advised me to clearly establish my own boundaries and to help the family to do the same. At this point, the problems were so severe that I referred the family to the family therapist in our group, who then began treatment of Mrs. T and her husband.

In both of these situations, several concerns of my own were stimulated, including the pull on me in my own family to become overinvolved, particularly around the issue of my father's drinking behavior (see Figure 13-2). For many years, I perceived myself as the one who had the responsibility of solving that problem. In addition, there had been much conflict with the organized church among members of my own family. The combination of the church connection of Mrs. T's friend and Mrs A's inordinate amount of talk about, and focus upon, religion drew me into the arena quite readily. Presenting this case to the group allowed me to see the comparisons with my own family and to set appropriate limits and boundaries with this family.

The most important facilitative factor in this case was the presentation of Dr. B's own family. It made this and other cases more understandable and allowed the group to provide more effective consultation to him. Countertransference issues are extremely common in daily medical practice, but physicians are often unaware of their presence, despite their major impact (Gorlin & Zucker, 1983; Smith, 1984). This is particularly true in the more difficult cases and in problem families that consume a great deal of the physician's time and energy. Having a group of peers with whom to share these difficult cases can help identify how the physician's own conflicts are part of the difficulty. The following case illustrates how the group helped to explore the effect of the provider's nuclear family on patient care.

FAMILY FURY WITH THE PHYSICIAN: A CASE EXAMPLE FROM DR. C

Mrs. L is a 75-year-old widow whom I have treated for several years in my practice as a family physician. Her health had been gradually failing, and she had a mild reactive depression. For several months, she had been considering selling her house and entering a nursing home. She was quite ambivalent about it and had changed her mind on several occasions. She was then hospitalized with a mild myocardial infarction. Though there was no change in her functional status after recovery from the heart attack, Mrs. L then decided to go into a nursing home after discharge from the hospital. Unfortunately, there were no beds available and she returned home for a short period of time.

Mrs. L's niece (and only relative), who had been trying for several

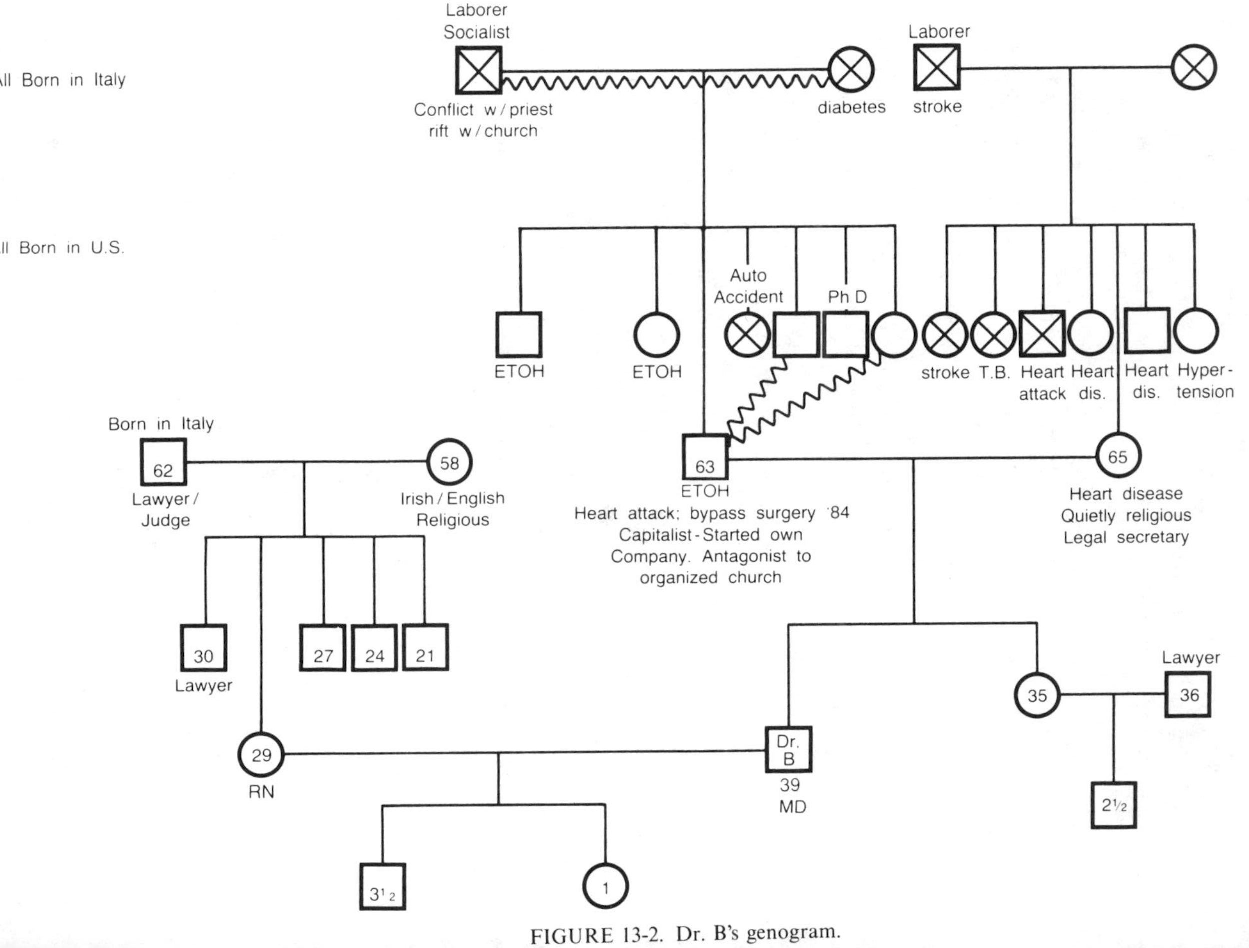

FIGURE 13-2. Dr. B's genogram.

months to get her into a nursing home, had become quite upset during the hospitalization. She insisted that her aunt could not to go home, and accused me of thwarting previous attempts at nursing-home placement and of not taking adequate care of her aunt. I was quite distraught as a result of these accusations and presented them to the group. The group first explored the anger of the niece, which had been displaced from her aunt onto me. Yet it was apparent that my reaction to the case remained unusually strong. During further discussion, I realized that I was particularly sensitive to the niece's accusations because of my own unexpressed anger at my wife's physician, who I felt had not taken adequate care of her medical problems. My identification with the niece's anger made it difficult for me to respond effectively as a caretaking physician.

The group helped me to explore these conflicts and to determine what aspects of the difficulty were due to countertransference. The group was also able to help me understand my own feelings toward my wife's physician and how to deal with that situation. I was then able to understand and tolerate the anger of my patient's niece and proceed with appropriate discharge planning.

Physicians, even those trained in the psychosocial aspects of medicine, may tend to focus more upon the patient and family than on the treatment system and its impact on the patient. The treatment system includes the patient and/or family, physician, consulting physician, and other members of the health care system, but it can also include other individuals or agencies in the community, such as schools, social service agencies, and government agencies. Being able to understand and optimally utilize this broader treatment system is an essential but sometimes neglected skill in clinical medicine. The following case illustrates how the group acted as a consultant with the treatment system.

IS THERE A DOCTOR IN YOUR HOUSE?: A CASE EXAMPLE FROM DR. D

This case involved a consultation request to me, an internist with expertise in pain problems, from Dr. W, a urologist serving as primary physician. The consultation began at an unplanned meeting following a hospital conference. Dr. W said that he had been meaning to talk to me about a patient he was admitting the next day; I wonder now if he would have made the consultation if he had not happened to meet me that morning. (Personal, informal access may make it easier to overcome resistances some physicians have in asking for help. Our group may perform a similar function by offering an ongoing structure that allows for personal, informal, easily obtainable consultation.)

Dr. W described with some intensity and more than customary detail the following complex history: Richard, a 43-year-old, married, restaurant manager, had been under Dr. W's primary care for 3 years. This patient initially had been referred to Dr. W for consultation by another physician. Richard's original problem was a worsening of chronic, intermittent bladder pain that, when medical and X-ray evaluation were unrevealing, Dr. W suspected was a "functional" disorder. In fact, I was not the only consultant on the case: Dr. W had begun as a consultant and had gotten personally mired in this complex situation. He had, perhaps, behaved in an overly responsible fashion, early on taking too much of the primary responsibility for medications and advice, and then ending up as the primary physician. I thought that some of the irritation he displayed may have been directed at himself, as well as at the first primary doctor for allowing the transfer of a very difficult case. Given this history, I expected to be pulled toward becoming overresponsible as a consultant, as had Dr. W, and perhaps ending up with a covert transfer of care in the same way as this case had begun.

This presentation also speaks to the issue of whom one chooses as a consultant. One of my own problems as a physician is that of overresponsibility regarding professional duties. Dr. W may have appreciated this similarity between us, making consultation easier for him but more complex for me. The stabilizing presence of the group, therefore, was very important to me. This issue of whom the primary physician consults is multidetermined; for example, one can choose a cardiologist who favors medical as opposed to surgical management of coronary disease. The final choice can reflect an unspoken hope that the consultant, with his or her authority, will complement and reinforce the opinions or approach of the consultee.

This patient's symptoms abated until about a year later when he returned to Dr. W after 3 months of a different type of pain. This time a carcinoma of the bladder was found. A resection of the tumor was immediately performed, but two positive lymph nodes were identified at operation. On hearing the diagnosis and the surgical findings, Richard became withdrawn and "unreasonably" insistent that he was terminal, according to Dr. W. The patient then became depressed, developing intractable postoperative pain that required high doses of narcotic analgesics. He became so dependent upon these that Dr. W confronted him with concern about addiction and insisted on psychiatric consultation. Richard, using the physician customers of his restaurant as his own consultative group, eventually agreed to see a therapist. He went briefly to one psychiatrist and then to another of his own choosing, but there was little improvement. In the face of his continuing bitter complaints of pain, a noninvasive exam was repeated. About 6 months after the first diagnosis of cancer, a "second look" operation to rule out recurrent tumor was performed. No tumor was found.

Gradually the symptoms remitted until 3 months before Dr. W's consultation request to me, at which time Richard developed severe nausea and vomiting, weight loss, and stabbing pain. A CT scan showed enlarged lymph nodes around the spine, and Richard was hospitalized for the third time in a year and a half. Although the house staff physicians thought that the symptoms represented a serious, recurrent carcinoma, Dr. W insisted that the man "didn't ever react the way you'd expect." He thought the problems were primarily psychosomatic and scheduled a lymph node biopsy.

I met Richard for the first time in his hospital room several days before the biopsy. He was an extremely well-defended, sociable man who was fairly certain the cancer had recurred and that his pain would not be adequately controlled. He also spoke of his concerns about Elsa, his second, much younger wife, who he said was very emotional and easily depressed. Plans for me to meet with Richard and Elsa as well as my recommendations about Richard's pain medications were welcomed by the house staff. Dr. W worried about the patient's addictive potential and appeared to have only limited interest in my assessment or recommendations. He did, however, institute the changes.

I was frustrated and a bit perplexed. Surgery had been performed when Richard was depressed but physically well; now that a cancer recurrence seemed likely, his doctor seemed reluctant to acknowledge it. It was time to present the case to the consulting group. I realized that part of the problem was Dr. W's special investment in this case, but I knew little about this physician or why this might be so. My request to the group was for a consultation on my consultation. The group allowed me to ventilate and supported me in my difficulties in engaging with Dr. W. They also pointed out that there might be value in asking Dr. W to review with me the history he had obtained of this complex case, for they suspected that this review might unearth missing information. A similar tack was regarded as potentially useful with the patient. The group suggested that I act as interested historian, listening to the story and occasionally asking such questions as: "What would you have hoped to happen if you'd done this?" The group also thought it was important to convey a sense of the difficulty and sadness implicit in these events for anyone involved.

In addition to these concrete suggestions, important associations relating to my own family of origin came out of the group's discussion. I was able to appreciate the resemblance of my difficulty in communicating with Dr. W to difficulties I had in communicating with my own physician–father. The group's exchange and the nonjudgmental acceptance of my presentation served to defuse this potential block to a productive consultation, and their specific suggestions provided a strategy.

After this group consultation, I arranged a meeting with Dr. W at his office to discuss the case. Almost spontaneously, Dr. W began reviewing the events, his interpretations, and his impressions from the beginning of his relationship with the patient. Any observations, questions, or comments by me seemed to distract him. During this 40-minute meeting, Dr. W mentioned for the first time that review of the original films had, in retrospect, shown an area suspicious for a tumor nearly a year before the diagnosis of cancer had been made. Treatment then might have been curative. This revelation certainly made some of Dr. W's behavior more understandable. The meeting ended with clear agreements on the roles Dr. W and I would play, plans for ongoing adjunctive psychotherapy for the patient and his family, and, for myself, a sense of satisfaction at having been helpful.

This consultation remains ongoing and has had subsequent ups and downs, as would be expected in the multidisciplinary medical care of any human suffering. The group continues to serve as a consultant's consultant. The group's capacity to connect with me vis-à-vis Dr. W allowed me to connect with Dr. W vis-à-vis the patient. This has been a valuable resource in a system in which people are likely to distance themselves when stressed. It further illustrates the unexpected complexities and benefits of having doctor(s) in your house. An additional aspect of this case was its value in stimulating a productive theoretical discussion about many subtle dimensions of medical consultation in general.

IS THERE A FAMILY THERAPIST IN YOUR HOUSE?: A CASE EXAMPLE FROM DR. E

The following is an example of a single consultation by the group on a case I had been treating in my family therapy practice for about 10 sessions. The case involved Hope, a 16-year-old patient who had cerebral palsy that had resulted in very poor vision and required the use of crutches. Hope denied her disability (never acknowledging in school that she could not see the blackboard or the markings on the chemistry beaker) and suffered greatly because she felt different from her peers. She was referred by a psychiatrist who had treated her as an inpatient on the three occasions when she attempted suicide by overdose. Hope reported great distress to me about family problems, especially the well-being of each of her parents, their marriage, and her older brother Terry. She reported that her suicide attempts were due to these family frustrations as well as to her inability to make friends at the exclusive private school where she was the only physically handicapped student in attendance. Hope had many of the usual concerns about leaving home, compounded by worries about her parents and fears about independent living. Though she was quite vocal in her complaints about her mother's overprotectiveness, Hope was not independently performing such tasks as getting herself up in the morning. She managed her peer relations by trying to deny her handicap (and her dependency needs), avoiding lunch because she would have to ask someone to carry her tray. She suffered from her lack of relationships. Even though she was the youngest, she functioned in her family as a parental child, making the family's distress explicit and being unusually insightful and psychologically minded.

Hope had two older brothers. Bill, age 24, had severe learning disabilities and had been away at boarding school or college since age 8. Hope described him as a "visitor" when home. Terry, the only child not labeled as having some handicap, was a gifted artist, but was seen by the family as rebelliously antiestablishment. He was heavily involved in the adolescent New Wave culture, much to his mother's horror. In sessions he appeared quite depressed, and his parents had what seemed to be well-founded concern about his possible drug abuse. Hope felt that she and Terry had a close and special relationship.

Mr. and Mrs. P both came from wealthy families, Mr. P's family having made millions through industry and Mrs. P's family having been wealthy for generations. Mrs. P appeared emotionally labile, often depressed, and quite concerned about her children. She complained of being the "heavy" with the children and her husband, and of carrying a large burden because of Mr. P's constant drinking. Mr. P appeared to be a kind, even-tempered man who refused to set limits with his children or himself. He accommodated his wife and tried superficially to pacify her. Neither adult worked outside the home. While the family appeared to be fairly well-off financially, much anxiety was expressed about Mr. P's having lost considerable money several years ago in a business venture. At that time, their lifestyle changed in that they fired their servants. Mrs. P said that Mr. P's drinking increased at that time as did other family problems.

When I presented this case, I felt somewhat stuck and worried about both Mrs. P's and Terry's depression. Hope had confided in me that Terry beat himself with chains when upset. Hope seemed less depressed but still in an over-responsible position, having made only small progress in developing relationships with peers. In presenting the case to the group, I hoped to receive some support and, in particular, a better understanding of the role of the cerebral palsy in Hope's dynamics. I told myself: What better group to explore both the physical and emotional aspects of cases.

I presented the case with an embarrassingly sketchy genogram. I could not recall Hope's oldest brother's name nor her parents' given names, which was quite unlike my usual case presentation. When the group began to ask specific questions about the family, I had to answer, "I don't know." While some biomedical aspects of the case and their psychological ramifications were discussed as I had requested, clearly this was not where the action was. More to the point, I became aware of my overidentification with Hope, because I too was the one in my family who was responsible and parental as well as the one who protested and tried to make family problems explicit. This identification contributed to the stuckness in the therapeutic system so that I did not adequately work with all members of the family, gather appropriate information, or really work with the subsystems in the family. In something of a role reversal (at least at the beginning of this group), the consulting group chastised me for my lack of family information and my lack of a systems approach to the case. This feedback unhooked me from my covert coalition with Hope and I was able to move forward with the family and treat them successfully. So much for my need for the group's "medical" advice!

This case also illustrated to me my own view of myself as somewhat handicapped in the group because I am not a family physician. I reacted to this at times much like Hope, by withdrawing and not requesting help, and only offering help to the group from a position of expertise. While the group had been very helpful on other kinds of cases, the mutuality involved in this particular case consultation was especially satisfying and important in helping me to feel more connected to my fellow faculty members.

CONCLUSION

This consultation group serves many functions for its members—ventilation, support, diagnosis, treatment planning, and an assessment of the larger treatment system. Among its most important functions is the development of strategies for managing issues arising from the interlocking triangles of the patient family, the provider family, and the treatment system. These sessions can offer consultation at many different levels of the system, from biomedical to community levels. At times, the consultee may be unsure why the case is disturbing him or her and then a multisystem assessment takes place. Commonly, the consultation will identify gaps in the data gathering, recommend more or less family involvement in the treatment, or suggest strategies for working with other colleagues around a case.

Recently, we have begun to examine the difference between cases brought to the group for consultation and those resolved by more traditional individual consultation. To explore this issue further, we plan to present some cases we think we might not typically bring to the group. We all agree, for now, that our most disturbing or emotionally draining cases are brought to this forum. The group consultation is likely to be more personal and more loosely structured than is standard in a formal medical consultation with an individual specialist. Furthermore, some individual consultations are obviated because of the existence of the group.

Another topic of recent interest has been the resistances we can identify in ourselves to presenting difficult cases to the group, for example, conceiving the problem as primarily biomedical, fearing not enough family information has been gathered to enable the group to consider the case effectively, fearing the group will recommend strategies that will be time-consuming, and fearing personal issues will again have to be confronted. Also, the fact that the group members have ongoing, close contact with each other as faculty members affects what each one is willing to share, sometimes with more disclosure and sometimes less than in an individual consultation or a different kind of group. We all have experienced these resistances at one time or another, but have not found them to be major impediments to the functioning of the group. Each week, at least one person has wanted a consultation, and often more than one person has issues about which they want help.

We have all found the exchange and consultation offered by a group of colleagues to be a rewarding experience, both personally and professionally. A well-functioning group can provide a much-needed forum to articulate and understand the complex way in which different systems affect health and health care delivery. Inevitably, as health care professionals, we carry a number of difficult cases. When it is a question of complex pathophysiology, traditional medical consultation often is helpful in providing appropriate patient care. However, patient problems are seldom limited to pathophysiologic processes alone. The care provided can be more effective if one takes into consideration the broader issues of the biopsychosocial model. A systems-oriented group can be of assistance in providing comprehensive care by offering valuable insights into potential impediments such as complex family dynamics, countertransference issues, or dysfunctional relations among the interfacing systems. Such insight benefits both patient and health care provider alike. In addition, we have found the group to have improved our abilities to teach a family systems approach in the medical training programs.

This group has extended the meaning of consultation beyond the usual boundaries found in the medical system to include rewarding personal and professional support as well as education and development. The format has much to offer.

ACKNOWLEDGMENTS

We would like to acknowledge the helpful comments and suggestions about this chapter given by two former group members no longer at the University of Rochester, Carl Osier, MD, and Stephen Taplin, MD.

REFERENCES

Balint, M. *The doctor, his patient, and the illness*. New York: International Universities Press, 1957.

Engel, G. L. The need for a new medical model: A challenge for biomedicine. *Science*, 1977, *196*, 129–136.

Engel, G. L. The clinical application of the biopsychosocial model. *American Journal of Psychiatry*, 1980, *137*, 535–544.

Friedman, E. *Generation to generation: Family process in church and synagogue*. New York: Guilford, 1985.

Gorlin, R., & Zucker, H. D. Physicians' reactions to patients—A key to teaching humanistic medicine. *New England Journal of Medicine*, 1983, *308*, 1059–1063.

Guerin, P., & Fogarty, T. Study your own family. In A. Ferber, M. Mendelsohn, & A. Napier (Eds.), *The book of family therapy*. Boston: Houghton Mifflin, 1972.

Guerin P., & Pendagast, E. Evaluation of family system and genogram. In P. Guerin (Ed.), *Family therapy*. New York: Gardner Press, 1976.

Krakowski, A. J. Doctor–doctor relationship. *Psychosomatics*, 1971, *12*, 11–15.

Rudd, P. Contrasts in academic consultation. *Annals of Internal Medicine*, 1981, *94*, 537–538.

Smith, R. C. Teaching interviewing skills to medical students: The issue of "counter transference." *Journal of Medical Education*, 1984, *59*, 582–588.

14

THE FAMILY THERAPIST AS SYSTEMS CONSULTANT TO MEDICAL ONCOLOGY

DAVID K. WELLISCH
UCLA School of Medicine
Los Angeles, California

MARIE M. COHEN
Private Practice
Los Angeles, California

Currently, one of three Americans can expect a diagnosis of cancer in their lifetime, and three out of four American families will have to confront and live with a diagnosis of cancer in a family member. However, three of every eight people with a cancer diagnosis at present will live 5 years beyond diagnosis (American Cancer Society, 1983). Thus, cancer is no longer the "absolute death sentence" that it was considered to be for so many decades. However, living longer with the diagnosis of cancer creates new adjustment problems for patients and their families.

This chapter is about family-oriented systems consultation in a university-based cancer center. This setting differs in two major ways from a private hospital: The university hospital is primarily a teaching hospital, and it has a very complicated hierarchy of health-care deliverers, especially among the physician group. Both of these factors are absent in the private setting.

The context of our consultation in the University of California at Los Angeles (UCLA) Cancer Center is triadic in nature (see Figure 14-1). Many cancer patients and their families are seen by us in the inpatient cancer center's medical and surgical oncology units. Although medical and surgical oncology are geographically contiguous, each has separate faculty attending physicians, separate house staff, and separate nursing staff. On a completely separate floor is the Bone Marrow Transplant Unit (BMT), which is a small, unique unit where a member of our service sees every patient and family for extended consultation as a matter of established protocol. This unit has a separate nursing staff, with only physicians at the rank of Fellow in Oncology caring for the patients, and with separate faculty attending physicians from the regular cancer center units. Thus, we actually consult to separate units with unique personnel, and each of these three units provide care for cancer patients with very different diagnoses and, hence, prognoses. For example, unlike the other two units, the BMT Unit treats only end-stage patients with leukemia or aplastic anemia.

Defining a family-based systems consultation in the cancer center must be done first in terms of who is the consultee. For purposes of medical–legal protection and hospital protocol, the formal consultee is always the treating physician, usually the intern or resident. However, in reality, the staff nurses often are far more perceptive and acute observers of family interactional difficulties, communication problems, or family pathology. We are the agents of the ward staff and not primarily agents of the family about whom we consult. Our working definition of the consultation is: the necessary intervention(s) needed to enable the patient and his or her family to deal with the phase of the illness or treatment in the most optimal way and in the most constructive interaction pattern with the ward staff.

Consultation–liasion is both diagnostic–therapeutic and instructional in function. Consultation is heavily oriented toward offering the staff a treatment plan to deal with the family and also to broaden the staff's understanding of (1) the stressor currently experienced by the family; (2) the family interaction pattern; (3) how and what the family is able to communicate, especially about the illness; and (4) how the staff affects the family. The staff's ability to hear meaningful discussion of item 4 is often our greatest problem. This type of consultation differs from a therapy contract in that (1) we routinely do not undertake a plan to effect broad changes in families; (2) it is usually limited to the hospital stay of the patient and often is for just one or two sessions; (3) it is often diagnostic or crisis-reducing, with the goal of effective containment of conflict, if possible, during the patient's hospital-

FIGURE 14-1. Consultation sites in UCLA Cancer Center.

SITE I	SITE II	SITE III
Surgical Oncology Inpatient Unit	Medical Oncology Inpatient Unit	Bone Marrow Transplantation Unit
Surgical Oncology Outpatient Unit	Medical Oncology Outpatient Unit	Bone Marrow Transplantation Alumni Group (Outpatient)

ization; and (4) extended family therapy, if needed, is arranged by referral to outside agencies or practitioners.

The role of the family-oriented systems consultant in the oncology setting is self-defined. There are advantages and disadvantages to being nonmedical practitioners. As nonphysicians we are less likely to become enmeshed in biologic ways of defining and solving problems. Our biopsychosocial framework enables us to place the physician's requests regarding a patient in a larger context—the family or the ward system. Our solutions create change of a more lasting nature than an antianxiety agent might (see the second case example). The disadvantages of being a nonphysician include the likelihood that physicians may initially perceive the psychologists as unable to understand "medical" problems and unable to offer quick, medical (e.g., pharmacologic) solutions. In fact, we, as psychologists, have become versed in medicine from exposure and reading and are able to "join" with the physicians. If pharmacologic interventions seem appropriate as part of the overall solution, the psychologist can swiftly ask the consultation psychiatrist for suggestions or else may confer with the appropriate physicians who can order tests and/or prescribe new medications.

The ward staff usually views our team (consisting of psychiatrists and psychologists based in the Department of Psychiatry and Biobehavioral Sciences) either as behavioral managers or pharmacologic consultants. The staff members call us most frequently when a patient has "hit the fan" and they wish us to calm him or her down quickly. The staff is highly task oriented and, naturally, expects the same from us. Our usual response is to combine family intervention with behavioral and/or pharmacologic recommendations. Quite often the ward staff, with the noteworthy exception of the BMT unit staff, do not see the family system implications that we see and choose to address. Two situations exemplify this point:

Two major losses: A case example. A 50-year-old man with metastatic melanoma was in the hospital for chemotherapy consolidation treatment. While this man was an inpatient, a private detective delivered a report to him that his wife was having an affair. The patient became severely agitated, stood by his fourth-floor window, and would not calm down. The oncology attending physician and house staff called our service to request the best medication to sedate the patient. We helped with the medication issue and then offered the staff and patient the option of marital evaluation to see if we could plan to prevent further episodes such as this one. Both patient and staff agreed. The evaluation was carefully undertaken over several weeks time, and it revealed a chronic, long-established cycle of mutual infidelity and, more important, a mutual emotional abandonment at critical times of need. The patient's wife acknowledged her wish not to support her husband in the upcoming course of his illness. The couple separated; the husband was offered individual, supportive therapy outside the hospital, which he accepted. He died reasonably peacefully several months later.

Silencing grief: A case example. A Mexican-American patient died of breast cancer on the surgical oncology service unit early one evening. Her family was present, and one sister began to wail in a high-pitched voice. The surgical oncology resident panicked, called our service to say that this sister was having a psychotic episode, and asked us to come at once. Upon arriving, the consultant was asked by the resident to arrange sedation of this woman. The consultant instead (1) assured the resident that this sister's behavior was culturally appropriate; (2) asked the resident to join him in meeting with the family; (3) assembled the family. The sister quieted immediately when the resident and consultant sat with the family. The sister was helped by the family to voice her concerns: Did her sister feel pain when she died? Who will care for the children? Some of these questions were answered by the resident; some were answered by the family as a group. Clearly, the resident had felt as much panic as the sister, and conducting a structured discussion helped the family to help the sister. We try not to sedate panic in house staff by giving medication to family members or patients.

Mental health professionals consulting to oncology services in the past have utilized a variety of approaches, usually not family oriented. For example, attempts have been made to use formal psychoanalysis with cancer patients in the hope of reversing unconscious conflicts that were theorized to have an impact on the course of the disease (Renneker, 1957). Interestingly, this individualized approach to the repressed conflicts of the cancer patient has been resurrected in the form of attempts to use mental imagery for remission of disease (Simonton, Matthews-Simonton, & Sparks, 1980). Behavior therapy to deconditioned learned responses to chemotherapy has been frequently utilized by consultants focusing on "targeted" symptoms in the patient (Redd, 1982). The biological–pharmacologic approach to cancer consultation has been extensively utilized because it is often most congruent with the medical mode of the wards where cancer patients are treated (Holland, 1973). Finally, the liaison model has at times been used in cancer programs, with the consultant dealing with the emotional stresses and concerns of the caregivers as a way of affecting the ward milieu (Klagsbrun, 1970).

Since 1974, when the UCLA Cancer Center was formally organized, we have attempted to combine several models of consultation. When conflict is evident, we take an overall systems approach, carefully evaluating the triadic structure of the patient–family–staff interaction. We often must include pharmacologic interventions and may choose to do straight liaison work with the staff. None of this, by definition, diminishes our basic commitment to the concept that effective coping with cancer is a family-based phenomenon. Our basic conceptual approach to family consultation on the unit is structural in nature, but is an abbreviation of the Minuchin model (1974). Sometimes we have been able to facilitate very rapid changes in the relationships of family members and open up previously closed territory when the family homeostasis is disturbed by the crisis of a cancer diagnosis, cancer recurrence, or death. The following was an example of this:

Leaving home, part two: A case example. A husband of a woman with hypernephroma presented with a near psychotic depression. He was jointly seen with his wife, the patient. The relationship was one of an overly maternal wife and an irresponsible, naughty son. Each held the other's role firmly in place. The knowledge of her impending death plus well-articulated, shortterm marital work enabled him to grow out of adolescent behavior and enabled her to stop reinforcing his naughty-boy behavior. When she stepped out of the maternal role, she began to grieve about her impending death and got support from the consultant for this. Also, the husband mirrored the consultant in providing her with support.

THE ENGAGEMENT PHASE

The official request for consultation to the medical and surgical wards and to the Bone Marrow Transplant Unit is made by the medical house staff, the Fellows (in oncology), or the attending physicians on the ward or unit. The responsibility lies primarily with the physician most closely associated with the case, usually the intern, who is also the least sophisticated person in the ward hierarchy with regard to knowing when a consultation is appropriate. Nurses cannot make a formal request for a consultation. But often the contact person, that is, the physician, is not the one who actually desires the consultation.

Among ward personnel, it is the nurses who spend the most time with patients and their families, and they may identify problems earlier than do the physicians who more narrowly delineate their treatment function as prescribing medication, diagnosing problems, and doing medical procedures. These tasks treat the patient's disease, not necessarily the patient. Although the nurses are in a position to recognize the need for a consultation, they have to relay their observations and informal requests to the primary physician, who may not have the time, energy, or inclination to follow through on any recommendation. It may happen that a resident or Fellow sees a problem but has difficulty convincing the attending physician of the need for a consultation. On the other hand, we have often observed attending physicians who recognized the need for a consulation even though their house staff minimized the serious nature of the problem.

Physician numbness: A case example. During morning rounds on medical oncology, an intern presented one of his patients—"a 15-year-old Hispanic male with acute myelogenous leukemia who lives with his mother. But there's no problem." The attending physician turned to him and said, "What do you mean this 15-year-old has no problem? Get the psych people in there." The intern had become numbed to this aspect of the tragedy; it was all too routinely a part of his day. From a greater distance, the attending physician could recognize the tragic and nonroutine nature of the illness for this adolescent and his mother.

The consultee, one of the ward physicians, may approach us to request assistance with several kinds of problems. On the BMT unit, a liaison consultation at the time of admission is a routine part of the total-care package. On the other units, requests are more episodic and include (1) behavior management issues, which often mean patient "noncompliance"; (2) family–staff conflicts in which the family battles a staff member or the staff as a unit over who will take care of the patient; and (3) interstaff issues that include doctor–nurse conflicts, low ward morale, depression and/or turnover among the nursing staff. The latter issues are often brought to us by one or more of the nurses, rather than by the physicians. Patient noncompliance is illustrated by the following case:

Taking the medicine: A case example. The medical oncologists became quite angry at Linda, a 15-year-old girl with acute myelogenous leukemia, who began getting oral candida infections because she refused to use the Nystatin lozenges prescribed for her. She further enraged the staff when they discovered that she was throwing away her other oral medications, including several chemotherapeutic agents and broad-spectrum antibiotics. We were called in to "make her take her medications, damn it!"

After interviewing the patient and her family, we learned that the family had begun to fall apart under the impact of this adolescent's illness. The father had begun to spend increasing amounts of time in the numerous bars near the hospital. His wife felt betrayed and abandoned by his unusual behavior and displaced her anger onto her daughter and, to a lesser extent, her two sons. In turn, they blamed their sister for uprooting them from friends, Little League games, and their local hangouts. It was Linda's conclusion that if she died, her family would no longer be so angry at her or so unhappy. Thus, she stopped taking her medications. As a result of several successive family interviews, sometimes including staff, we were able to restore the marital pair's functioning and, in turn, their ability to care for their daughter, who then began to "comply" with her doctor's orders and soon went into remission.

Staff versus family conflicts often result in the staff labeling the family a major nuisance and impediment to the delivery of good patient care. When we are asked to step in and mediate, we often find family members who perceive their spouse, sibling, or child as worsening under the staff's care. (In fact, chemotherapy, surgery, and the whole transplant procedure often make a sick patient sicker for quite some time.) In a panic, the family picks fights with nurses or challenges a doctor's procedures. The family's own brand of care has been invalidated by the onset of the disease, and the highly skilled care necessary to restore the patient to health is clearly beyond the family's ability. Or, staff members may decide that a family (all or part) is obnoxious and avoid him/her/them. Suddenly the staff is too busy charting or doing other tasks to help the family. This avoidance and anger is picked up by the family, which then feels alienated and more insecure. Our interventions have included helping the staff and family devise patient-care rituals that only the family can do, and that simultaneously relieve the staff of some of the more time-consuming, noncritical care. We also have sat down with the "pariah" family members and taught them how to "manage" staff members without alienating them.

Oncology and BMT units are all too often in a state of mourning for patients who have died. In such times of intense, draining emotionality, it is not uncommon for the nurses, who cannot rotate off service every six weeks as the house staff does, to bicker with each other, to call in sick for several days in a row, or simply to resign with a minimum of notice. During our weekly psychosocial rounds with the nursing staff, we attempt to monitor these events and to translate the anger into the underlying grief and depression. When the bickering spills over into nurse–doctor interactions, we try to assist the involved parties to air the details of the actual problem. When the ward is taxed by a heavy load of sick patients, all of whom require intensive nursing and medical care, physicians or nurses can feel that the other professional group is asking more of them than is possible, or is asking them to do things that properly belong to the other's domain. Boundaries need to be redrawn and roles need to be redefined, while the attention of both groups needs to be drawn to the fact that stress can obliterate the usually clear lines of task and role definition.

Every consultation is reviewed by at least one of us on the consultation team. Most requests are accepted. Those that we decline are handled by redefining the problem presented to us. For example, is an emergency consultation requested because of a staff member's emergency or a patient's?

In the former case we may not see the patient, but will speak with the staff person in crisis. If one has skillfully joined the organization, it is easier to decide which requests should be honored and which declined, and the staff members also make clearer requests of us. Staff members come to the consultant because, like a family, they have been struggling with an issue (be it patient, family, or other staff) for some time. In their attempts to cope, they have overfocused on the problem area and are using stereotyped responses (Minuchin & Fishman, 1981). Initially, the consultant gets into the same boat as the ward staff and then has to earn the right to be the temporary helmsman. As such, he or she has to accommodate, seduce, submit, support, direct, suggest, and follow in order to lead (Minuchin & Fishman, 1981).

Getting into the ward's boat means becoming a part of the crew on an ongoing basis, not just drawing alongside a sinking ship at the last moment and sailing away right after the rescue. Thus, our approach to joining the organization includes coming on working rounds with staff several times a week, routinely checking in with the clinical nurse-specialist and head nurse, and being visible and available to families at the weekly multifamily groups that meet on all units.

With input from us and the support of the nursing staff, weekly psychosocial rounds were initiated prior to the opening of the medical oncology unit. The main purpose of the rounds was and is to provide nurses and physicians with a forum in which to discuss along psychological dimensions their own needs, as well as those of their patients, in meeting the ongoing challenge of work on a cancer ward. Because of our individual and collective visibility and availability to staff and families, we have been accepted as regular members of the staff, although we are not located directly on the ward. Families perceive us as a useful support system rather than as the infamous "men in white coats." It is also helpful that several of us have continued to consult to these services since their inception almost 10 years ago. We are perceived as seasoned veterans who "know the score." This experience with some staff members, and with the units, create powerful linkages. Only because of such joining can one help to restructure a troubled family, be it a patient and immediate family, or the larger family of the ward staff.

ASSESSMENT OF THE SYSTEM

The official unit of consultation is that of the ward (medical and surgical oncology) or unit (BMT). In actuality, the consultation unit might consist of any of the following dyads or triads: patient–house staff; patient–staff; patient–nurse; attending physician–patient; patient–family–staff; or any permutations thereof. Furthermore, the nature of the dyadic or triadic interaction is dependent upon the ever-changing cast of characters in those roles: the nurse assigned to each patient; the house staff during the 6-week period; the attending physician; and the families.

Behind the presenting request there is usually another implicit request. One must differentiate between the "presenting" problem and the "real" problem. Again, one must ask who the "real" consultee is not only who the official one is. In order to ascertain what the request is, one must have a sense of the subcurrent themes on the ward (Newton & Levinson, 1973). These themes are defined as ways in which enduring and recurrent concerns are expressed, directly and indirectly, in the ongoing life of the group-treatment team (Newton & Levinson, 1973). These authors' formulation of a theme elucidates both the manifest concerns that arise as the group sets about its work, and the preconscious or unconscious imagery, fantasies, and feelings associated with them. They arise repeatedly in the course of the group's life and are observable to outsiders. But if group members cannot see these problems because they are so enmeshed in group process, the themes can become woven into the fabric of group life to the extent that they are taken for granted. The need to decode the request behind the request is especially important in those frequent requests to assist the house staff in having a patient "comply" with his or her prescribed treatment. The treatment may involve being subjected to painful procedures that are somewhat experimental in nature because this is a research setting. The patient may refuse to cooperate at some point, saying that he or she is tired of being a "guinea pig." Here, the presenting problem is the patient's refusal of a procedure, which is interpreted by the staff as jeopardizing the management of his or her case. Because we have worked in this clinical and research setting, we know from experience that one of the dominant themes is a mixed message: "Research comes first, but so does clinical care." The first underlying problem is that the patient is interfering with the orderly progress of a research project, and the principal investigator is going to be unhappy. The second underlying problem is that ward personnel are not going to be happy if they cannot deliver good clinical care.

The request behind the request is also affected by issues of structure and role. Structure and role interact because the role of the nurse may be to tend to the patient as a whole. If the structure of the ward is such that six seriously ill patients are assigned to one nurse, he or she will not be able to respond adequately to these emotionally needy, frightened people. Hence, those patients and families are labeled as "troublesome" when they make even small demands for attention from staff members who already feel overwhelmed. The explicit request to us is to "manage" the patient, but the implicit request is to relieve an overwhelmed nurse.

A request does not emanate from an amorphous setting; it emerges from a work group, in this case the ward team of physicians and nurses who carry out one or more organizational tasks, including clinical care, research, and teaching. The work group must be examined from the perspective of its social structure (Newton & Levinson, 1973), particularly the division of labor and the division of authority. Division of labor refers to the fact that different members carry out different parts of the total work of the group. There are formal positions that help differentiate one part of the task from others (attending physician, head nurse, intern) and informal, implicitly defined positions that emerge, for example, Nurse X is "really" in charge. There is a division of authority to the extent that the legitimate power and responsibility to make decisions are distributed unequally within the group (Newton & Levinson, 1973). The social structure and hierarchy of the work group tend to reflect that of the organization. Thus, in the ward hierarchy, doctors are at the top and nurses are at the bottom.

In our work on the unit, we examine the network of relationships between physicians and nurses, and between the treatment team and the patients and families. To understand the hierarchy, we must know who is the attending physician for the month. This helps to define what is said by whom about tasks on the ward. Our boundary issues consist of:

1. What can we say about how the staff is delivering treatment to the patients? Do we merely prescribe a behavioral intervention and/or psychotropic medications for a patient, or can we point out that the patient's distress is intimately linked to the fact that the staff is overworked right now and less tolerant of "deviance" in patients?
2. Can we assume the authority to call a staff conference about a patient or must the doctor on the case do it? It is clear to us that the social structure of the surgical ward is much more formal than that of the medical oncology ward and the BMT unit. We have learned this by observing the strict division of labor and the authoritarian division of authority. We cannot call a conference about a family on surgery (only the surgeons can), and dealing with patient–family issues is not perceived as an appropriate task. The boundaries regarding task division are more blurred on medical oncology. We do treat patients, but we are also implicitly invited to comment upon staff–patient interaction. There is more latitude in our task definition there.

Examining the division of authority on the wards alerts us to who is really in charge, that is, who actually wields power. We observe who makes the requests of us and who then carries out our recommendations. If our recommendations are dismissed or invalidated, that also indicates who holds the real power. Observing who supports us, as contrasted with who opposes us, can alert us to coalitions and triangles within the setting. In a patient–staff conflict, one can observe who lines up on which side. The power that the contact person, the physician, has to implement change depends on that person's formal and informal power. If such persons are high in the social structure and effective in the organization, and if they are in the organization to stay, as opposed to rotating off, chances are high that their power is considerable and change will be implemented.

Our consultee system has a culture, by which we mean there is a relatively enduring pattern of core values, assumptions, and beliefs that provide a framework for group development and action (Newton & Levinson, 1973). Thus, our culture is embedded in the larger culture of the hospital that, in turn, is part of the medical system and the context of the treatment of cancer. Within this culture are certain important rules and myths that we have learned about by listening to the metaphorical language of the ward, by observing which people are accorded status and respect and which are not, and by observing how we are given time or are interrupted with our consultees, whether with doctors, patients, nurses, or families. The belief systems are slightly different on the surgical oncology side of the corridor and on the medical oncology side; both are different from that of the BMT unit.

As with other groups who are caught up with issues of life and death (e.g., the military), the language and behavior of staff on cancer units metaphorically express and caricature emotionally charged, functionally understandable points of view.

On surgery, the doctor is always right; if he or she is wrong, no one talks about it. Similarly in surgery, the surgeons almost always "get the cancer out," whereas their brethren on medical oncology are not so assured. "People don't die" on the surgical oncology ward. They do on medical oncology. This reinforces the implicit belief of some surgeons that only by cutting out a tumor can one really cure a person. Because of the disfiguring effect of some surgeries, some medical oncologists view their surgical colleagues as carrying out cruel and unusual punishment on some patients. Chemotherapy is seen as more effective and less detrimental, although privately the doctors and nurses will refer to their armamentarium as including various poisons, for example, "Red Death" (Adriamycin). All of the units mentioned here call their patients "players" and patient data are carried around in doctor's pockets as the equivalent of baseball trading cards. The players are participants in what appear to be war games, an idea that perhaps derives from a national consciousness of there being a "war on cancer." One "blasts out" tumors that have "invaded" lymph nodes and tissues. On the BMT unit, the belief exists that a transplant is in a patient's best interest, but clinical care and research vie with one another for the right to define that interest. It is not always clear when patients are kept on a research protocol in order to produce data and when they are removed because it is no longer working in their best interest.

IMPLEMENTATION OF CHANGE

The contract we make with the consultee varies greatly with the nature of the presenting problems and the request. What we actually decide to do with a family and how often depends upon the nature of the problem. Sometimes we make a contract for crisis intervention with no plan for follow-up or lengthy intervention. At other times, it is clear that we must see this family for the duration of the present hospitalization, between hospitalizations, and during future hospitalizations. This decision is largely based on the assessment of the family in terms of (1) intensity of problems prior to the cancer diagnosis; (2) presence of current conflict; (3) interference with treatment objectives due to family conflict; and (4) diminution of quality of life due to family conflict. Two separate examples serve to illustrate our divergence of approach and differential contracting with families:

Informing family: A case example. A 44-year-old woman dying of malignant melanoma had been married only 4 years prior to the diagnosis. In the hospital she developed a psychotic reaction that appeared to be a hysterical psychosis. Phenothiazines were tried but there was little improvement.

In our interview with the patient, we discovered the following facts. She had lived with her elderly, Jewish parents in a small Texas town until she was in her late 30s, whereupon she left, came to Los Angeles, and met and married her current husband. Although she had been ill with melanoma for about 2 years, not only did her parents not know she was dying, they also did not know she had melanoma.

We decided that our intervention with this family would be circumscribed yet definitive. With this patient's permission we did the following in this order: (1) we contacted a family therapist where the parents lived in Texas; (2) we contacted the rabbi in the parents' temple; (3) we arranged for the rabbi and family therapist to meet with the parents, tell the parents what was happening to their daughter, and arrange for them to come immediately to Los Angeles; (4) we met with the parents and patient jointly when the parents arrived on the ward 2 days later, also utilizing the services of the campus rabbi who participated in the family session. The patient's psychotic reaction cleared almost instantaneously when the parents arrived and when she saw that they knew and could bear the reality of her condition. We did not again intervene with the family. The patient was calm when she died approximately 1 week later.

A demanding case: A case example. A 49-year-old woman with metastatic breast cancer was presented by her harassed medical oncologist for treatment of her extreme nervousness and agitated demandingness. Her daily calls to him for "information" were thinly veiled pleas for emotional help. The patient was asked to bring her husband to the sessions, which she did each time.

It was evident from the onset of the consultations that this couple was locked into an "intruder-rejector" pattern previously described by Napier (1978) as a chronic, marital dysfunctional style. This pattern predated the cancer diagnosis but had grown worse during the patient's illness and decline. Her demands for caretaking by her husband and two daughters were limitless. She would never permit herself to be left alone in her bedroom, but would torture her caretakers in a frigid room where the air conditioner was kept going full blast. The husband responded by getting two jobs, which effectively kept him out of the house 16–20 hours per day in order "to be able to pay for all of this." The daughters and the patient's mother became caretakers for her endless needs. It emerged in treatment that the husband had fathered a child with another woman during this marriage, thus confirming the patient's worst fears. Space does not permit a full description of the treatment, but the contract with the oncologist and this family extended from the time of referral to the patient's death a year later, and beyond into bereavement work with the family.

Several shared goals exist between us and the ward staff, some explicit, some implicit. On the explicit level, one of the three general goals are usually on everyone's mind when we are asked to consult with a family in the Cancer Center. These are (1) solving the presenting problem *if*, after evaluation, we feel it is a problem and we can do something about it; (2) restoring order, which usually means attempting to patch up a rupture in the staff–family relationship; and (3) facilitating family-based decision making about treatment. Often, there is an impasse about going on with treatment. We will be called to facilitate functional staff–patient–family communication and patient–family interaction around such circumstances. This can help to dissolve the impasse and bring about the necessary family-based resolution either to stop or go on with treatment.

Opting out: A case example. A very attractive, athletic 18-year-old male was diagnosed with acute myelogenous leukemia. He could not be put into remission with chemotherapy, hated the confinement of the hospital, and accepted the reality (including likelihood of death) of his disease with surprising dignity and equanimity. He was offered admission to the Bone Marrow Transplantation Unit and given the four-page, informed consent form with all of its rigors pointed out. He decided to opt out of the BMT and go home. His family was horrified at his decision while at the same time realizing the BMT was no panacea. We facilitated a vigorous family–

patient discussion, with the family hearing the patient's real inability to tolerate the hospital. He did not return to the hospital and died at home.

Implicit shared goals between us and the staff break down into two areas. First, when asking us to help a family with a specific problem, the staff always hopes implicitly that we can enable the family to live more effectively with the stresses of the cancer. Second, the staff members want to help with their own feelings in dealing with the patient and family. They know they can and often do get lost in their own countertransference with families and need help for their inability to "see the forest for the trees." The following is a good example.

A deadly disease: A case example. A nurse fell into an intense and confusing relationship with a dying, 55-year-old leukemic woman and her husband. This patient was initially the focus of great curiosity and concern by the staff. Early in her hospital stay, while she had multiple IVs in each arm, she was found in her room with a screwdriver, having taken the cover off her air conditioner. Her explanation was that she needed to check the filter of the air conditioner to see if it was clean enough for her. Our team did not feel she was mentally ill but rather that she was frightened of the loss of control her illness imposed upon her. This was her unique way of regaining control. In addition, she told us from her first day on the ward that she would never allow her disease to take her life and that she already had pills saved at home in case the need arose. Her husband was not frightened or upset by her statements or behaviors. Rather, he seemed accepting of them as part of her need for control. This obviously was an aspect of her with which he had been quite familiar in the course of their marriage. The nurse's ultimate difficulty arose when this couple asked her for more exact information on how the patient could commit suicide. She found herself beginning to tell them without thinking of the potential consequences for herself or them.

Two steps were taken by our team in consulting with this nurse and the couple around the suicide issue. First, we attempt to help the nurse examine her feelings and her relationship with this couple. She was able to see that her connection to this couple revolved around her perceiving them as approving parents for her; her own mother had not been approving. Second, we asked for and received support and intervention from a senior faculty member from our department who is a world authority on suicide. We did this for several reasons. One was that we genuinely needed his input on how to handle the issue of suicide with this couple. Another was that we saw that this nurse and our own team had slipped into a transference–countertransference mode of being "perfect children" and the couple being accepting, grateful parents. We believed we needed the authority and seniority of the faculty member to reestablish a functional perspective and professional position vis-à-vis this couple. The senior consultant did lend perspective. He enabled the patient to think of ways of being in control at home while she was dying; he also cautioned the nurse and our team of the potential for disaster in aiding suicide, especially with regard to guilty and ambivalent surviving family members possibly instituting legal action against staff members. The patient, in fact, did not take her own life, but did die in the comfort of her own home.

Goals that are not shared with the consultee can include facilitating a change in doctors or a change from the university hospital to the private sector for the patient and family. These changes are rare but have been known to happen when the patient and family were being hampered by the rotation of physicians in the university hospital setting and obviously needed one case-manager physician to provide emotional stability. Another implicit goal is to help the family understand and accept the behavior and feelings of the physicians, which at times may be confusing, provocative, and counterproductive. This obviously would be important to share with the physician in question but at times cannot be done, especially if the physician is a senior faculty member.

The issue of our being "go-betweens" for the staff and patient–family bears directly upon transmission of information. Our role is never to be the primary transmitters of medical information; this is as true for the psychiatrist members of our consultant team as for the psychologists. To do so might result in being co-opted by the medical team in an inappropriate attempt to reduce their anxiety about their role as medical information givers. Our job is to help the patient and family cope and deal with the emotional impact of the medical information they have received. Conversely, we often struggle with how much of what we learn in our consultations with families legitimately should be shared with the medical and nursing staffs and how much should not be discussed or, as important, should not be written in the patient's medical record. There is no clear-cut solution to this problem. Our general stance is to relate and write in the chart those family issues that directly bear upon the patient's current hospital course or discharge planning. Thus, we do not feel bound to relate all the family secrets but do feel it necessary to relate serious covert conflicts that may interfere with the family being able to cope emotionally with a dying family member at home. At times we have recommended that the patient beset with family conflicts be discharged to a local hospital or hospice for terminal care rather than be sent home. It is often our experience that the family feels relieved rather than undercut in such a situation.

Our general method of intervention is structural in nature but also oriented toward crisis intervention. Both approaches are important because we must attempt to obtain rapid change and rapid resolution of symptomatic problems. We move into engagement with a family that is paralyzed with anxiety or fear and must facilitate change in several areas. We work to enable them to talk to one another about the illness, to make decisions that cannot be avoided in regard to cancer treatment, and to feel comfortable and effective in their ability to handle the patient at home. Crisis intervention sometimes becomes important, as in the previously mentioned case where the patient's parents were brought from Texas. Here, family supports were mobilized and the family members were given structure that enabled them to work through a specific impasse. Very often crises in Cancer Center families parellel developments in the disease, for example, during diagnosis, recurrence, or the realization that treatment is over. All of these developments call for decision making that becomes a crisis if the family cannot interact enough to make decisions. Sometimes our structural and crisis intervention work flows together, as in a situation where an adult child and a cancer patient parent must change roles for the first time, with devastating effects on both. Here, we sometimes need to facilitate the *reverse* of what Minuchin (1974) has described, with the child in the executive position, the parent in the child position, and a clear boundary between.

Resistance is an interesting, though relatively rare, phenomenon in work with Cancer Center families. In general, resistance is more common in work with families in which cancer is not the main issue. Cancer Center families can often be so frightened and in need of a direction that they will do anything that is suggested and, indeed, become overdependent. At times, however, spectacular resistance crops up and defies our best efforts. This is generally present where severe family problems predated the cancer. The following case example highlights the problem of resistance:

Gourmet meals and misbehavior: A case example. A 16-year-old boy with aplastic anemia presented severe behavior problems on the BMT unit. He had been manageable until the parents stopped coming to the hospital. They stopped coming for two reasons. First, they had seemed able to visit when they thought he would die; they stopped coming when it was apparent that he would leave the hospital and live for a time. Second, the BMT unit serves gourmet meals to its patients. This boy could not eat them, but his parents, both morbidly obese, ate them nightly. When the nurses canceled these meals, the parents stopped visiting. The father was noted by one appalled nurse to have stated, upon observing his son acting out: "I'd like to beat the shit out of you, but your platelet count is too low." We realized that successful efforts to change this family interaction in a fundamental way had a low to zero probability. Therefore, we elected to take a very task-oriented, educative approach. We tried to equip the parents to deal with their son medically and situationally at home, potentially reducing one aspect of their resistance and anxiety about him. He, in turn reduced his complete noncompliance with treatment, was able to go home, and died a few months later in a community hospital.

Probably the most common resistances we see in families involve those regarding talking about cancer directly with the patient or with younger children of the patient. We are straightforward in our dealing with this, sitting down with the patient and family and modeling how to talk with one another directly. It is never helpful for us to tell the family to do this; we must do it with them.

Insuring the durability of change can be done in two ways. One way is to follow up the family after discharge from the hospital. Another is to serve as a liaison with the staff members and work through them. This can be done with team conferences and with meticulous notes in the patient's chart about what we believe is going on and needs to be done with the family. The staff is eager for information about the families and will often reinforce the changes and new patterns once they are begun by us.

TERMINATION OF CONSULTATION

The decision to terminate a consultation depends on several factors. If the contract has been fulfilled to all parties' mutual satisfaction (including the patient and family), the consultation is over. If the problem is not being resolved to the satisfaction of the official consultee, the physician, then a consultation may be terminated on a one-sided basis, leaving the possibility of our being called upon in the future. Here the decision can be taken out of our hands because the patient becomes more upset, firmly refuses all treatment, or becomes quite intransigent vis-à-vis his or her treatment team. It is also possible that we can be fired by the patient, who may see us for one visit to placate the physician but will not go beyond this, or by family members who dislike the results of our restructuring their interactions even though the patient may have become more individuated and effective. The cancer itself may fire us; a patient suddenly may go "sour" and be too ill to see us, or die.

The process of termination is accomplished by various procedures and rituals. There are formal good-byes to patients if all went well, and even if it did not (i.e., we were fired). We bring the staff members up to date on what we did and invite them to call upon us next time (if all went well). If it did not, we try our best to have them tell us what went wrong and why they decided to take us off the case. When we are fired, we sometimes learn more about the culture, social structure, and social process of our client ward than when we are successful. For example, did we help the depressed, passive patient become too assertive so that he or she challenged the physicians about too many professionally sensitive aspects of care? This may have upset the hierarchy of the ward—patients have the least authority, doctors have the most. Termination may result when the patient is medically improved even though our interventions are incomplete when the patient is discharged. Death may also terminate our involvement on a case, and then the ritual may include attending the patient's funeral or in some more informal way acknowledging our loss.

EVALUATION OF CONSULTATION PROCESS AND ITS OUTCOME

We tend to assess the consultation in terms of its impact on the family unit. We want to enhance the family's ability to communicate and to plan in regard to the illness and to reduce the patient's depression and/or anxiety. These changes cannot be facilitated, in our experience, without intervention into the patient's family.

Consultees tend to assess the usefulness of the consultation quite differently. They are much more patient oriented and work directly in the context of the medical/biological model. They tend to note only whether the patient is less symptomatic or less of a treatment and management problem. They are vaguely aware that the family is somehow changed, but tend either to minimize or ignore the importance of this or its impact on the patient's changes. Our conclusions and comparisons, therefore, can differ greatly from those of the staff in regard to what has happened and why.

We have very definite and profound limitations and constraints on what we can do. Sometimes the staff reacts with acute discomfort to what are obviously lifelong family interactions such as infantalizing symbiotic ties between family members. We caution the staff about the realistic possibility of our changing such interaction. As alluded to earlier, we can be constrained by the attitude of an omnipotent senior physician or nurse who is making things harder and is simply not available for feedback. A classic example of this follows:

Refusing to consult: A case example. A 45-year-old man was dying of acute myelogenous leukemia. He had a wife and two children. The nurses observed that his wife was "falling apart" and believed that the couple was not talking at all about the children or about their own feelings. They pressed the man's physician, a very senior faculty member, to write an order for psychological consultation, especially for the patient's wife. The physician balked. Finally the physician and consultant talked by phone about the physician's hesitation. The physician asked the consultant: "Why should his wife feel so bad about his dying? What's so bad about dying? I wish I were dead half the time myself."

Family-based consultation to cancer patients and their families can have very gratifying unexpected benefits and opportunities. The crisis of cancer is a severe destabilizer of family homeostasis and equilibrium. It is just the emotional TNT needed to blast many families loose enough to interact differently. It is very easy to get them to see that time is running out and to seize the opportunity to interact, take risks, reach out, and express previously withheld feelings, both positive and negative. A lot can happen in a short time. The silver lining in the dark cloud can be rapid change, mobilization of support, and much more positive bonding in families than was previously present. This, needless to say, can be gratifying for the family therapist consultant.

SUMMARY

We recommend the following for family therapists attempting to consult with families of cancer patients:

1. Do not assume that the work will be only morbid or depressing.
2. Expect the possibility of real change in many situations.
3. Do not assume that the staff or treating physician is sufficiently aware of the family issues to tell you what is going on.
4. Expect that the course and events of the illness will significantly control the family emotions and interactions.
5. Engage the staff members directly in the family work because they often value dircction and role modeling on how to proceed with families.
6. Do not accept family resistance to talking about the cancer directly with the patient. Once this resistance is overcome, anxiety in all family members is usually much reduced.
7. Do not minimize or ignore the impact of cancer and patient death on the staff, which often becomes "part of the family" and needs support and attention as much as the actual family.

REFERENCES

American Cancer Society, Inc. *Facts and figures*. New York: Author, 1983.

Holland, J. C. B. Psychologic aspects of cancer. In J. F. Holland & E. Frei (Eds.), *Cancer medicine*. Philadelphia: Lea & Febiger, 1973.

Klagsbrun, S. C. Cancer, emotions, and nurses. *American Journal of Psychiatry*, 1970, *126*, 1237–1244.

Minuchin, S. *Families and family therapy*. Cambridge, MA: Harvard University Press, 1974.

Minuchin, S., & Fishman, H. C. *Family therapy techniques*. Cambridge, MA: Harvard University Press, 1981.

Napier, A. Y. The rejection–intrusion pattern: A central family dynamic. *Journal of Marriage & Family Counseling,* 1978, *4,* 5–12.

Newton, P., & Levinson, D. The work group within the organization: A socio-psychological approach. *Psychiatry,* 1973, *36,* 115–140.

Redd, W. H. Behavior analysis and control of psychosomatic symptoms of patients receiving intensive cancer treatment. *British Journal of Clinical Psychology,* 1982, *21,* 351–358.

Renneker, R. Countertransference reactions to cancer. *Psychosomatic Medicine,* 1957, *19,* 409–418.

Simonton, O. C., Matthews-Simonton, S., & Sparks, T. F. Psychological intervention in the treatment of cancer. *Psychosomatics,* 1980, *21,* 226–233.

15

FAMILY-ORIENTED CONSULTATION IN PEDIATRICS

STEPHEN MUNSON
University of Rochester School of Medicine and Dentistry
Rochester, New York

Pediatrics is a medical specialty that increasingly is becoming concerned with a focus of health care broader than individual children and their physical illnesses. Green and Haggerty (1977) summarized the scope of child health care by describing three constituencies of child health services: children, their families, and the larger community. In particular, they described pediatrics as "inherently a family focused specialty." The pediatrician's concern for the child's welfare is expanding to include behavioral and psychological aspects of development in addition to those biomedical physical problems that have been the traditional focus. Many pediatricians set aside several hours of their weekly schedule to meet with patients and their families and to discuss issues of psychological and physical development. In addition, many group practices employ mental health professionals to assist in diagnosis and treatment of patients.

The pediatrician is in a uniquely advantageous position to detect emotional difficulties in children because of the longitudinal nature of the relationship with his or her patients. When that relationship is positive, the pediatrician is also a professional to whom families turn for advice about other problems.

As pediatricians increase their sophistication about children's emotional needs and appreciate the relation of these needs to the family context, they turn to mental health specialists with increasingly sophisticated questions. In answering these questions, the family therapist offers a point of view that is well matched with the evolving philosophy and practice of pediatrics. However, the needs of the pediatric patient are often unique and require the family therapist to expand in point of view to encompass elements of the patient's context that are beyond his or her usual concern.

These unusual elements include the effects of physical illness on individual children, the challenges that hospitalization presents to children and their families, and the transactions between medical professionals and the family in both inpatient and ambulatory settings.

CONSULTATIVE TASKS IN PEDIATRICS

PRELIMINARY TASKS OF THE CONSULTANT

In answering a request for a family-oriented consultation in pediatrics, the consultant faces a number of potential tasks. First, he or she must understand and clarify the questions of the consultee. To do so, the consultant should be familiar with the nature of pediatric medical practice as well as the more specific approaches used by the consultee/pediatrician in solving problems. Almost always, direct communication between the consultant and the pediatrician is necessary.

In some cases, the consultation has originated with a request from someone other than the child's pediatrician. As part of clarifying the questions to be answered, the consultant should identify the person or persons who have asked the questions, and should understand the relationship between the consultee and the rest of the child's caretaking system. Furthermore, it is very important for the consultant to consider the consultation question in relation to the specific medical context of the index child. The consultant must question the pediatrician about the nature of the child's illness and the possible ramifications of this illness for the child's mental status. It cannot be assumed that the pediatrician has already clarified this question. The consultant and the pediatrician must agree whether it will be the consultant's task to answer this important question, or if the pediatrician will answer it. If the index child is hospitalized, a careful review of his or her chart will help the consultant to assess the nature of the medical problem.

Second, the family-oriented consultant may be asked to provide services at many points in the pediatrician's decision-making process. In some cases, the pediatricians are uncertain of their diagnosis and are asking, "Is there a psychological problem here that is influencing the diagnostic picture?" In other situations, pediatricians feel secure with the diagnosis and are asking the consultant to corroborate their impressions and elaborate on the nature of the existing psychological problems. In still other cases, pediatricians may have evaluated the child and begun a program of psychological treatment; they may then ask the mental health consultant to assess their therapeutic work with the family and make suggestions about further therapeutic interventions.

With each kind of request, a dialogue between the consultant and the primary medical caretaker creates an opportunity for clarifying the services that the consultant will offer. Often the harried pediatrician wants and expects the consultant not only to answer diagnostic questions and make suggestions for treatment and disposition, but also to take responsibility for arranging and providing a component of the treatment. While it is often not possible to predict in advance how far along the road from assessment and diagnosis to treatment and disposition the consultant will travel, it is important that the boundaries of the consultant's role be specified from the beginning as part of an ongoing process of negotiation that will be useful throughout the consultation. The pediatrician and consultant should agree on how the consultation will be presented to the index child and the family. The family may be confused about the reasons for the consultation. This confusion can be reduced if the pediatrician carefully orients the family to the consultation and if the consultant is in agreement with the pediatrician about the reasons for the child being seen.

The pediatrician and the consultant should also agree in advance about which members of the child's family will be included in the evaluation. While many pediatricians are very concerned about family relationships and their impact on the child, few have direct experience with conjoint family meetings. The consultant should therefore be explicit about who should expect to be included in evaluation sessions and why their presence is important.

Before beginning the consultation, the consultant should also consider those elements in the child's life outside the nuclear family that may be influencing the clinical picture. A child hospitalized for treatment of a medical illness enters a complex community of medical professionals with whom he or she begins to have important relationships. The hospitalization alters not only existing relationships with schoolmates, but also the relationship with the extended family and even the primary physician. In order to provide the most accurate assessment of the child's problems, the consultant must identify those aspects of the various interlocking systems of the context that are dysfunctional. Almost always, there is dysfunction at more than one point, and a systematic evaluation of each element of the child's context is necessary.

MEETING THE FAMILY

Once the family-oriented consultant has accomplished these preliminary tasks, arrangements to meet the family must be made. It is important for the consultant to make these arrangements directly with apropriate family members. Arrangements made through the pediatrician's secretary or through the index patient are often misunderstood, resulting in missed appointments and absent family members.

The approach the consultant uses with each family should be attuned to the specific questions raised for that consultation. If the consultant has been asked to assist in diagnosis, the approach will be gently exploratory, summarized by the proposal: "Let's look together for possible problems and concerns." Here the consultant's role is to help the family and the pediatrician develop hypotheses about family responses to and influences upon the index child's illness. While many families will engage willingly in this exploration, others will resist. The consultant's role when families reject a psychological approach to understanding the child's situation is one of support and acceptance of the resistance, as long as ambiguity about the basis of their concerns remains unresolved.

On the other hand, if the referral for family consultation has been made after the existence of psychological problems has already been recognized, then the consultant's goal is to explore the nature of these problems: "There are problems in this child's situation which seem to affect the illness. What do you think they are?" Again, some families eagerly engage in this exploration, and others resist. Certain families conspire to present a healthy appearance to the mental health consultant, defying him or her to discover an emotional problem. They defend against their anxiety by continuing to focus on the child's medical problems, and to insist that another medical test will uncover the "real" problem.

If this form of resistance to psychological exploration occurs, the family therapist should not challenge their defenses by attempting to coerce them into seeing their difficulties. Rather, the consultant should insist on helping the family explore their medical concerns further with the pediatrician. A joint meeting of the family, pediatrician, and therapist is usually helpful in this situation.

In this meeting, the role of the pediatrician is to reinforce his or her earlier recommendation for psychological inquiry by further explanation and review of all medical evidence that previously has been collected. The family consultant's role is to encourage the family members to ask more questions of the pediatrician and to help them to be more articulate about their concerns.

At the conclusion of this meeting, the decision must be made whether to continue with more medical evaluation or to return to the difficult work of the psychological evaluation of the child in his or her family. For some families, even diagnostic exploration is anxiety provoking, and the presence of the pediatrician is necessary throughout the consultation as a means of maintaining the family's focus on the task.

THE CONSULTANT AS EDUCATOR

A central component of the consultation is the difference in viewpoint brought to the clinical problem by the consultant. While such a difference in perspective is essential to the process, it may also hinder it. If the consultant's observations and recommendations make no sense to the family or pediatrician, then there is little likelihood that the family will make any progress toward a creative solution to its problems. The consultant should make every effort to explain his or her findings in terms familiar to all participants. However, it is usually necessary to help the family, and often the pediatrician, to see the problem in a new way before they can accept the consultant's observations and recommendations.

Thus, an essential role of the consultant is one of education. The education process may include approaches that are common in family therapy, such as broadening the family's understanding of the factors influencing the identified patient's behavior, discovering other sources of distress in the system, and labeling the sequences of transactions that complicate conflict resolution. In all circumstances, the consultant must take special care to orient the family about the relevance of these observations to the specific questions under consideration. If the consultant is successful in the education of the child, the family, and the pediatrician who requested the consultation, then the transition from evaluation to appropriate intervention will be a smooth one.

THE CONSULTANT AS FACILITATOR

An integral part of the consultation process is the facilitation of the family's transition from evaluation to treatment. Most families are confused by the array of therapeutic alternatives and need help in assessing which professionals and which settings will be most appropriate.

Seeking the family's permission to share clinical information with the professionals responsible for treatment will emphasize continuity between the consultation and therapy. The consultant should take the initiative in contacting the agency or individual who will be accepting the family for more intensive evaluation and therapy in order to help that agency avoid unnecessary redundancy in the beginning of work with the family.

SPECIAL ISSUES WITH HOSPITALIZED CHILDREN

A substantial number of consultations are requested while children and adolescents are in the hospital. In part, this is because of the intensity of the medical problems that have necessitated hospitalization. In addition, the context of the hospital provides additional points of stress and possible conflict for the child and family and these may be expressed through symptomatic behavior. When responding to consultation requests about hospitalized children, the family-oriented consultant must be very careful to consider each of the interlocking subsystems of the hospitalized child's context as a possible source of difficulty.

THE PROBLEMS AND EXPERIENCE OF THE HOSPITALIZED CHILD

Before requesting consultation, the pediatrician most often has noticed disturbing behavior in the child patient. Therefore, it is logical for the consultant to begin the inquiry about those aspects of the child's emotional difficulties that are a function of direct physiological effects of the illness on the child's central nervous system. There are also psychological effects of many treatment regimens as exemplified by the effects of high doses of the steroids used in treatment of inflammatory illnesses.

An obvious example is the experience of the child who sustains head injury in a motor vehicle accident and subsequently develops delirium. The resulting confusion, agitation, and emotional disinhibition are always alarming to family members and often become a management problem for the ward staff. Thus, the consultant must look for and recognize the signs and symptoms of nervous system dysfunction before providing suggestions for appropriate management.

An understanding of the child's feelings and thoughts about illness and hospitalization is essential for the consultant. The daily routine of hospital care involves multiple and often painful medical procedures that are frightening and difficult for the child to understand. While it is natural for hospitalized children to feel annoyed and frustrated, it is difficult for them to express these feelings directly to physicians and nurses who appear so powerfully in control in the hospital setting.

Many children displace their anger onto those who are more familiar and less dangerous. The loving parent who becomes the object of this frustration may not understand or appreciate this fact. In attempting to help the parent deal with the child's reaction in this situation, it is important for the consultant to be aware of the realities of the medical regimen as well as the child's experience of it.

The consultant must also be aware of the history of the child's illness prior to the current hospitalization. The return to the hospital may rekindle anxiety and sadness that were associated with earlier hospitalizations, but defended against successfully during illness-free periods in the child's life. Similarly, children sometimes feel a sense of defeat and failure when hospitalized for an acute episode in a chronic illness. They may become depressed when they realize that the illness has not been cured. Rehospitalization may bring awareness that the illness is chronic and likely to be fatal. In many instances, their thoughts and feelings are expressed indirectly through withdrawal or aggressive, uncooperative behavior. Questioning of the parents and staff about how the child is viewing this illness and hospitalization as well as direct discussion with the child will provide useful insight into this important aspect of the child's emotional experience.

THE FAMILY OF THE HOSPITALIZED CHILD

In the early and middle portions of this century, in Western cultures, children who were hospitalized were kept in isolation from their families. As a result of the important investigations of Spitz (1946, 1950), Bowlby (1973), the Robertsons (1953, 1971) and others (Fagin, 1966; MacCarthy, Lindsay, & Morris, 1962), the 1950s and 1960s produced a dramatic change in the involvement of families with their ill children in the hospital. It is now commonplace for a member of a young child's family to stay with the child nearly continuously during the hospitalization.

This more extensive involvement of the family in the child's medical and psychological care has proved extremely beneficial for the child. However, it also results in dramatic change in the family's ecology, and challenges the family's traditional homeostatic patterns. At the most obvious level, there is a strain on the family's financial resources. Beyond the medical expenses are transportation, motel, and food expenses, as well as babysitting costs for the children who remain at home. In an era when many couples share the responsibility for financial support, parents are faced with the choice of reducing their income or leaving the child in the hospital without adequate family support. Even routine, simple tasks, such as meal preparation and laundry, may become disrupted.

The combination of anxiety about the child's illness and the stress of adapting to the practical difficulties presented by the hospitalization leaves little time for parents to experience intimacy with one another. Thus, the child's hospitalization becomes a time of increased stress on the marital relationship and decreased mutual support between the parents. For those parents with strong and flexible relationships, this temporary loss of pleasure and solace becomes an unfortunate but surmountable problem, the resolution of which may increase the strength of the relationship. However, for many parents, the stress uncovers weaknesses in their relationship, further compounding the problems they face.

A case example. Lucy J, a 3-year-old girl, was hospitalized for treatment of fever and suspected bacterial septicemia. During a previous hospitalization, her doctors had diagnosed and begun treatment of acute lymphocytic leukemia. The initiation of treatment had been successful, and her parents and physicians had developed an attitude of cautious optimism. Lucy's fever and subsequent return to the hospital were the first major complications of her illness and treatment.

When Lucy returned to the hospital, her mother decided to remain with her, and her father returned home to care for Lucy's siblings, Tommy, age 6, and Alice, age 2. Mr. J arranged for his mother to spend the day with Tommy and Alice, which allowed him to return to work.

Lucy's illness progressed rapidly after her hospitalization and she became seriously ill in spite of intensive medical intervention. Mrs. J spent most of her time at Lucy's bedside and was in close contact with her physicians and nurses. She soon realized that Lucy's mild fever had developed into a life-threatening illness, and her optimism about Lucy's future began to fade.

Mr. and Mrs. J spoke with each other nightly by telephone, but the distance between home and hospital prevented Mr. J's traveling to visit Lucy except on weekends. In their phone conversations, Mrs. J took heart from Mr. J's natural optimism and task-oriented coping style and shared little of her own increasing discouragement. She felt an obligation to protect Mr. J from her depression and therefore did not emphasize the negative aspects of Lucy's illness. Although she did not share her worries with her husband, Mrs. J did share her sadness and sense of impending loss with one of the staff nurses.

When Mr. J visited the hospital for the first time since Lucy's admission, Lucy's condition had improved somewhat. In part because of relief, and in part because she had not seen her husband for several days, Mrs. J greeted him with an outburst of tears. Mr. J was baffled by his wife's behavior and brusquely pushed her aside, reminding her not to show so much emotion in front of Lucy. Mrs. J made an excuse to leave the room and sought support from the nurse who usually comforted her. Mr. J focused his attention on Lucy who, although surprised at her mother's emotions, was delighted to see her father.

The nurse to whom Mrs. J had turned had witnessed Mr. J's apparently unsympathetic response to his wife and shared Mrs. J's anger at him. When Mr. J approached the nurse later, seeking information about Lucy, the nurse was unhelpful and referred him to the intern who was on call for the weekend. Although the intern attempted to answer Mr. J's questions, he was unfamiliar with Lucy's day-to-day care and reflected the optimism that the temporary improvement invited. When Mrs. J later attempted to discuss her concerns with her husband, Mr. J interpreted her worry as just another example of her tendency to coddle the children.

When Mr. and Mrs. J parted at the conclusion of Mr. J's visit, both felt alienated and confused. Mr. J could not understand his wife's highly emotional and depressed state, and Mrs. J was contemptuous of her husband's apparent insensitivity to their daughter's critical illness. In an attempt to deal with her confusion and anger, Mrs. J sought consultation with the social worker who was part of the pediatric oncology team.

In her role as a family-oriented consultant to Mrs. J, the social worker first met with Mrs. J to provide the support that she had been unable to find elsewhere. Mrs. J spoke with the social worker for over an hour, expressing her anger, and later her sadness, and finally, her anxiety about Lucy's illness as well as her deteriorating relationship with her husband. At the end of their meeting, the social worker asked Mrs. J if she would be willing to meet again with her husband present. Mrs. J expressed some willingness, but pointed out that her husband was very busy and probably would not be able to take time from his many responsibilities. The social worker offered to talk with Mr. J directly, and when she called him, he readily agreed to attend a joint meeting.

During that meeting, the social worker supported both husband and wife as each expressed their loneliness and isolation, as well as their wish to keep their feelings from one another in order to protect each other. The social worker then suggested that both parents meet with the oncologist to discuss Lucy's medical condition. The social worker participated in the meeting, encouraging both parents to be open and direct in their questions about Lucy's care and prognosis.

This case example is typical of many families in which the mother spends more time than the father in the hospital with the child. In the course of the hospitalization, the mother becomes familiar with the staff and their terminology; she is there when the physicians make rounds and she is able to keep track of the course of her child's illness. Her husband's understanding of the hospital course is often less complete, having been developed through conversations with his wife or with the physicians who are on call in the evening and who are less familiar with the child's care. Under these circumstances, the husband and wife often develop difficulties in supporting one another. The mother's developing understanding of the seriousness of her child's illness may lead her to experience significant feelings of sadness and loss. These feelings will be incomprehensible to her husband, whose focus on his daily routine at work and maintenance of the family functioning at home encourage a different impression of the child's progress. Such differences in understanding can be perceived by parents and the medical staff supporting them as a sign of serious dysfunction when they may in fact be situational in origin and relatively easy to correct.

In the case example, the social worker served as a direct consultant to Mrs. J, answering her plea for emotional support. She assessed the causes of

Mrs. J's unhappiness and brought the larger system together to assess its strengths. It became clear that referral for therapeutic intervention was not warranted. Rather, an opportunity for the parents to reestablish communication and to support one another was enough to resolve the crisis. Often the consultant can effect change in the system by merely initiating a process that the family continues.

In the case described above, it is likely that the father's infrequent visitation was the result of practical considerations, such as distance from the hospital and demands of work and family. However, the consultant should also be aware that the mother's intimate contact with her daughter and the father's complementary distance from the situation might have been an example of the family's general pattern of conflict resolution and relationship. Hospital staff are keenly observant of family visits and are aware of the transactional patterns that occur when family members meet at the patient's bedside. Their observations can be extremely useful to the family-oriented consultant in developing hypotheses about family structure and function. However, the case example illustrates the importance of meeting with all family members to discuss the reasons for the observations that are reported.

Minuchin, Rosman, and Baker (1978) have focused attention on the role family functioning may play in the maintenance of symptoms of certain illness in children. They developed an open systems model of psychosomatic illness, in which the child's symptoms play a role in the maintenance of family stability and are thus likely to persist.

While it is clear that family dysfunction does not cause such illnesses as asthma and diabetes, it is equally clear that certain family constellations can make more difficult the management of such emotionally responsive illnesses. It is therefore important for family-oriented consultants to consider the role of family dysfunction in those illnesses that are unresponsive to usual medical treatment.

In describing the characteristics of families of children with intractable psychosomatic disease, Minuchin *et al.* (1978) stress the importance of certain observable qualities of family interaction. Among these are poor conflict-resolution skills, enmeshment, rigidity, and overprotectiveness. The latter three qualities represent one end of three spectra of interactional characteristics that can be thought of as (1) the degree of the family's emotional closeness, (2) the amount of flexibility in their interactions, and (3) the extent to which they attempt to protect one another from painful experiences. Observation of these characteristics in a family should lead the consultant to suspect that the family's troubles are affecting the child's illness. In addition, if a family's tradition of interaction falls at extremes of any of these continua, the child's adaptation to illness and hospitalization may be threatened.

EMOTIONAL CLOSENESS

In a family whose relationships are extremely close, the boundaries separating individuals become blurred, and parents may identify with their child's anguish to an extreme degree. When it is necessary for the child to undergo a painful or anxiety-provoking procedure, parents may become overwhelmed by shared emotion and unable to provide appropriate support. Such parents may even cry in the child's presence when a procedure is described. In such circumstances, the child's experience of the parents' anxiety compounds his or her own feelings of insecurity and helplessness, leading to a sense of panic and inability to cooperate with the medical staff.

Since it is always true that children reflect to some extent the emotional state of their parents, an anxious and distressed child should lead a consultant to suspect that the parents are also experiencing anxiety and frustration. These feelings are most likely to be framed in terms of the child's illness and associated events. In many cases, the family has not presented these concerns to medical staff and is relieved to express them to a sympathetic listener. However, given the opportunity to discuss these issues, families often reveal other areas of concern that go beyond the immediate stress, and the consultant must be prepared to expand the focus of the discussion in response to the family's needs.

At the other end of the continuum of emotional involvement are those families who seem emotionally disengaged from one another. For some families, the anxiety of hospitalization and physical illness leads to withdrawal of their usual sensitivity to one another's needs. Such families can appear callous and unresponsive to a child's request for assistance and support. Such families respond quickly and gratefully to supportive intervention that focuses on resolution of their questions and concerns about their child's illness and treatment and provides information about appropriate ways that they can participate in the child's care.

Those families that are already disengaged in their characteristic relational style represent special problems for their hospitalized children. Sometimes, such families will be seen sitting in the child's room preoccupied with television or conversing with other parents, while the child, in obvious distress, is calling for assistance. These family members seem narcissistically preoccupied and unable to attend to each other's emotional needs. When a consultant discovers that such a pattern of disengagement is characteristic of a family, he or she will need to assist the ward staff in providing compensatory attention to the child while also attempting to use the child's illness and expression of need as a focus for building affective communication in the family.

INTERACTIONAL FLEXIBILITY

It is obvious that acute and severe medical illnesses require a high degree of flexibility from the family of the patient. Many families have difficulty adapting to the rapid flow of information and the unpredictable changes in treatment plans that characterize acute medical care. Such families will become increasingly anxious as their need to follow predictable patterns and routines in their day-to-day living is repeatedly challenged. Some families may become increasingly rigid in their adherence to a familiar routine, while others may become chaotic in response to mounting and destructive uncertainty and anxiety.

At the most dysfunctional end of this spectrum, in those families whose patterns of interaction appear chaotic, the parents may be heard telling their child that they will return in 10 minutes whereas they are actually leaving the hospital for the night. They visit the child at unpredictable intervals and often miss meetings with physicians and staff members. Even those children who have adapted to such patterns of parenting outside the hospital have difficulty responding to unpredictable support when they are ill. Families who respond to stress in a chaotic fashion require special attention and energy from medical staff. These families are especially likely to anger the child's medical caretakers. Such anger, even if subtly expressed, may aggravate the family's anxiety and chaos. These families need special assistance; for example, they often respond positively to written schedules and telephone reminders of important meetings with physicians and staff. The selection of a staff member who can meet with such families at a predictable time on a regular basis can provide a source of comfort and support.

PROTECTIVENESS FROM PAINFUL EXPERIENCE

Although the term "overprotectiveness" is usually used to characterize parental relationships with children, in many families overprotectiveness is a characteristic of affective relationships throughout the family. In such families, even the children attempt to prevent suffering in other family members. Everyone in these families is apt to keep disturbing events and feelings a secret. The parents attempt to keep children anxiety-free for as long as possible by avoiding discussions with the child of anxiety-provoking aspects of the illness.

Such overprotection becomes a problem when children are denied information that would be useful to them. For example, a parent who brings a 7-year-old son to the hospital for a scheduled admission without telling him that he will be staying in the hospital creates for the child an atmosphere of betrayal and uncertainty. The anxiety that accompanies the sense that anything can happen at any time may pervade this child's experience throughout the hospitalization. In a similar fashion, children who protect their parents from their own anxiety about their illness and the possibility of dying isolate themselves needlessly from their primary supportive alliances. The diagnosis of an overprotective pattern can lead a family therapist to help construct more appropriate support systems.

In direct contrast to overprotective parents are those who seem oblivious to the effects of emotionally disturbing comments. Such parents do not adjust their conversations about hospital procedures and mortality to fit the experience and developmental level of the child. They may engage hospital staff in brutally direct questioning and conversations in the child's presence under the mistaken impression that there should be no secrets and that everyone should know everything. It is possible for a child's anxiety to intensify either from knowing and expressing too little or from hearing and knowing too much.

The family therapist as a consultant to pediatric inpatient units is often asked to assess the family's ability to raise its children appropriately. In many community hospitals, as well as tertiary medical centers, the pediatric inpatient service often serves as the triage point for decisions about adequacy of parenting. In its most extreme form, this question centers around evidence of child abuse and neglect. In addition to assisting the medical authorities in their attempt to judge the family's competence, the family consultant may also provide valuable direct assistance to the family. It is difficult for such family members to feel supported by a medical staff who has reported them for child abuse and are arranging to remove children from their custody. As an outsider, the family consultant can establish an alliance with the family and help them seek rehabilitative help from appropriate social service and mental health agencies.

PROBLEMS IN THE CARETAKING SYSTEM

When a child and family enter the hospital, they begin a series of transactions with the community of health professionals in the hospital. The family therapist as consultant must look beyond the usual focus on the child and family and assess the characteristics of the caretaking system because the index child's emotional problems in the hospital may be related to dysfunction in the caretaking team.

Within the medical-care hierarchy there may be significant problems with communication and lack of problem-solving skills at all levels. There may be problems within professional groups as well as between and among professional groups. The intensity and complexity of such difficulties seem to be proportional to the complexity of the medical problem and the number of medical consultants attempting to formulate the diagnosis and the treatment plan. Consulting physicians frequently offer their opinions and observations to the patient and his or her family before conferring with their colleagues. Under these circumstances, physicians themselves often feel confused about who is the physician in charge and who is responsible for coordinating the flow of information within the team and to the family.

A case example. Joe C was a 7-year-old boy who, along with his mother and father, was involved in a serious motor vehicle accident. His injuries were extensive, involving a compound fracture of his left femur, internal injuries including a ruptured spleen, and head injuries. Although his father escaped injury, his mother was hospitalized because of compound fractures of her tibia and fibula. Joe was treated by orthopedic, general, and neurosurgical teams. In addition, general pediatric house staff followed his care, at first in intensive-care units and later on a general pediatric unit. Joe's injuries required initial emergency abdominal surgery as well as subsequent orthopedic surgery.

Because of her injuries, Joe's mother was confined to her room in a separate wing of the hospital. She was emotionally distraught following the accident, and required much of her husband's attention. Mr. C was also preoccupied with accident-related arrangements with insurance companies and attorneys, and he had little time to spend with his son.

Joe's recovery from his injured femur was complicated, and the orthopedic surgeon decided that further surgery was necessary. Joe was informed of the decision the night before the operation was to occur. After the surgeons left his room, Joe became uncontrollably angry. He thrashed about on his bed, and several staff members were required to restrain him. An emergency consultation was requested from the child psychiatry unit to help calm the patient and discover the cause of the outburst.

In talking with Joe after his anger had subsided, the Child Psychiatry Fellow discovered that Joe had been surprised by the orthopedic surgeon's plans for a surgical procedure the following morning. Joe had asked his general surgeon earlier in the day if more surgery was planned and had been told there would be no more operations. Joe's father had been unable to visit that day because of other obligations, but he had called Joe and reiterated the reassurance that there would be no more surgery. He had heard this reassurance in a conversation with the pediatric house staff whom he had seen earlier in the day.

Both the general surgeon and the pediatric house officers had spoken with the orthopedic surgeons 24 hours earlier, and all had agreed that no more surgery was required. The pediatric house staff had been informed of the need for surgery after their contact with Mr. C but, it was discovered later, they had assumed the surgeon would contact the family. The surgeons had assumed the house officers would make those arrangements. All the physicians had assumed someone else would inform the child and would help him to deal with the information.

In his conversations with Joe, the child psychiatry consultant discovered that Joe had a close relationship with one of his primary nurses. The consultant was able to arrange for that nurse to meet with Joe informally every day to listen to his experiences and provide the support his family could not. The nurse became Joe's advocate in the medical system and was able to assist medical staff in coordinating their plans and communication with Joe. When Joe's father became more available, the consultant helped the primary nurse include Mr. C in the support and advocacy role, thus returning the family to a more adaptive and customary pattern.

In the case example, the child's anxiety following severe trauma and multiple surgical procedures was complicated by his concern about his mother's health and his father's inaccessibility. The medical caretakers' inability to function in a clear and focused manner further added to the child's distress by confusing him and presenting contradicting information about factors that directly affected his care. At a time when his defenses needed support, he was abandoned, with predictable results.

Just as children tend to mirror anxiety and confusion experienced by their parents, families often mirror the confusion and frustration of the medical system attempting to help them. It is therefore important for the family consultant to use an understanding of systems to assess the caretaking system and its transactions with the family and the index patient. In particular, the consultant must assess the lines of authority and the points of discord within the system. Also, he or she must discover who provides for the informational and emotional needs of the family and the child. Such an assessment will provide the therapist with a better understanding of the experience of the familiy and child while in the hospital. It will also provide important information about how to gain leverage in helping the family deal with its difficulties.

When the family consultant discovers that the patient's problem results from significant strife within the health care team, he or she must help the team resolve its difficulties. Often pediatric wards have regularly scheduled interdisciplinary meetings that are designed to solve such problems. If this resource exists, the consultant should attend the meeting to enlist the aid of staff members in solving the child's problems. If there is no regularly scheduled forum for such a discussion, the consultant may use the child's illness and emotional difficulties as a focus for a meeting of relevant staff. Such ad hoc consultation to the health care system is a necessary and useful part of many mental health consultations in pediatrics.

PROBLEMS OF HOSPITAL STAFF–FAMILY INTERACTION

Specific transactional problems between families and staff members are worthy of special note because of their relative frequency and the ease with which they are overlooked. Because of the length of their hospitalization, certain children with chronic illnesses develop a special relationship with nursing staff. Some of these children are in families that find it difficult to visit them on a regular or frequent basis. The ward staff begins to assume the role of parents to these children, thus inviting them to experience a particularly difficult form of loyalty conflict.

To compensate for what staff members perceive as inadequate parenting, some of these children are overindulged and given special privileges on the wards. They are given nicknames and described by the nurses as "my boyfriend" or "my special little girl." Parents often sense the rivalry but feel helpless and confused. The children wonder why their family does not treat them with the special attention lavished on them by the ward staff and often express their unhappiness directly to their families. In their confusion and frustration, family members may become hostile and be seen as difficult and harmful to the patient's well-being.

When such situations arise, the consultant may be asked to help the staff control the "difficult parent." However, the staff is often oblivous to the role they are playing as they compete for the index patient's attention and affection. Once the consultant has discovered the nature of the problem, the solution requires considerable skill in supporting all parties in the conflict before a resolution can be sought.

Transactions between hospital staff and families become particularly complex when there is a disagreement between the family and the physicians who are managing the child's care. The possible causes of disagreement are many. As a result of their anxiety, the family members may find it difficult to listen to physicians discuss their observations, diagnostic impressions, and treatment recommendations. Almost all parents give the impression of hearing and understanding the doctors' words, but after the consultation is over, many find they have not really understood, or have questions and doubts about what they understood. The physician's busy schedule and the general aura of competence of the ward staff inhibit many parents from pursuing their questions adequately. Their doubts linger and their anxiety increases, making fruitful discussion less and less likely.

For their part, many physicians feel uncomfortable with diagnostic and treatment situations that are ambiguous and unclear. They feel that it is necessary to present a positive and assured stance to the family, and find questions and observations about the ambiguities of the situation anxiety provoking. This anxiety and defensiveness on the part of both physicians and family is but one of many possible causes of unrseolved conflict in this subsystem.

When such a conflict occurs, members of the ward staff occasionally form alliances with one side or the other and indirectly complicate the problem. For example, the child's primary nurse may respond to the parents' complaints about a physician's lack of availability by agreeing with the parent and saying, "Many parents have that experience with that doctor. I know how you feel." The ward staff's own unresolved feelings toward the physician then become a part of the conflict. The physician usually senses this alliance, and the resolution of the problem may become impossible. Once again, the consultant who enters such a system in response to a question about the individual child and his or her family is called upon to assess the larger system and help resolve its difficulties.

In summary, the family-oriented consultants who answer requests about children on an inpatient ward must systematically evaluate all the interlocking systems in which the children find themselves, from the individual status of the children through their relationships with family and medical staff, to the complex transactions among and between family members and staff. This assessment process should include individual meetings with the physician requesting the consultation, the nursing staff primarily responsible for a particular child, and the child with relevant family members. In most instances, a careful assessment of these transactional patterns will lead to a clear plan of action.

SPECIAL ISSUES IN OUTPATIENT CONSULTATION

The child referred from an outpatient practice is a member of a complex social system that is less visible than the inpatient system of ward staff, attending physicians, and anxious family members. Nevertheless, the family systems consultant must apply the same broad scope to the investigative process. Most of the same principles described above remain applicable, but it is often easier to persuade the family to participate when the child is hospitalized than during an elective outpatient assessment. Families are less likely to be concerned and motivated to take part in outpatient consultation.

Another problem faced by the outpatient consultant is the difference in the pace of clinical work for the pediatric practitioner and for the mental health worker. An outpatient consultation may require several meetings, spaced over a few weeks, before a clear recommendation can be made. The pediatrician and the family may wonder what is taking so long, because the usual pediatric evaluation occurs in the space of a few minutes in the pediatric office. Frequent contact between the consultant and the pediatrician to explain the progress of the assessment and the reason for further meetings will facilitate the evaluation, and the pediatrician will be in a better position to support the process.

Evaluation of complex psychosomatic cases often takes place in the outpatient setting. Close cooperation between referring physician and consultant is essential in these cases because of the likelihood that the evaluation itself will exacerbate the medical condition under investigation. In such cases, the consultant should make specific arrangements to meet with the family at a time when the pediatrician will be readily available in person or by phone in case the child's symptoms become more acutely severe.

A case example. Jon was a 15-year-old boy with chronic, severe asthma. In spite of competent medical care, his asthma attacks were increasing in severity and frequency. In the 3 months before referral, Jon had been hospitalized twice and had required intensive medical support on both occasions. Medication after discharge included both experimental drugs and high doses of steroids, which produced significant side effects. Although the pediatric pulmonary specialists had suspected an emotional component to Jon's illness, there was no clear evidence for it, and the family had strongly resisted referral for psychiatric evaluation. The complete failure of appropriate medical treatment to prevent life-threatening asthmatic episodes led the physicians responsible for Jon's care to insist that the family receive an evaluation to "rule out" a psychological component to his illness.

At the evaluation interview, Jon was joined by his mother, a nurse employed part-time in a nursing home; his father, an attorney for a major corporation, whose duties took him away from the family for prolonged intervals; and his 19-year-old sister, home from her first year at college.

The consultant found the family to be intelligent, cordial, and charming. However, they seemed unable to discuss even the most trivial differences among one another. As the consultant was nearing the end of an unproductive hour, Jon's sister began to weep quietly. With much support from the consultant, she began to express her concern that her parents were near the point of separation or divorce. As their daughter's distress became more intense, the parents became noticeably anxious, fidgeting in their seats and attempting to divert her from her expressions of anxiety and sadness.

At the point when it appeared that Jon's father was about to lose patience with the entire endeavor, Jon began to wheeze audibly. Jon's mother noticed his labored breathing and called it to everyone's attention. Within a matter of minutes, Jon was having serious difficulty breathing and the focus of all present was on the problem of his illness. The family's affect changed dramatically from anxiety and discomfort to a calm, focused attention to Jon's care.

The consultant called his colleagues in the Pulmonary Division of the University Medical Center and arranged for Jon to be treated immediately. At a follow-up meeting that included the family and the referring physician, the consultant was able to share his observations of the events leading up to Jon's attack and the dramatic change in the family's affect once the focus was taken off the problem of the marriage. While the family members were anxious to downplay the consultant's observations, the physicians were impressed with the evidence. With the consultant's encouragement, the physicians devoted several subsequent meetings with the family to an explanation of the physiology of stress and its relationship to asthma. At the conclusion of those meetings, the family accepted a referral for family therapy.

In the case example described above, the close relationship of the consultant with his medical colleagues was useful in two ways. First, he was able to recognize the seriousness of Jon's asthma attack in his office and arrange for prompt treatment. Second, he was able to use the occasion of that attack to support his colleagues' impressions of Jon's illness and help them convince the family of the probable value of therapy. A less sophisticated consultant might have misunderstood the severity of Jon's problem and focused instead on the family's response, with possibly tragic consequences. For their part, the pediatricians understood the possibility of an exacerbation of Jon's illness by the consultation and were prepared to treat it if necessary.

HELPING THE PEDIATRICIAN IN HIS OR HER OWN WORK

Many family therapy concepts are fully applicable to the pediatrician's office practice. While most pediatricians counsel families about routine adaption to developmental changes, some are incorporating brief family therapy sessions into their practice schedules.

Karofsky, Keith, Hoornstra, and Clune (1982) have reported results of a follow-up investigation of the treatment of 15 children with school problems or behavior problems. Fourteen of these families readily accepted the role of the pediatrician and nurse practitioner as family therapist. In training pediatricians in family therapy principles, it is important to focus on issues of family diagnosis and assessment of the family's suitability for brief intervention. It is useful for the pediatric trainee to observe family consultants in interaction with patients and their families. Through the process of mutual observation and discussion, pediatric trainees and family consultants can develop an understanding of each other's language and therapeutic style.

The process of mutual education that develops naturally in a training program is also important in later consultation with pediatric practitioners. Early in a consultative relationship, it is important for the consultant to arrange to observe the pediatrician at work with his or her patients. This can occur most easily in the pediatrician's office, but many pediatricians are willing to accompany families to the consultant's office as well. In the absence of a clear understanding of the pediatrician's conceptual knowledge and interactional style, the consultant who gives advice, even when it is based on a direct observation of the family in question, runs significant and obvious risks. The novice practitioner may seize upon a technique and overuse it as a potential panacea. Alternatively, the sophisticated pediatrician may regard the suggestions offered by the consultant as patronizing and unhelpful.

In summary, the consultant who wishes to help the pediatrician use methods of family counseling and therapy should first establish a close and well-informed relationship with the pediatrician upon which later, informed collaboration can be based.

SUMMARY

The family therapist serving as consultant to pediatric professionals is consulting to health caregivers who are sophisticated and well educated about emotional problems and family issues. Nonetheless, the need for the pediatrician to focus primarily on the often-complex medical problems of his or her patients may obscure the psychological issues. In particular, the complex interaction of medical staff and medical treatment with the patient and family may be impossible for the participants to discuss. The family therapist as consultant is in a uniquely useful position to untangle the complexities of these interactions and help both pediatric and family systems to mesh and function more effectively. Most important, the therapist must consciously look beyond the family for problems in the larger system in order to be optimally helpful.

REFERENCES

Bowlby, J. *Attachment and loss* (Vol. II, *Separation*). New York: Basic Books, 1973.

Fagin, C. M. R. N. *The effects of maternal attendance during hospitalization on the posthospital behavior of young children: A comparative study.* Philadelphia: F. A. Davis, 1966.

Green, M., & Haggerty, R. J. Child health services and the clinician. In M. Green & R. J. Haggerty (Eds.), *Ambulatory pediatrics* (Vol. II). Philadelphia: W. B. Saunders, 1977.

Karofsky, P. S., Keith, D. V., Hoornstra, L. L., & Clune, C. A follow-up study of the impact of family therapy in the pediatric office. *Clinical Pediatrics*, 1982, *22*, 351–355.

MacCarthy, D., Lindsay, M., & Morris, I. Children in hospital with mothers. *Lancet*, 1962, *1*, 603–608.

Minuchin, S., Rosman, B., & Baker, L. *Psychosomatic families: Anorexia nervosa in context.* Cambridge, MA: Harvard University Press, 1978.

Robertson, James. Some responses of young children to the loss of maternal care. *Nursing Times*, 1953, *49*, 382–386.

Robertson, James, & Robertson, Joyce. Young children on brief separation. *Psychoanalytic Study of the Child*, 1971, *26*, 264–315.

Robertson, Joyce. A mother's observations on the tonsillectomy of her four-year-old daughter, with comments by Anna Freud. *Psychoanalytic Study of the Child*, 1971, *11*, 410–433.

Spitz, R. A. Anaclitic depression. *Psychoanalytic Study of the Child*, 1946, *2*, 315–342.

Spitz, R. A. Anxiety in infancy: A study of its manifestations in the first years of life. *International Journal of Psycho-Analysis*, 1950, *31*, 138–143.

Editors' Commentary on Consultation in Medical Contexts

The chapters in this section have focused on systems consultation in different spheres of the medical community, from oncology to family medicine and pediatrics. In this commentary we shall note some important issues regarding medical consultation that are implied but not fully addressed in these chapters.

WHO IS THE CONSULTEE IN A MEDICAL CONSULTATION?

Medical consultation has its own tradition and rituals known to today's primary care physicians and their consultants. Generally, primary care physicians call on specialists for their expertise, while specialists rely on primary care physicians for their livelihood. Despite this interdependency, case-focused consultations often take place without direct personal contact between the primary care physician and the consultant. Rather, the patient may set up the appointment after it is recommended by the primary care physician, or the referring physician may send a letter ahead of the patient. After the consultant has diagnosed and/or treated the specified problem, the patient may return to the primary care physician, with the consultant writing a letter or perhaps making a phone call to report the results of the consultation. Most medical consultation procedures are in keeping with a biotechnical medical approach and have been streamlined to the barest essentials for the sake of efficiency. Many times these procedures work; sometimes they do not. A systems approach would predict that the likelihood of incomplete communication or misunderstanding is quite high. Available research supports this prediction by citing the frequency with which medical consultants and consultees disagree on the value of a consultation and even on what the consultation question was. "Breakdowns in communication are not uncommon in the consultation process and may adversely affect patient care, cost effectiveness, and education" (Lee, Pappius, & Goldman, 1983).

The convention for medical consultation described above reveals the ambiguity and confusion that can exist around the question, "Who is the consultee?" Is it the primary physician or is it the patient and the family? In some circumstances, a patient may phone a family therapist or other consultant at the suggestion of a primary care physician, set up an appointment, and directly communicate the consultative question. The consultant/specialist may then diagnose and/or treat the patient/family, and then give them the information that has been requested. At other times, a consultant may work with both the physician and the patient/family, or only with the consulting physician. This range of approaches is illustrated by the chapters in this section. Munson describes direct consultation with patients and families on a pediatric service, and Wellisch describes a similar approach to consultation with patients in an oncology service. Sluzki, giving a case example from family medicine, works with the consulting physician and the family together. The chapter by McDaniel, Bank, Campbell, Mancini, and Shore and the chapter by McDaniel and Weber describe a consultation format in which the consultant works directly with the consulting physician only.

When a consultant sees a patient or family directly, there is a great variation in the amount and quality of communication between consultant and primary physician. Sometimes, it is left unclear whether a consultation has been requested; perhaps the physician is the consultee, or perhaps a referral has been made for transfer of care to the specialist. Such situations obviously are ripe for difficulties. Consultants complain when they receive no information from the primary care physician prior to seeing a patient, and primary care physicians complain when they do not receive immediate or useful information from the consultant at follow-up. (Physicians say that psychotherapists are particularly negligent on this score.) Either of these problems may be the result of triangulation among the patient/family, the consultant, and the primary care physician.

From a systems point of view, we believe that it is most useful and clear to view the primary care physician as the consultee and the patient as the subject of the consultation. This conceptualization emphasizes the centrality of the consultee's concerns and the need for direct communication between the consultant and the primary physician. At times, a patient may also act as a consultee, asking the primary care physician to recommend a consultant. This situation might be termed a consultation within a consultation. Here, the consultant actively solicits information from the patient after having spoken with the referring physician, and then renders an opinion directly to the patient as well as having direct contact with the referring physician. This situation is consistent with the consultations described by Munson in his work with pediatrics. Other consultants may choose not to relay results to the patient, so that the information flow remains primarily between the consultant and the primary physician. In both situations, the patient pays for the consultation needed by the primary care physician to carry out treatment adequately. In all circumstances, maintaining a clear view of the roles of consultant, consultee, and patient/family diminishes the possibility for ambiguity and misunderstanding.

CONTRACTS AND AMBIGUITY IN MEDICAL CONSULTATIONS

One solution to the ambiguity described frequently in the chapters on medical consultation is an explicit contract or agreement to minimize misunderstandings and maximize outcome. This approach is alluded to in some of the case reports in these chapters; however, many physicians feel overt, negotiated contracts between specialists and the referring physician are too time-consuming. The current model of letters and occasional phone calls focuses on the patient's problems rather than on the consultee's difficulties with the patient and family. The system is designed for efficiency, but, as discussed above, there is ample potential for the consultant to be unaware of what the primary physician wants or is doing. The contracting phase of medical consultations is often implicit and can leave unclear, for example, what exactly the consultation is for; who initiated the consultation; and who will carry out the intervention. Clarification of these issues is important especially in the mental health field, where there is some substitutability of skills and providers. The fact that treatment, in addition to assessment, may occur in the context of a medical consultation makes these clarifications important.

Clarification of the request itself is also important, whether in a primary care context or a mental health context. For example, "family consultation, please" is a frequent request from a busy physician for a consultant to see a family. Clearly, discussion is needed with the consultee to clarify the exact nature of this request. In one case, this request translated to mean: "This family is in crisis, constantly calling me for reassurance, and I'm not sure how to deal with them." In another, it was: "This hospitalized patient is the 'healthiest' member of the family. With her hospitalization, the family is in trouble. Please evaluate and refer, if appropriate." In these cases, the consultees seemed to be asking both for advice about the case and for advice about their own interactions with the family. As with many consultations, a central question for the consultant is: "How do you pass the anxiety back in a manageable form?"

THE INTERPERSONAL DYNAMICS OF MEDICAL CONSULTATION

Krakowski (1972) has suggested that while a physician's overt request to a mental health consultant is "to gain better information about diagnosis and treatment," the most common personal qualities wanted in consultants were "kindness and empathy" for the physician handling a difficult situation. In systems terms, the initial, covert request may be to give support and provide a new perspective on the interpersonal relationship between the referring doctor and the patient/family. The standard medical model approach to consultation may not always effectively fulfill both the overt and covert requests. This is well illustrated in the examples in the McDaniel *et al.* chapter on using a group as a consultant. A collaborative approach to consultation in which consultant and consultee directly negotiate and contract regarding the goals and the final effects of the consultation may avoid the complications and pitfalls of the traditional model and, in the end, be more efficient.

Krakowski (1971) also described the general reluctance of many physicians to request consultations, psychiatric or otherwise. Part of any reluctance to request consultations may be a recognition of the triangulation that can occur among consultant, consultee, and patient. Physicians worry about other physicians "taking over" their patients, or they fear that a consultant will in some other way undermine their position with the patient. "The consultee may be ambivalent, for though the support may be helpful, it may at the same time lower the consultee's self-esteem" (p. 15). There is general agreement in the medical community that one needs to choose one's consultants carefully. The art of being a consultant involves providing the requisite knowledge and competence while supporting the consultee's self-esteem and relationship with the patient. Many of these issues, as well as the controversy over who is the consultee, also are concerns of the field of consultation–liaison psychiatry.

CONSULTATION-LIAISON PSYCHIATRY

The field of consultation–liaison psychiatry provides vivid examples of conceptual and practical opportunities and difficulties that can arise within the field that we broadly call systems consultation. By and large, the participation of family therapists in consultation–liaison psychiatry has been recent and fragmentary. The most appropriate model for consultation–liaison psychiatry is hotly disputed between those in the field who emphasize "liaison" and those who focus on "consultation." Although some authors use the terms "psychiatric consultation service" and "psychiatric liaison service" as synonymous (Krakowski, 1973), these usually have been described as models with distinct differences. These contrasting viewpoints can usefully be sketched to help clarify issues that we discuss in this volume. The hyphenated term "consultation–liaison psychiatry" represents various amalgamations of the two approaches (Lipowski, 1974, 1984).

The liaison model has been most clearly developed by George L. Engel and his colleagues at the University of Rochester (1957). Education of nonpsychiatric physicians to assist in their becoming more skilled in dealing with psychosocial issues has been a central feature of this approach. In addition, in the Rochester model, the liaison professional is well trained in the specialty in which the service is taking place. For example, a liaison person on an obstetric–gynecology service might be board certified in that specialty and hold a faculty appointment in the department. In addition, this liaison staff member may have had special training in psychosocial medicine and/or psychiatry. He or she is then able to interweave ideas stemming from a broad systems-oriented biopsychosocial model (Engel, 1977) into the care of specific patients and into the organization of service teams, most commonly on inpatient services. This approach is similar to the concept of liaison that is described by Landau-Stanton in the first chapter of the next section, in that a specialist becomes a permanent team member in the work of another clinical specialty. Optimally, the liaison staff member commands respect both as a competent practitioner in psychiatry and in the nonpsychiatric specialty. However, as the rigors of specialty training have increased, relatively few persons are able to become competent and stay expert in both psychiatry and another medical specialty.

Much of the work of the medical–psychiatric liaison specialist does not involve diagnosis and management of specific cases. Instead, broader issues in what can be called program consultation in an educational and treatment setting have been more central to this approach. A systemic point of view has been more widely accepted in liaison psychiatry than in traditional, individually oriented psychiatry. Within this type of liaison, when consultation on specific problems takes place, the consultant has the advantage of background experience in seeing recurrent patterns of staff functioning. Ideally, then, the liaison relationship provides a framework for consultation that can go beyond specific cases. This can also help the consultant make sure that the consultee/physician builds rather than loses competence. However, confusion sometimes has arisen when consultants with these broad medical–psychiatric liaison goals have been asked to carry out psychiatric diagnosis and treatment on behalf of the referring physician; direct patient care then is central to the consultation request.

Some persons who use the term "liaison psychiatry" have emphasized more strongly the therapeutic component (Greenhill, 1977, 1980). From this vantage point, the liaison psychiatrist is "an active interventionist in determining the treatment programs in the psychiatric care of the medically sick" (Greenhill, 1980). When liaison with active intervention is attempted but the service has not accepted this approach, such efforts at education of the nonpsychiatric physician in psychosocial issues by the liaison person may well be regarded as arrogant and intrusive. It should be stressed that this is quite contrary to the model of collaborative medical–psychiatric liaison developed and advocated by Engel and others.

Still more oriented to direct patient care is the approach called "psychiatric consultation," with the "liaison" concept dropped. For example, Thomas P. Hackett (1985) defines consultation as "expert diagnostic opinion on a patient's mental state or behavior and advice on patient management given at the request of another physician." He regards psychiatric consultation as patient-oriented and liaison psychiatry as systems-oriented. Clearly, we do not subscribe to this distinction. Rather, we contend that consultation (as well as liaison teaching) should be systems-oriented, with the patient/family as a key subsystem that also includes the referring physician and treatment team.

The controversies among psychiatrists about "consultation" and "liaison" approaches need to be understood by family therapists who attempt systems-oriented consultation in medical facilities. Similar difficulties are likely to develop for systems consultants in defining functions that can range from staff education about family systems to case consultation with specific families. A consultative tradition for family therapists in medical settings remains to be developed. It often is initially unclear whether the family therapist as consultant is being asked to provide therapy for a series of families or to address broader educational issues under the umbrella of psychiatry, psychology, and behavioral science.

The hazards of misunderstanding are compounded because family therapy consultants and psychiatric consultants may be perceived as having overlapping functions. Nonpsychiatric medical consultees are more interested in receiving management suggestions from psychiatric consultants than they are in obtaining psychiatric diagnoses (Mackenzie, Popkin, Callies, & Kroll, 1983). In contrast, medical consultations most often lead to a series of confirmatory or exploratory diagnostic studies. A systems-oriented consultant will make use of systems principles to become cognizant of the overall treatment context, as well as the context of the family, before making treatment recommendations, providing treatment, or providing education that may or may not fit with what is wanted by the consultee, the patient, and the family, all of whom may have unclear or conflicting requests.

The systems consultation that has been discussed in this volume calls for more attention to the context of the family and the treatment team than is usually considered in medical case-treatment consultations. Educational functions are compatible with systems consultation, but are not essential. Most systems consultation terminates after a brief, task-oriented contact, but may be renewed with the consultant over a series of new cases or problems, thus creating a consultant role that is similar to that of the liaison psychiatrist.

CONSULTATION AND THE ECONOMICS OF HEALTH CARE DELIVERY

An important issue neglected for the most part in these chapters is the changing economic scene for health care delivery and its probable impact upon medical consultations. Bloch is the only author in this section to pose the issue, but even he does not make predictions or recommendations. In the medical system, cost containment is the name of the game. Some prepaid plans now literally charge the primary care physician for any consultations he or she orders, making clear the issue of "who is the consultee" from an economic standpoint. On the other hand, many patient advocates feel that patients should have the right to consult with specialists directly without requiring a referral from a primary care physician. Even with the model of the patient as consultee, a collaborative relationship between providers will provide the most effective care for the patient. The economics of health care delivery in the '80s are changing so rapidly that the consequences for consultation are difficult to predict. Research is needed to show whether systems consultation may be, in the long run, cost-effective.

THE MD VERSUS THE NON-MD CONSULTANT

A final issue of interest to many systems consultants working in a medical context is that of the non-MD who consults with MDs. Certainly some prejudice can exist, whether on the part of a MD who only consults with other MDs or on the part of the non-MD who refuses to work in medical contexts or passively shows resentment about the power of a physician in the context. A medical context, like the military or a large business, is organized around certain rules and rituals that distribute power and obligation. Non-MD consultants, unaccustomed to such rituals, may feel like outsiders on foreign territory and may inadvertently transgress the rules. MDs may naturally trust other MDs who are insiders and who they feel will play by the same rules.

For example, one of us, a PhD, consulted with a family about their son, who had an attention deficit disorder. The consultant recommended that the boy be evaluated for drug treatment and suggested that he follow new strategies for learning in school. The family, which was in the military, also consulted with their military pediatrician. He advised the parents that the child was normal and needed no intervention of any kind. This represents a common situation, in which two consultants make contradictory recommendations. Even with a call from the PhD consultant to explore the possibilty of collaborating with the pediatrician for the benefit of the family, the pediatrician maintained his original position and explicitly questioned the competence of a non-MD consultant.

Some such situations are not resolvable. However, many times the most pressing need for a physician as consultee is the need for a competent consultant. Clearly many non-MDs have been successful systems consultants in medical contexts, as demonstrated by Wellisch and Cohen and others in this volume. (Three of our six chapters on medical consultation include contributions by non-MDs.) Once a systems consultant, whether MD or non-MD, makes clear his or her areas of expertise, many physicians will be pleased to call upon such a resource.

Whether MD or non-MD, frequently a systems-oriented consultant in a medical context may need to initiate, or urge a primary care physician to initiate, a meeting of professionals involved in a case. Multiple consultants who disagree and are not in communication with (or even aware of) each other can be a major problem in complicated medical cases. Coordination and leadership of a treatment team is essential for these families who often are already highly stressed to begin with, especially in the treatment of chronic diseases, such as schizophrenia, or terminal diseases, such as cancer, where treatment may be partial or inadequate at best. In these cases, a consultant such as a systems consultant or an oncology consultant, may become the de facto primary therapist who must coordinate treatment if a primary care physician is absent. How such roles can best be integrated is an example of the many challenging issues that are ripe for consideration in the area of medical systems consultation.

REFERENCES

Engel, G. L. The need for a new medical model: A challenge for biomedicine. *Science*, 1977, *196*, 129–136.

Engel, G. L., Greene, W. A., Reichsman, F., Schmale, A., & Ashenburg, N. A graduate and undergraduate teaching program on the psychological aspects of medicine. *Journal of Medical Education*, *32*, 1957, 859–870.

Greenhill, M. H. The development of liaison programs. In G. Usdin (Ed.), *Psychiatric medicine*. New York: Brunner/Mazel, 1977.

Greenhill, M. H. Therapeutic intervention in liaison psychiatry. *Psychiatric Journal of the University of Ottawa*, 1980, *5*, 255–263.

Hackett, T. P. Concept of liaison psychiatry seen as harmful. (Report of an address.) *Psychiatric News*, 1985, May 3, pp. 7–8.

Krakowski, A. J. Doctor–doctor relationship. *Psychosomatics*, 1971, *12*, 11–15.

Krakowski, A. J. Doctor–doctor relationship II: Conscious factors influencing the consultation process. *Psychosomatics*, 1972, *13*, 158–164.

Krakowski, A. J. Liaison psychiatry: Factors influencing the consultation process. *Psychiatry in Medicine*, 1973, *4*, 439–446.

Lee, T., Pappius, E. M., & Goldman, L. Impact of interphysician communication in the effectiveness of medical consultations. *American Journal of Medicine*, 1983, *74*, 106–112.

Lipowski, Z. J. Consultation–liaison psychiatry: An overview. *American Journal of Psychiatry*, 1974, *131*, 623–630.

Lipowski, Z. J. History, definition and scope of consultation–liaison psychiatry. In L. Grinspoon (Ed.), *Psychiatry update* (Vol. III). Washington, DC: American Psychiatric Press, 1984.

Mackenzie, T. B., Popkin, M. K., Callies, A. L., & Kroll, J. Consultation outcomes: The psychiatrist as consultee. *Archives of General Psychiatry*, 1983, *40*, 1211–1214.

IV

CONSULTATION WITH COMMUNITY GROUPS AND SERVICE SYSTEMS

Within communities there is a wide diversity of institutions, agencies, and groups that frequently need assistance from consultants. The chapters in this section reflect the diversity of these community organizations and their consultation requests, the contrasting strategies employed by systems consultants, and the striking similarities in emphases among consultants despite these differences in strategies.

In describing her consultations with a variety of community groups, Landau-Stanton outlines her model of "transitional mapping," which she finds adaptable to both therapeutic and consultation contexts. Singer discusses the consultation approach she has used with the many families who have sought assistance when family members have become involved with cultic groups, including pseudotherapeutic "human growth" organizations. The difficult problem of domestic violence is addressed by Anderson and Goolishian. In consulting with agencies dealing with this problem, they underscore the importance of maximizing the potential for change by avoiding "side-taking" in a system where there are many conflicting beliefs. Wynne and Wynne, as co-consultants, report on their work with the family court system. As the divorce rate has climbed, there has been an increasing need for collaboration between the legal and mental health systems in helping families with deeply entrenched custody and visitation conflicts. Weber and Wynn examine the process of consulting with the clergy, often the first community professionals turned to by people in trouble. In reviewing consultation with the school system, Fisher describes how his conceptual model includes both family-based systems theory and a model of group-relations theory. Finally, Imber-Black presents her work in consulting with the "big business" of human-service-provider systems, an approach based on the Milan systemic model that attempts to introduce flexibility into systems that tend toward rigidity.

16

COMPETENCE, IMPERMANENCE, AND TRANSITIONAL MAPPING
A Model for Systems Consultation

JUDITH LANDAU-STANTON
University of Rochester School of Medicine and Dentistry
Rochester, New York

The model for consultation presented here has evolved from engagement in this kind of work since 1963. It is oriented toward prevention, having developed from a community and social-medicine perspective (Caplan, 1965; Kark & Mainemer, 1977; Kark & Steuart, 1962). It was developed in concert with my approach to family therapy (Landau, 1981, 1982; Landau-Stanton, 1985, in press), and in many ways the two are operationally inseparable. This model has been used in consulting in such diverse contexts as community, self-help, business, educational, medical, religious, and legal groups.

The view that one takes of the families one treats is inescapably reflected in the approach assumed when undertaking systems-oriented consultation. The two are isomorphic. There are at least three features of the present model that warrant emphasis: *competence*, *impermanence*, and the use of *transitional mapping* to guide the intervention.

COMPETENCE AND IMPERMANENCE

A major contribution of most current family therapy approaches has been their recognition of a family's inherent competence and integrity—the realization that the family does not need a permanent guardian functioning in the role of therapist. Like many brief therapies, and unlike some individual approaches, these family therapists hold that, if one believes the family is competent, one does not enter its domain with the idea of long-term residence. Instead, one supports family members, restructures, builds on strengths, and attempts to leave them with the tools to continue, unaided, into the future. Likewise, one should enter a consultative relationship with the belief that the system at hand is intrinsically sound and possesses the competence to right itself, perhaps with only a little help from a friend. Thus, the consultant serves more as an agent of growth, and works under a time-limited contract. If consultants are effective, they succeed in obliterating their function and their position in the system.

I generally find it useful to start a consultation with parables and metaphors drawn from the area of competence of the person or people consulting me. This is then translated into a potential action within that area (a procedure that is very empowering), and then generalized to the subject or system about which consultation is requested. I encourage the consultees to design a course of action in their own way, even if it is not the way I would have done it. This design is then transferred to the system in question. Such approaches (1) take advantage of both the consultees' general knowledge and knowledge of the system, (2) reduce resistance because the adopted plan is primarily their own, and (3) allow them to accept primary credit for any beneficial change that does result.

There certainly are ways *not* to empower that will make the consultation a failure. For instance, the student learning to provide consultation frequently makes the classical error of attempting to enter as an "expert," saying, "The only way to handle this particular problem is my way, and you've made catastrophic mistakes so far." A related error is for the family-oriented consultant to believe that only he or she has the answer and, for example, to assert: "This is a specific family problem that only family therapists can resolve. Whenever you hit this particular problem, you will have to come to me because I'm the family consultant." A better approach would be to say, "You must see these problems over and over again. I'm sure you've learned an awful lot about how to deal with them. What are the things you've managed to do and what are the problems you've run into?" This approach immediately removes blame and relabels the problem as generic rather than specific. The more generic it gets and the more one identifies the consultees' particular areas of expertise, the more one empowers them, and the more able one is to exit rapidly.

The position taken thus far is different from what some family therapists consider to be "consultation." However, this may simply be a matter of terminology. Some forms of "consultation" may be more aptly termed "liaison." *The American College Dictionary* (1953) defines liaison as "a connection or relation *to be maintained* between . . . units, bodies, etc. [italics added]" (p. 702). In a liaison relationship, the specialist becomes a permanent part of the system, providing it with input from his or her own special area of expertise—like the neurologist who provides ongoing case advice to a cardiopulmonary unit. While a legitimate and often essential activity, liaison is obviously different from a consultation model aimed at getting in and out with the least amount of effort over the briefest period of time.

A major and unfortunately all too common error that a consultant can make is to imply that "I'm the only one who deals with this kind of problem, and you're going to need me forever." When I hear somebody imply that he or she expects always to be the consultant to a given service, or state that "I have been their consultant for 10 years," I think, "Why are you still there?" Optimally, one should be able to say, "I *was* a consultant to that group. They may, rarely, call me at intervals only when they get stuck with something new, and I say, 'Oh, this is a new problem. Let's see what you've done in the past and what we can add now.'" In other words, the error is in taking on long-term consultative commitments and presuming that one will be needed again and again. In fact, after a truly successful consultation—one in which the consultee has been provided with all the tools necessary to resolve new situations—the consultant should hope and expect never to be called again.

There is a parallel here with the sort of cradle-to-grave commitment that some therapies seem to espouse. If the consultant attempts to assume the decision making or the executive functions of an organization, that consultant has exchanged his or her original role for the role of executive or therapist. The concept of consultation implies a time-limited, temporary engagement, in which one enters and then departs. If one remains permanently inside, one has abused or abandoned the consultant role. A good therapist does not do that. One's first therapy session should begin with something like "Let's talk about the problems and how you see them, and how I see them. Let's see whether we want to work together, whether we're going to like each other. You are the experts on your own family. I'm a relatively uninformed stranger. Because I came from outside, I may have some ideas that you can use. But the strengths and ideas for change lie within your family." A tack such as this is easily transposed to a consultation relationship.

An important advantage of this type of consultation should be noted. If a consultant "consults" with an agency or system over an extended span of months or years, his or her capacity to affect and influence positively more than a very few agencies or systems is limited. A brief, impermanent approach, on the other hand, allows the consultant the time and freedom to help a considerably larger number of systems, thereby having a much more widespread impact on the society within which he or she works.

TRANSITIONAL MAPPING

Along with the presumption of system competence, it is usually helpful to recognize that the system to which one consults has a history, a future, and a legitimate raison d'être. While such notions are perhaps self-evident, holding them in mind can help one begin to determine what the system is having to contend with at present, where it is heading, and, therefore, how it may be most effectively helped. It is always legitimate to ask why the group, agency, or system is requesting consultation at this time. Why not 6 months ago, or 2 years hence? Where did it, or they, get off track? What changes have occurred to make things different? Are there subsystems in conflict and, if so, in what different directions are they moving? As answers to these questions materialize, the consultant can begin to implement a plan to get the system back on track—to mobilize its resources so it can continue at a more efficient level of functioning and in a direction of its own choosing.

It was in response to questions such as the above that I began to develop the approach of *transitional mapping* (Landau, 1982; Landau, Griffiths, & Mason, 1981; Landau-Stanton, 1985). Transitional mapping is a generic technique for both diagnosing a system and suggesting where the key point(s) of intervention might be; it is applicable to both therapy and consultation and is based on what I have called "transitional theory" (Landau-Stanton, 1985, in press), which concerns the intrasystem change from one status or state to another. A sociological example is the change from an agrarian to an urban society, with families moving from an extended to a nuclear form. This can happen instantly in some situations—either as a result of precipitous change or natural evolution—and it can happen slowly in others. When there are disparate rates of change among subsystems, with resulting asynchrony, dysfunction often results. Disparities develop between elements, that is, between individuals or subsystems, in which certain elements are not changing as fast as others. Thus we may get disparity between the individual and the family, or between the family and the context or culture.

Transitional theory is readily applicable to organizational consultation. For instance, if new managers come into a business system with a whole set of their own ideas and fail to look very carefully at the system (in a sense, fail to map it and work out who relates to whom, what the projected trends in the business are, what the level of financial return might be), they will be asking for trouble. If they do not clearly discern these processes, attending instead only to goals of their own that are totally different from those of others, they are going to get acting out, a possible breakdown of the system, and loss of profit. On the other hand, if they go in and analyze exactly how the system components are interrelated, assessing where the system is coming from and where it is going along all possible significant trajectories, they have a chance of success. Unless one knows the transitional pathway and the actual directional trend, "stuckness" will result. One needs to allow the system, or certain of its elements, to move backward a bit, and then perhaps forward, connecting both extremes simultaneously, because all movement in natural systems is in both, or many, directions. When one gets tremendous asynchrony, one gets huge pendulum swings from one polar extreme to the other, rather than natural growth. In a way it is like the stage of leaving home in the family life cycle (Haley, 1980) in which the parent pulls back and the young person desperately rushes out and fails. The movement is extreme and oscillatory, rather than gradual and recalibratory.

In this approach, one constructs a clear structural and directional map of the group with whom one is consulting, not just in terms of the families or groups that form the units of the system, but in terms of how those families or groups relate to each other, how they fit into the larger system, what the hierarchies are, and what the trends are. Whether it is a closed community, a surgical ward, a transplant system, a school system, a state service, or whatever, one maps it in terms of its transitional trends. How did that particular system originate and where is it heading in terms of service, of growth, of philosophy, of ideals? This model shares elements with some of the approaches used in sociology and anthropology. It asks: What are the basic modes of relating and the basic ideals, philosophies, and motivations of the group? What are the trends of change, and how did the group originate? Where are the ideals likely to take it? How much is this group influenced by its larger context? Is the cultural context pushing it in a particular direction? Is it a question of a new group evolving in a larger system? Where is the larger system going? How does the direction of the larger system affect this particular group?

The transitional map should encompass the whole organization as to subsystems, power structure, history, development, and culture. Both intended and potential directions for change are also indicated. Rigid or conservative and progressive or pioneering elements are included—these usually denote who is ready to change, who is in the transition between change–no change along the various trajectories, and so on. While there is not space here for a full explanation of transitional mapping (the reader is referred to the aforementioned references), a simplified example will be given in the section on "countering insularity."

APPLYING THE METHOD

INITIATING THE PROCESS

My general approach is not to seek consultation, or to reach out for it, but rather to wait for the system to make the first move. When I am contacted, there is often discomfort on the part of the requester, as if he or she feels embarrassed at not being able to solve the problem alone. My inclination at that point is to put the person at ease, assuring him or her: "This is a really tough situation that you couldn't be expected to deal with . . ." or "It's not surprising that you feel this way given how unreasonable the expectations are . . ." Essentially, I want to eliminate any notions the person may have that he or she is stupid or incompetent. I want him or her to feel supported and empowered because then he or she is more liable to take a chance on doing something different, if that is appropriate.

There are times when I break my rule about not reaching out. This usually occurs when I get a number of similar referrals from a particular person, agency, or neighborhood. In the first and second cases, this may indicate a dysfunction within the treatment system. The third case may be indicative of a problem in a community, neighborhood, or school system. In such instances I may contact the people running the system and bring the pattern I have observed to their attention. This must be done tactfully, and in a joining way, so that it can be perceived as helpful rather than critical. An example of such a situation with a mastectomy group is given later in this chapter.

INCLUSIVENESS

While there is often a natural tendency for the consultant to deal primarily with the person requesting consultation, the systems consultant should be aware of the myopia that can occur with this approach. Frequently the person with the "complaint" is at the nexus of competing, counterpulling subsystems within the overall system and has become immobilized. Dealing with this person exclusively is analogous to trying to treat a severely symptomatic member of a family alone—progress is difficult or impossible to make and is, at best, very slow. This person is not empowered by the system and is unable to empower others, remaining stuck and impotent to effect change. For this reason, I find it more efficacious to expand the system immediately, bringing in as many of the cast of characters as possible, in network fashion (Speck & Attneave, 1973). All are then included in the mapping process and the problem solving. Consulting with a group or a team in this way gives much more valuable information, allows a wider range of interventions, and introduces flexibility in terms of the kinds of change that may be possible. In particular, the consultant should beware of being exclusively linked to a "system pariah" who is unfavorably situated within the overall organization, because any moves the consultant makes from that position will invite the same reaction incurred by the pariah.

THE LINK APPROACH

Even when one does deal primarily with the requesting person, it is not always necessary to deal with a large group or a team. If one gets a proper sense of the system, one can approach the consultation with an adaptation of the *link therapy* approach (Landau, 1981, 1982; Landau-Stanton, 1985, in press). In this approach with families, the system is mapped and a "transitional" member—one who has access to all the subsystems and power leaders but is not firmly planted in one camp—is selected with whom to work. This person is then coached as a therapist or agent of change to his or her family.[1] The link concept can also be used with an organization.

Coping with mastectomy: A case example. A surgeon specializing in cancer called me and said, "I'm worried about a woman who has had a mastectomy and doesn't seem to be coping." I asked to meet with him about the case and then proceeded with psychotherapy. Subsequently, however, two similar cases were referred and, although I also commenced treatment with them, my antennae had, by that time, shot up. I requested a meeting with the surgeon, at which time I told him the trends I was seeing. Identifying with him, I asked, "What are you up against in your practice? What are your colleagues dealing with? What are the other resources that you use? Could we meet with the cancer association and see what they're providing for mastectomy patients?"

The surgeon and I then met with the person conducting a mastectomy group and all the other surgeons in the city who were doing mastectomies. We invited the radiotherapist and the head nurse from each inpatient unit, and we all considered what action might be indicated with this particular group of people. What they had been doing up to that point was convening a mastectomy group where the women sat and moaned to each other once a week. We redesigned the whole system, moving it into a multifamily group mode. We looked at what could be done in terms of helping prevent emotional difficulties around mastectomies. We first had to make the service people competent because they believed that these women were a dead weight and that there was nothing to be done with them and their classical, postmastectomy reactions.

After careful consideration, I decided that the surgeon was in a transitional position within the larger body, agreeing with aspects of both extremes, refusing to be pushed into a rigid position, and relating well to all concerned. At a meeting of the professionals and paraprofessionals, it became evident that this surgeon would serve best as leader of the group. I coached him as I would a link therapist (Landau,

1. See Landau-Stanton (1985) for a discussion of the clear differences between this approach and that used by Bowen (1978).

1981), to work with a team of selected representatives from the professional and paraprofessional groups involved in the treatment of mastectomy patients. I did some coaching beforehand and some of it in the meeting, as I would in family therapy, encouraging the surgeon to take charge and slowly coaching him until he took over. I did not have to go to all meetings. I was already empowering him and his group and moving myself out so that they could continue without me. What he then did was to get the others to decide what they would feel most competent doing. How could they work with this group of patients and feel really good about it? What did he and each of them dread about this mastectomy group? What was the pain of the group? What were the problems that were draining them? Each problem was then positively reframed so that it became more obvious what both the professionals and the mastectomy patients could do to become more competent. For the patients this meant bringing in their families and making a contribution to other cancer patients. From the multifamily group, a whole community service evolved, oriented to other groups of patients with cancer, laryngectomies, ostomies, and so on. By the time this had happened, I was out of the picture.

RETROGRESSION AND PROGRESSION

In the application of transitional therapy with families (Landau, 1982; Landau-Stanton, 1985, in press), one option is to attempt to move the families ahead in a "progressive" way vis-à-vis the overall society or context, for example, to get them to accept more flexibility in curfew hours for their teenagers, to learn the language in a new culture, and so on. The other major option is to help such families reconnect with the "old" ways, for example, by adhering to the time-honored prescriptions of their culture for dealing with problems. This is the "retrogressive" approach. It is sometimes chosen by rigid families because they feel safer with it. Later on, they may rise up, shake themselves, and move forward, perhaps going forward and backward through several cycles. By reconnecting them with both their past and their possible future, one enables them to make a choice. Usually they end up going in the direction that is most "natural" to them. However, whatever direction is selected, in the end the family must make the choice. A synchronization of the subsystems must occur. If the therapist arbitrarily attempts to select the final direction, perhaps even imposing himself or herself at the head of the system, he or she will be extruded by the family and efforts to bring about change will be ignored.

The decision to foster retrogression or progression—whether initially or at later stages in treatment—usually requires an understanding of the system in its broadest terms. Otherwise, the therapist can slip into a miscalculation. For example, sometimes in applying a structural intervention, the restructuring on its own may look absolutely perfect, and yet it does not take effect. In isolation, the intervention may appear appropriate, but it may not have been applied at the right point and in the right direction. This is particularly likely to happen if the family is not permitted to participate in the choice. When one constructs a larger map that includes more of the multiple systems involved, as well as details of where they have come from and where they may be going, that particular restructuring may be against the overall direction of change or contrary to the history and future of the transitional pathway. Thus the restructuring does not work. The same holds for consultation. Where the person most directly related to the potential change is not properly empowered, one tends to get many people, each feeling responsible for change, working at cross-purposes and creating a transitional conflict in which they actually heighten the asynchrony in the system. Without a proper overview, the consultant may err toward precipitating exactly the sort of symptomatology that one sees in a dysfunctional family system.

It is my experience that, in contrast to working with families, consultation with communities and large groups does not result in the selection of a retrogressive option. While they certainly have elements and subsystems that prefer retrogression, and such an option may be explicitly proposed by the consultant, progression finally wins out. This may be because, in consultations of this sort, I have endeavored to use the whole system, while specifically avoiding consultation with a particular individual. Where everyone is included, perhaps progression is the inevitable choice when the survival and well-being of the total system is at stake.

Death and dying: A case example. In 1967, I was asked to consult with a diverse group of clergy about death and dying. They had been feeling very hopeless as to what they could achieve. In the first meeting, I talked with them about the way they were handling this in their communities. They were still at the stage where death was handled as an isolated thing, where the minister counseled the family separately from the patient. As the discussion continued, it became more and more clear that the context of that particular community made an enormous difference in these clergymen's readiness to carry out a more systemic kind of consultational counseling around issues of death and dying.

I decided to map each aspect of the context separately with them—the historical development of the religious group, the way that they saw their role in society, the extent to which they had formed an isolated group, the direction they were moving, and so on. (At that time, the ecumenical movement had become infused with new vigor, and whether certain individuals were seeing themselves as moving more in an ecumenical direction made a tremendous difference, being reflected in the way that they were prepared to treat the individuals within a family.) As the process unfolded, the clergymen became enthusiastic and, by the end of the session, they had coalesced and decided to continue together as a group. They gained strength by understanding each other's philosophies. They became able to provide hope more easily and to define family goals that could be meaningful to the people they were counseling.

Interestingly, those people within the group who were moving toward an ecumenical bias were more amenable to working systemically in their own counseling systems.[2] The less ecumenical and more traditional members observed with interest what the others were doing, but shifted only slightly, generally holding to their previous position. Being able to observe without feeling judged themselves, however, allowed them to open up a bit and to understand what the others, whom they regarded as very radical, were doing.

As the meetings continued, several members initiated multifamily groups on death and dying. In response, the more traditional members tended to exclaim, "This is not for me. It's ridiculous. It's taking away all my power. You can't do this. It's like a circus. Dying is something between man and God." But they were still prepared to work with multifamily groups instead of dealing with members separately. This was preferable to feeling scared and incompetent. They did not shift as much as the more ecumenical group, but they did shift to including family members and persons from the community. Rigidity often results from a feeling of incompetence. If the helping leaders do not feel competent, they take on far more responsibility than is necessary. They almost become family members. However, once they see their own position in a broader context and in a context of change, rather than "this is where I'm stuck and I'm going to be stuck for a long time," they are able to move into a broader helping mode in which they use community resources and require less detailed control. Broadening and empowering them allows for change.

COUNTERING INSULARITY: SOME EXAMPLES WITH SELF-HELP GROUPS

In consulting with self-help groups in such areas as learning disabilities, postoperative cancer, inherited disorders, substance abuse, and mothers of twins, certain features stand out. One of these is the insularity that can develop. This can reach such extremes that dissolution of the group, or a major change in its charge, may be the most healthy result. Let us take the Mothers of Twins Association as a somewhat amusing example.

2. In the ecumenical movement, diverse churches share community activities, educational programs, clergy, and interdenominational fellowship. Frequently their efforts are directed toward overall social change.

Mothers of Twins: A case example. I attended the inaugural gathering of one of these groups as their guest of honor, being privileged to have twins myself. I found they were regarding themselves as some sort of rare, unique group. The feeling I had, in fact, was very similar to what I had experienced at the initial meeting of the Inherited Disorders Association—a semiprivileged, semipunished group. What struck me about both of these, and subsequently about a lot of other self-help groups, was their self-perception both of being a particularly prized piece of the community and also of being damned. In both ways, they felt isolated from the community. Being prized or being damned made them different, something of which they felt both scared and very proud. Such groups often start similarly. Commonly, one or two people feel that they are not coping. Hence they get together and make themselves special in order to compensate. Generally, though, they do not feel so special that they truly believe they are coping.

I never became a member of any of these groups. I remained a consultant. With the Mothers of Twins group, I was very careful not to join, but rather to say, "I have twins, but I don't feel the need to belong to a special group, because twins are also children," which was a small beginning toward moving them back into the community. These mothers had been emphasizing their differences and ignoring their similarities. In consulting with them, the thrust was toward first getting the people who had originally formed the group, the ones who were feeling (as with any other group) both empowered and incompetent, to become truly competent. These mothers could then aid the other members to be competent and reassimilate with the community. Up to that time, they had been involved in activities such as getting together and having their twins play with other twins, very much like the muscular dystrophy groups sometimes get their kids to play with other children with muscular dystrophy. My tack was to encourage them to come out of the isolation to which they had let their uniqueness carry them. The transitional choice these families were making was whether to continue the pathway toward dysfunction or to select a different direction. Consequently, I got them to question why had they come there, and to map out where they had come from and what some other alternatives might be in terms of a transitional pathway. Should they be making an impact on the community by asserting, "Look, we have twins. We therefore are unique and must be helped"? Or should they be working toward dispersion of their group and mobilization of larger parts of the community, which would both provide a service to others and fulfill their own needs? More specifically, to help the Mothers of Twins become aware that they had a choice of direction, and did not have to continue blindly along one route, I primarily used mapping, drawing a huge map on the board, and asking: Who are the people in this group who started the organization? Why did you do it? What were you hoping to gain from it? What were you scared of losing if you didn't have it? What are your fears and hopes? How do your parents and grandparents feel about it? What do you think your great-grandchildren are going to experience?

Where do you want it to lead? I did a lot of restructuring and reframing around the possible trend, drawing out the trajectory they were on and asking: What does this mean? Were the people who started the group specifically people who had felt they had a mission because they were producing twins like great-grandmother's twins? In some ways, this intervention amounted to a form of graphic consciousness-raising, forcing the whole group to come to grips with where they came from, why, and where they might (or should) go.

Mapping a Leader's System

For simplicity, rather than mapping the entire system of the Mothers of Twins (MOT) group, I will concentrate on the founder and show how her family's transitional conflict affected the group and its evolution. Because the map I arrived at illustrated some personal conclusions about the founder, this was generally not what I drew for the group, but rather the map I constructed for my own use in order to understand the system.

The group was essentially started by a clergyman's wife, who, it was later determined, had been using the group to maintain balance within a system that included her family and her husband's family, as well as the larger church community which he served. The stated goals of the group were fellowship, support, education, and making a contribution to future mothers of twins. The hidden agenda was to share the feeling of "specialness" and also to find an accepting peer group in other parents who struggle similarly. The clergyman's wife's personal agenda included creating an "elite" society in order to find acceptance outside of the congregation (her husband's) that had rejected her.

The stated purpose for the consultation was to teach the members how to raise twins, for example, by lectures and through being available to advise on child-raising decisions. The hidden purpose was for the group to have access to a professional who had already "coped" with raising twins. It was also anticipated that the consultant would fulfill the role of mother/grandmother to the group, and provide them with a stamp of understanding approval for their "not quite coping."

I projected several possible future directions (some of which were shared with the group):

1. Continuation of current direction: Group stays together forever. Clergyman is free to adapt to his own congregation with wife occupied elsewhere and not competing with him. Clergyman's wife helps him move into other sectors while she has her own area where she is both in authority and accepted. Consultant stays on forever as new members join and old members remain.

2. New direction by the wife: (a) Clergyman's wife is ordered by hus-

band to devote more time to their own community and she leaves the group, which collapses without her leadership. (b) Clergyman's wife drops out, but another strong leader with equal needs emerges and takes over—leading to a status quo situation of the group.

3. New group direction: Clergyman's wife and the rest of the group review their agenda, map out where they came from (how the group arose) and where they may be heading. This may lead to: (a) occasional lectures on educational topics; (b) occasional consultations on immediate problems; (c) moving the twins and their mothers back into the larger community; and (d) taking responsibility for helping new mothers of twins fit into the larger community so they no longer need an isolated group or regular consultations.

In obtaining a historical overview of the group and its primary leader, it was learned that the clergyman had moved from another country where he had been schooled by the traditional, patriarchal "Mother Church." When he arrived in this new environment, it was unclear whether he fit into the culture, what his place was within the church hierarchy because of his youth and inexperience, and how his philosophy meshed with or differed from that of his congregation. In addition, he and his wife had met and married soon after his migration. The congregation refused to accept the wife, who dressed in a very old-fashioned way with covered head and long-sleeved, high-collared garments. Her attempts to fit into the congregation also failed because she was seen, ironically, as too self-willed and modern in behavior. When their twins were born, the clergyman, feeling deprived of his wife's attention and unsure of the congregation's acceptance, diverted his energies to a new ecumenical movement. This left the wife feeling even more isolated, and she embraced the MOT movement wholeheartedly.

Thus, both the clergyman and his wife were caught in the transitional conflict between, on the one hand, rigid clerical traditions upheld by a conservative board of trustees, and, on the other hand, their youth and desire to become part of the ecumenical movement by dropping many of the traditions and becoming less insular and more modern. In addition, the clergyman's wife felt dissatisfied with her role as a patriarchal wife and wanted to join pioneering groups for women's rights. In her attempt to be accepted by her own community, she covered her head, hid her body, and appeared to be very religious; at the same time, she resisted her husband's authority and made a move to join a more open society. Thus, she oscillated between the extremes. The twins were both a burden and special, and they also provided a link to an admired great-grandmother who had had twins. They gave her the perfect justification for moving out toward a different group.

Regarding the MOT group, the members of the group, each with her own agenda, may have been seeking group support, forgiveness, and acceptance for producing a relatively unusual phenomenon. In some ways this is similar to people with a particular illness who band together against the world. The consultant should be careful not to encourage this. Instead, it is better to help the group create natural support networks within their extended families and communities—to mobilize the natural support system rather than create a permanent, artificial one, with its attendant consultant.

By mapping the trajectories of sociocultural change (e.g., movement toward matriarchy or parental equality in a traditionally patriarchal culture) as well as the trajectories of the clergyman's family, it became apparent that there were three possible outcomes: (1) more of the same, (2) retrogression for the clergyman's wife, with either more of the same or dissolution of the group, or (3) a shift by the clergyman's wife and family and by the group toward normalization and greater community contribution. These possibilities were presented to the group. The group, not the consultant, made a choice, opting for the third possibility. (As with most groups, and families, once the map is clarified, the third option is generally selected.) In this particular case, I subsequently learned, the clergyman and his wife moved still further along the transitional pathway and are now in partnership in business together. The group continues to meet occasionally for educational purposes.

As another example, I recently consulted to a group of service providers in substance-abuse programs in Holland who were undergoing a consolidation of state and city services. There was confusion and anxiety as to who was going to provide the services and how the two systems were to mesh. Eventually, the situation became so complicated that there had been talk of discontinuing the service altogether. We proceeded by mapping first the major system, then the people within it and their directions of transition, and finally by looking at how one could help them reach synchrony before the merger. We determined that when they merged, people should fit into a matrix rather than continuing the dysfunctional behavior that had led them to consider a merger in the first place. I later received a letter from the group informing me that they had managed to get the plan adopted and that it has been working.

In family treatment, once the family has made a transition and moved on, there is usually little reason to continue the therapy. Consulting with self-help groups is very similar. In contrast, the self-help group itself usually needs to implement a membership recruitment process with built-in continuity. Otherwise, the group will continue primarily to serve its original members, which would eventually lead to decline and dissolution.

INTERVENING AND EMPOWERING

Once one has derived a transitional map, one can design a specific kind of intervention aimed at the point of transitional conflict—the locus where the transitional conflict patterns keep repeating. This intervention must, of course, be tailored to the system and be the sort that less sophisticated leaders in the system can apply. As an example, the aforementioned cancer group was a collection of women who were feeling unloved, unwanted, and mutilated, and, therefore, not able to provide mothering and loving for their families. A simple strategic intervention here might be to assert to them that they themselves needed to be cared for before they could provide caring to others and that, therefore, their families, their community members, and their health workers should take extensive care of them. One "compresses" (Stanton, 1984) the "caring" to the point where they can say, "Hey, this is enough. I'm not a baby. I don't need to be an infant. I'm going to start providing for myself and others." Meanwhile, one has mapped out how the leaders (in this case the professionals) can help the consultees to minister to the community. The map gives one an overall perspective and aids in the choice of the point of intervention.

Regarding one's posture vis-à-vis the organization, it is strategically wise not to be seen as a "member." Better that the consultant remain an outsider so as not to be easily pre-empted or co-opted. In fact, the consultant would be well-advised to refer to himself or herself as a "stranger" rather than an "outsider," because the former term more readily connotes a need to learn.[3] Too often, consultants enter an organization to teach. I believe that *one can consult more effectively if one enters to learn.* For instance, in consulting with organizations such as the Catholic and Mormon churches, I immediately phone the appropriate bishop or archbishop as soon as a case is referred. My purpose is to ask for help and direction: What does he think is going on with this family? What should be done? These requests elevate this key person and establish his authority clearly. After all, he is going to have to deal with this and similar instances after I am gone. While I might make suggestions about what I think might work, I leave the decision up to him.

Making sex education infectious: A case example. I was consulted by the director of health for a large region. He had been asked to redesign for the schools the sex

3. The senior editor has told me that he and his wife developed a reputation for being skilled and understanding in dealing with black families primarily because from the beginning they emphasized their lack of knowledge and their need to learn (L. C. Wynne, personal communication, April 1984).

education and family-life curricula, topics that lay well outside of his areas of expertise. He had become director of that system because his particular field was infectious diseases. In such instances, one has to recognize that by the time somebody approaches one for consultation he or she is often feeling incompetent enough to request a consultation. However, like all of us, he or she is often very reluctant to admit incompetence. Similarly, it is not uncommon for students, when they are starting to consult, to compete with, rather than to empower, those with whom they consult.

In this particular case, I asked the director, "If you were having to set up a system for teaching in schools, or developing an education system around infectious diseases, how would you do it? Who are the people you would bring in to teach? Which of your staff would you use? Would you use the parents? How much of the community would you use? Would you use the kids and ask what their perceptions are?" I thus encouraged him to do his initial mapping in an area in which he was competent. This gave him confidence and he was able to transfer the vast knowledge that he already possessed to this new arena. From there, his final plan only needed a bit of fine tuning before the implementation process began.

This example readily illustrates the principles of competence, impermanence, and transitional mapping. The end result is that the consultee, and the system, are empowered. To empower or not to empower is never the question. For successful consultation, one must always empower. No system needs a permanent consultant. It primarily needs *itself.* The consultant who knows this can both eliminate and prevent dysfunction.

REFERENCES

The American college dictionary. New York: Harper, 1953.

Bowen, M. *Family therapy in clinical practice.* New York: Jason Aronson, 1978.

Caplan, G. *Principles of preventive psychiatry.* New York: Basic Books, 1965.

Haley, J. *Leaving home.* New York: McGraw-Hill, 1980.

Kark, S. L., & Mainemer, N. Integrating psychiatry into community health care epidemiologic foundations. *Israel Annals of Psychiatry and Related Disciplines*, 1977, *15*, 181–198.

Kark, S. L., & Steuart, G. W. *A practice of social medicine.* Edinburgh: Livingstone, 1962,

Landau, J. Link therapy as a family therapy technique for transitional extended families. *Psychotherapeia*, 1981, *7*, 382–390.

Landau, J. Therapy with families in cultural transition. In M. McGoldrick, J. K. Pearce, & J. Giordano (Eds.), *Ethnicity and family therapy.* New York: Guilford, 1982.

Landau, J., Griffiths, A. J., & Mason, J. The extended family in transition: Clinical implications. *Psychotherapeia*, 1981, *7*, 370–381.

Landau-Stanton, J. Adolescents, families and cultural transition: A treatment model. In M. D. P. Mirkin & S. L. Kolman (Eds.), *Handbook of adolescents and family therapy.* New York: Gardner, 1985.

Landau-Stanton, J. *The family in transition: Theory and practice.* New York: Guilford, in press.

Speck, R. V., & Attneave, C. L. *Family networks.* New York: Pantheon, 1973.

Stanton, M. D. Fusion, compression, diversion, and the workings of paradox: A theory of therapeutic/systemic change. *Family Process*, 1984, *23*, 135–167.

17

CONSULTATION WITH FAMILIES OF CULTISTS

MARGARET THALER SINGER
University of California, Berkeley

In recent years, families have sought help for a new problem—what to do when a son, daughter, or other relative appears to have undergone a relatively rapid and often drastic personality change as a result of affiliation with a group suspected of having unduly influenced that person (Clark, Langone, Schecter, & Daly, 1981; Delgado, 1977; West & Singer, 1980). Broadly speaking, these groups can be called cults. According to *Webster's Third New International Unabridged Dictionary* (1966), the term "cult" may convey one or more possible meanings: (1) a system for the cure of disease based on the dogmas, tenets, or principles set forth by its promulgator to the exclusion of scientific experience or demonstration; (2) great or excessive dedication to some person, idea, or organization; and (3) a religion or mystique ordinarily regarded as spurious and unorthodox. By "cultic relationships" we refer to those relationships in which a person intentionally induces others to become totally or nearly totally dependent on him or her for almost all major life decisions, and inculcates in these followers a belief that he or she has some special talent, gift, or knowledge.

In the late 1960s and the 1970s, parents were seeking help because a relative had entered one of the cultic groups often referred to as "New Age" or "New Movement" groups. More recently, families have been troubled about relatives who appear to them to have been drastically influenced by one of the human-growth or group-awareness organizations (Cinnamon & Farson, 1979; Ofshe, 1983; Singer, 1983; Tipton, 1982). Still others have relatives who have become enmeshed in pseudotherapy groups or involved with a person or persons who appear to be wielding undue influence over them (*SCP Newsletter*, 1984; Singer, 1983; Temerlin & Temerlin, 1982). Added to these are relatives concerned about young children who are being reared in cultic organizations. These relatives are primarily grandparents and separated or divorced spouses who have left the organization. Yet another new group includes whole families that have emerged from cultic organizations. By far the largest number seeking consultation are those families who have become alarmed at seeing a somewhat abrupt and marked shift in the social identity of a family member. They report noting a sudden personality change; a drastic change in goals, such as leaving school, a job, or a relationship; sudden attempts to transfer funds or personal possessions; or, more dramatically, the relative has dropped out of sight (Addis, Schulman-Miller, & Lightman, 1984; Clark *et al.*, 1981; Delgado, 1977; West & Singer, 1980).

These situations call for appraisal and consultation with families in order to help them realistically and legally deal with what they think has occurred. The term "therapy," which originally meant to nurse or cure, implies the presence of a condition that needs treatment. In contrast, the term "consultation" historically referred to a "gathering together" in order to seek technical or professional advice before planning or deciding something. The families of cultists usually do not seek family therapy. They are not asking for treatment of an internal condition but, rather, aid in dealing with an external organization or situation. Thus, they are seeking consultation, including information and advice, about their options and the reality of their concerns. The first stages of consultation are the gathering of factual information and observations from those involved and then helping them to define and understand the situation. This process will be outlined later.

SOCIAL IDENTITY AND INFLUENCE

A series of events in the past half century has highlighted how fragile social identity can be under certain circumstances and how easily human conduct can be manipulated under certain conditions. In brief, these events began with the Russian purge trials in the 1930s in which people were manipulated into both falsely confessing and falsely accusing. The world press expressed bewilderment and amazement at the phenomenon but, with few exceptions, soon lapsed into silence (Rogge, 1959). The late 1940s and early 1950s saw the effects of the Chinese revolutionary universities that subjected an entire nation to a thought-reform program in which millions were induced to espouse new philosophies and exhibit new conduct through psychological, social, and political coercion techniques (Chen, 1960; Hinkle & Wolff, 1956; Lifton, 1961; Mindszenty, 1974; Schein, 1961). Next came the Korean War, in which prisoners of war were subjected to an indoctrination program based upon methods growing out of the Chinese thought-reform program and combined with other social and psychological influence techniques. At that time the term "brainwashing" was introduced into our vocabulary.

Interest in human influence and manipulation subsided for the most part after a few years except for general academic curiosity and the ever-present reports of blatantly unethical or illegal influence techniques being brought to bear on persons in distant countries, or local frauds, confidence games, and undue-influence situations.

Then Charles Manson's diabolical influence and control of a group of middle-class youths shocked the world (Atkins, 1978; Bugliosi & Gentry, 1974; Watkins, 1979). Soon after, in 1976, the Symbionese Liberation Army kidnapped Patricia Hearst and manipulated and controlled her behavior (Hearst, 1982). By the mid-1970s, thousands of families in the United States were beginning to be puzzled and alarmed as they saw the influence of a vast array of new gurus, messiahs, and mind-manipulators on their offspring. On November 18, 1978, Jim Jones, through his controls and manipulations, led 912 followers to their death in a Guyana jungle (Reiterman & Jacobs, 1982). If Jonestown served no other purpose, it did serve to call attention to the extent of control one man could exert over his followers in the modern world. People could no longer ignore or downplay the existence and extent of such domination. They could no longer think that such control methods had existed only long ago or far away. Jim Jones's final hours of domination brought the concepts of influence, persuasion, thought reform, and brainwashing to the attention of the world. The many families who had sought help from state and national authorities because of the conditions they claimed existed within the People's Temple had not been listened to, for few people understood the totalistic control Jones held. One of the few who listened was Congressman Leo J. Ryan, who lost his life as a result of Jim Jones's last orders. Jones was not about to relinquish his mad control over the lives of those he dominated.

In the post-Jonestown world, thousands of families who had relatives in various other cultic organizations began to feel they might be heard when they described the control and influence they saw being wielded in various groups—religious, health, flying-saucer, and psychological cults. The first wave of families seeking consultation were primarily describing a phenomenon in which they had noted sudden personality changes in relatives who had become involved with some of the New Age religious and philosophical cults. But as Singer (1979a, 1979b) and West and Singer (1980) noted, throughout history the ever-present, self-appointed messiahs, gurus, and pied pipers appear to adapt to changing times. Thus we see a broadening of the possible realms into which persuaders will move.

More recently, families have been seeking consultation not only about cults but also for what, for lack of a better term, we shall call "cultic relationships," which include pseudogrowth and pseudotherapy groups, and "undue-influence" situations. An entirely new set of consultation problems are being presented by a number of families across the nation.

Here I am less concerned about whether or not a particular group would universally be labeled a cult. What is of interest are the properties of the relationship and the types of processes that go on between a group leader and his or her followers. In the past several years, families have been seeking consultation about groups and about relationships that cause them to question how much freedom of choice actually exists for followers, and how much initial information a new member was given about what would happen in the long run. Families are seeking consultation about the structure and impact of influence. As a shorthand convenience in this chapter, the terms "cult" and "cultic relationships," experiences in intensive indoctrination, and thought-reform programs will be used interchangeably.

The following case description illustrates undue influence in a cultic relationship situation that both resembles and differs from the more widely recognized involvement with established cults. This type of problem is becoming more frequent as the focus of requests for consultation from families.

A "diet cult": A case example. A young professional woman was asked by a casual acquaintance to participate in a "free, scientific, experimental weight control project." While vague, the description implied that scientists were providing new educational methods. Instead of attending lectures and continuing her independent life, she soon was flattered by the male and female leader into accepting their definition of her as a "natural clairvoyant healer" and "to go on course" with them. They induced her to sever ties with her family and friends, to leave her job, and to join their small "weight control program." Because she was not working, she eventually turned over her car, savings, and property to them in return for the "courses in natural healing" that they urged her to pursue with them.

Growing more obese by the day, as were the several other recruits, the woman moved with the group to an isolated small town where they lived with the two leaders and were persuaded not to write or contact families or friends who were said to be apt to "lower their consciousnesses" because outsiders were not privy to the "course." The course consisted of a 20-hour, daily routine filled with 4 to 5 hours of hypnosis and self-hypnosis exercises plus many periods of hyperventilation. She spent additional hours "in group" and she was taught to "speak in voices and to hear in voices." These were trainings in how to link, randomly but rhythmically, nonsense syllables into singsong patterns and to chant these aloud for interpretation by the female leader, who supposedly was "a natural knowing interpreter." After being given her interpretations for the day, the young woman was instructed to try to hallucinate what she had just heard as if it were coming from outside her head. That is, her remembrances of the "interpretations" were now to be "heard in voices." She was to learn to hallucinate and experience her own thoughts as if they were being heard through her ears. While attempting to accomplish this, she was berated, humiliated, and alternatively threatened with expulsion from the group or told she would have to "go on basic" again. While attempting to learn to hallucinate, she became psychotic. Her relationship with the group then ended and she was put on a bus with a ticket home to her parents.

The acute psychosis subsided after several days of hospitalization, but the woman remained in the hospital for 2 weeks. Her psychiatrist asked me to be a consultant during the hospitalization. He phoned the morning after her admission stating: "I've got a new kind of cult case. This group combines odd diets, speaking in tongues, isolation, sleep deprivation, hypnosis, and a lot of magical thinking. There is no religious angle; it's a diet cult." His description of what the patient had told him indicated that she had been in a cultic group and had been subjected to many stressful and bizarre processes. The psychiatrist asked that I meet with him and his patient to consult with them about the various activities of the group. He had told her that we had worked together on other occasions and that my knowledge of how various groups utilized Ericksonian-like trance-induction techniques and created verbal systems to block reflective thought might be of value. The psychiatrist had concluded that it was unlikely that the woman would have broken down if she had not been exposed to the stimuli of the group. In addition, he wished to hear me interview her and give my views. He told her to quiz me about my research to see if any of the studies of other groups applied to her experiences in her group. He wanted to use a consultant as a sounding board to test his perception of reality. Both the psychiatrist and patient wanted an analysis of the organization's techniques and contents and an opinion from me as to whether I thought the techniques might have contributed to her mental and emotional responses while in the group.

My role was a technical one—to learn directly from her more about the group's practices and to attempt to relate its procedures to my research on influence techniques if it seemed appropriate. As we proceeded, the psychiatrist commented on how much new material about the group she was providing, because the wording of my questions was helpful to her. He used consultation to help the patient see that her breakdown was understandable to him as her physician, and he hoped that it would be understandable to her as a kind of "reasonable" response to what she had been through. The consultant became a part of the "reality testing" her therapist was helping her to achieve. The many implications this use of consultation permits are vast and beyond what can be detailed here.

Upon release, the woman, her parents, and siblings were referred to me for further consultation. The psychiatrist told her family that it was his opinion that she would not have had a breakdown had she not been subjected to the bizarre routines and processes the group used. He further stated that he found the family to be warm and closely knit, "a kind of all-American family until she became involved with these diet-cult folks," and that he did not think that any of them needed treatment at this point.

Consultation with this family began by getting a clear picture of the woman's and family's immediate needs. All of them needed to talk about the cult because they were still in the dark about what had actually happened in the group. I joined in when needed to help explain certain effects. Further, the family had been frightened and bewildered at this woman's psychotic condition when she had been sent home by the cult. They wondered if it were all right to talk with her about her time in the group. Two meetings of 2 hours each, with the entire family (including two younger siblings), were held on successive days. During these sessions, the young woman explained details of many of the "processes" the leaders had used. The consultant helped this family understand the role of influence, hypnosis, and self-hypnosis in the change process to which the young woman had been exposed. The consultant also clarified for the family how her social isolation and dependency on the leaders after they had separated her from her past support systems had stripped her of her old identity. They had attacked her belief systems, both her belief in how the world operated and her own beliefs about herself and her values. Her past life had been "revised" by the cult leaders, who declared that her good relations with her family were to be denounced as "crazy dreams from your crazy childhood."

Consultation was an informational and educational process in which the woman and her family were assisted in discussing how the intensity and structure of her cult experiences appeared to have produced the exhaustion and dissociation that culminated in the acutely psychotic state she was in when the cult sent her home. Her mental state seemed to be a direct effect of the processes and combined stressors of the situation—including the beratings and her dependency on the cult leaders after losing her whole past view of herself and substituting their interpretations of reality. The consultant aided the family in making sense out of what had happened. The approach was to provide a transactional explanation rather than to ascribe her reaction solely to some inherent mental weakness.

The consultation closed with the young woman, the family, and consultant concluding that further therapy was not indicated at this time. This was in agreement with the thinking of the referring psychiatrist, who also felt that consultation, education, and finding a support system were preferable to further treatment.

After a period of time in which she greatly profited from sharing her experiences with other ex-cult members (a national network of persons who have been involved in one or another of the vast array of cults operative in the United States today), the woman again sought consultation. She reported that she was working in her profession, and was successful occupationally and socially, but that she was experiencing what she has termed "flashbacks." These appeared to be brief, dissociative episodes in which she felt depersonalized, dizzy, and anxious, that is, feeling as she often had while in the group. The fact that such episodes are a common aftermath of cult experiences was explained to her. Because she was soon moving to another part of the state and thought that the move might cause some unusual tensions, she was referred to a therapist in that area who was experienced in working with ex-cultists and those with dissociative problems.

A recent telephone call to her revealed that she had met with the therapist three times after she had experienced some periods when she "spaced out and got stuck"—her words for an Atypical Dissociative State (DSM-III, code 300.15; American Psychiatric Association, 1980) during periods of marked exhaustion and anxiety. The episodes were similar to those she frequently had had while in the cult. The therapist used behavioral and educational techniques analogous to those I, as the consultant, had offered to the woman. These taught her how to control the intensity and duration of the episodes so that they were only momentary phenomena and no longer caused her any alarm. She has now married, is functioning well in all areas of her life, and is a volunteer in a local cult clinic.

CONSULTATION OR THERAPY?

Reactions such as this woman's are not uncommon in persons subjected to similar treatment in cults and various intense indoctrination programs. Special approaches are needed in those relatively unusual cases in which the cult member has had a disturbed psychiatric history apart from the cult experience. Most often, the best treatment to effect a fast recovery for these people focuses on helping them properly attribute to the cult or indoctrination procedures the psychological and social pressures that overwhelmed them. They need to see that the behavior change or breakdown does not doom them to a life of fragility or a need to see themselves as weak or mad creatures. It is important to educate the ex-cultist and the family about how the indoctrination programs in intense confrontational groups produce the psychological and social effects that contribute to their changed behavior and occasional breakdowns. The focus is upon the impact and evaluation of such group processes.

This approach is not typical of the path taken in traditional therapy in which therapists wittingly or unwittingly assume that inherent, intrapersonal weaknesses of either a psychological or constitutional nature cause the breakdown or behavioral change. Such a therapy format demonstrates to the client that problems stem from internal needs and defects, and it directs the patient to seek hidden motivations and weak internal properties of the self without properly conceptualizing the context, the external factors, and the system within which the breakdown or behavior change occurred. A better perspective is that which has been effective in working with victims of many kinds—victims of kidnapping, violent crimes, natural disasters, and victims of thought-reform programs. Many victims of violence and coercion need help in seeing that their symptoms arose out of their responses to intense, external stressors. They should not leave the consultation or therapy feeling that they were uniquely fragile in the face of the duress or highly unusual circumstances that existed in a group situation.

Whether a family seeks consultation during the period of involvement or after a member has left a cultic relationship, some form of the general educational, consultative format described above is useful. However, few professionals or agencies have addressed these special needs of families of cultists. These families are faced with a perplexing and unusual problem that has arisen between them and an outside force. They seek specific information, concrete guidance, and advice. This outside influence has so affected one of their members that the conduct, demeanor, and personality of that person has changed to such an extent that they no longer know how to deal with him or her. Often that member may have disappeared and they have no knowledge of where to locate the relative. The majority of these families, until the entry of a member into a cultic relationship or organization, have been ordinary, normal families—not necessarily ideal or free of difficulties, but average families.

Therapists often ask: "How is consultation with families of cultists different from therapy with families in general?" This question requires several answers. The first is that therapy is a procedure therapists engage in with families who usually say, in effect, that something "internal" in our family system is not working; help us fix "our" system. The families of cultists are saying, help us deal with an "outside" system in which one of our family has become enmeshed. The families of cultists need a great amount of input from informational and assistance networks. Such information can be provided by the consultant, as well as by suggested readings and referrals to local, national, or international parent and ex-member networks, and to law enforcement and other agencies when indicated. The consultant is in the role of a broker or triage person. That is, based on the best available information, the consultant makes a tentative assessment, informs and directs the family to the next stage of procedures if they agree with the plan, and remains available for further consultation at different junctures in the subsequent efforts at problem solving, which may include ex-cultists and parents of ex-cultists if indicated.

Many professionals are unaware of cultic practices and thought-reform programs and falsely assume that anyone who becomes involved in these programs is merely acting out teenage rebellion or, if not, must have a severe personality disorder or an "ambulatory psychosis," or be some type of markedly impaired person. Such practitioners are both uninformed and harmful because they often delay families from locating proper help early.

Professional assessment failure: A case example. Two children, aged 10 and 12, were taken by a drug-using, bizarre, charismatic street person into his small cultic group. Their parents were told by three consecutive therapists that the children were merely "doing pre-teenage rebelling" and the parents needed to allow the children "to individuate." The parents were persuaded to embark upon couples therapy by each of these professionals. None directed the parents to the proper legal authorities. When this was done by a cult expert whom the parents contacted after several years had passed, swift and helpful action was taken and the children were located and restored to their parents by the police. Needless to say, by that point the children needed some appropriate professional assistance, which was provided along with consultation with the rest of the family.

The general format followed by cult consultants begins with a history-gathering period in which it is determined what group or persons the missing member is with, for how long, what contact, if any, has been made, how it went, what the family would like in the way of help at this point, and what their hopes and plans are. An outline is made of how they and the consultant and others will proceed. The consultant needs to have available reading materials on specific cults, lists of material available in libraries, bookstores, and from cult-information agencies. A general outline is made of the social and psychological influence mechanisms used in thought-reform programs and cultic relationships (Addis *et al.*, 1984; Hinkle & Wolff, 1956; Lifton, 1961; Ofshe, 1983; Schein, 1961; Singer, 1983; West & Singer, 1980). These group processes are discussed and linked to the concrete experiences that the family or former cultist has related. The family is helped to learn about psychological and social influence techniques that may have been involved in their relative's behavior. They are assisted in getting continuing network assistance, such as meeting with ex-members of the same group, who often have specific instructions about the best ways to communicate with persons in the group. When indicated, they are given addresses of local, national, and international parent-support networks and informational agencies.

The role of the consultant varies with each family, and the multiple contingencies that may arise cannot be delineated here. A thorough history of the cultist is always obtained to determine how stable or unstable that person had been in the past and what is known about their present physical health and mental status. For example, a mother described her adult son as severely malnourished, mute, and unable to leave her house. However, the cult leader was phoning the son and badgering him to return to the group even though he was reported to be too feeble to leave the house. The consultant recognized the emergency nature of the son's condition and put the mother in touch with a psychiatrist in her area who, upon making a house call, arranged for an ambulance transfer to a hospital.

Most of the above remarks describe my work as a single practitioner. A team approach is used by a Los Angeles agency that has developed a cult clinic for families (Addis *et al.*, 1984). Since early 1979, this clinic has primarily used teams of volunteers, psychiatrists, social workers, attorneys, ex-cult members, parents of present and former cult members, and a mental health administrator. A full-time professional conducts an initial intake interview with the family. This person assigns certain families to meet with individual volunteers if the problems of the family are severe. Otherwise, most families participate in group sessions. These sessions focus on education and problem solving. Staff ex-cult members and staff parents of cultists share their experiences with the new families. Cult recruitment methods and the processes used in inducing behavior changes are discussed. The objectives are to help the families gain perspective, understand what strategies and options are available, mobilize the family, and attract the cult member's attention. Addis *et al.*, (1984) point out that these objectives are achieved over a period of time and are not instant solutions.

The staff meets before each group meeting to share information about the families that will attend. This insures continuity and coherence. In the interval between meetings of the large group, individual contacts sometimes occur between a family and a staff person because of outside developments with the cultist members. The staff person shares this information in order to keep the group abreast of developments and to help direct the consultation–education meetings that ensue.

When local cult consultants are not available, it is useful for family therapists to locate a network of ex-members and parents of former members to co-consult with him or her and families of cultists. Reviewing the literature is also helpful for formats and techniques to use with families (Addis *et al.*, 1984; Andron, 1983; Clark *et al.*, 1981; Dellinger, 1982; Etemad, 1978; Goldberg & Goldberg, 1982; Singer, 1979a; West & Singer, 1980).

RECENT TRENDS

Earlier it was noted that changes have occurred in the type of cultic groups about which families seek consultation. In the mid-1970s, families sought assistance primarily in dealing with relatives who had become involved with new religious groups. Recently, there has been a burgeoning of occult, psychotherapy, and prosperity groups.

There has also been a shift in who is coming out of cults. Instead of young adults emerging after a period of time in a cult, we now have children, teenagers, and young adults reared in cultic groups who often emerge into the general society in need of special assistance. These individuals often have had limited age-appropriate contact and experiences with the larger society, or quite unusual experiences that may ill-equip them for life outside the group.

The aftermath of cult child rearing: A case example. One young man, taken into a group by his parents at an early age, ran away from the group at age 21. He hid out with other, older ex-members who were also afraid the group would seek them out and attempt to make them return. They helped him get a laboring job and suggested he see me. He was overwhelmed by his lack of knowledge about the outside world. He did not know how to rent a room, get a telephone, start a bank account, get a driver's license, and lacked knowledge of other simple skills. All these had been taken care of by the cult hierarchy. He was embarrassed to let his employers and new friends know that he was as "uninformed as a Martian," to use his terms. My consultant's role consisted of determining that he was neither seeking nor needing therapy. He needed education, explanations, and a support system. I helped him contact some ex-cultists of his own age who were glad to assist him and quickly walked him through all the new places and procedures he needed to learn.

Entire families are now exiting from certain cults with young children who have been taught habits far afield from the mores of the outer society. Some families have sought consultation in person; some have phoned for advice and guidance in how to retrain their children. Usually these families have left cults in which incest and child-sex activities had been practiced. Once out of the cult, the parents easily return to their precult behavior, but find themselves with young children who have seen and been taught behaviors that are taboo in the outer world. Consultation focuses on clearly delineating those behaviors that have been carried out in the cult but are not practiced outside. It is suggested that the parents tell the children that they had lived by the outside standards until joining the group Now they are bringing the children and themselves back into the outside world where the parents really want to live and have their children grow up. Out here there are different rules, and they are easy to learn. A clear-cut break with the cult rules and an avoidance of guilt-inducing explanations works well over time.

Siblings of cultists are a neglected group. When teaching and lecturing, I have asked certain siblings of former cultists to appear along with the ex-member and parents to inform other families of how neglected a sibling can feel during the months or often years that a family's attention has been focused almost solely on the cultist.

As social and economic climates have changed, so has the nature of some cultic organizations. Recently, families are seeking help in dealing with relatives caught up in psychotherapy cults in which either professionals have gone astray and have multiple relationships with clients and patients, or nonprofessionals start "therapy" groups. In both instances, cultic relationships have occurred and the therapists or pseudotherapists have become the landlords, employers, financial advisers, and lovers, having "patients" move in and live with them, perform household chores, and turn in pay checks to the leader (Singer, 1983; Temerlin, 1982).

A number of occult cults have sprung up. But with the tightening of the economy, the largest number of new cultic relationships that have appeared seem most to resemble purely financial scams. Somewhat charismatic schemers using a "psychological" or a "prosperity-minded" philosophical content entice young working adults to move into a group living situation run by the leader. The leader usually "psychologizes" about trust, integrity, and other virtues, using the vocabulary and experiential exercises of the human potential movement and encounter groups. These techniques keep members dependent on him or her in continuing relational and living arrangements. Eventually the conditions resemble those in the well-known cults. These cult members drop contact with their family and old friends, put all free time and money into the "group," drop their career, and work at low-level jobs with hours that permit more time with the leader and group and less with the outside world. The personality changes originally seen in members of exotic cults now are reported in these persons living in the smaller cultic groups.

OVERVIEW

The role of the consultant to families of cultists is first to assess the immediate informational and support-system needs of the family and to see that the family begins to receive this information and guidance.

Different approaches need to be taken in those instances in which the cult member appears to have had a poor psychiatric history before and/or since being in the cult. These families are relatively few and need special assistance. However, all families looking forward to the possible emergence of a relative from a cult need to begin to plan among themselves for their roles in assisting the reentry of the cultist into everyday life when that person exits from the group. Concrete issues such as where these persons will live, how they will support themselves, and what educational or vocational plans need to be considered ahead of time, should be dealt with by the consultant because families, in their haste to rescue a relative, may fail to plan ahead.

Without being a purveyor of doom, the consultant should also warn families that a certain number of cultists may never leave groups; this possibility should be considered as one possible outcome no matter what is hoped.

Because this is a new area of family consultation, it behooves the practitioner to know when to call on cult specialists. These specialists can usefully direct practitioners to selected readings and help them contact local, national, and international groups interested in research and consultation on cults, undue influence, and persuasion issues.[1] Generalists, it is hoped, will become more fully informed about group influence and cultic phenomena, and thus may become more able to consult directly and effectively with families of cult members or, alternatively, know when to refer these families to specialists.

REFERENCES

Addis, M., Schulman-Miller, J., & Lightman, M. The cult clinic helps families in crisis. *Social Casework*, 1984, *39*, 515–522.

American Psychiatric Association. *Diagnostic and statistical manual of mental disorders* (3rd ed.; DSM-III). Washington, DC: Author, 1980.

Andron, S. *Cultivating cult-evading: A teacher's guide.* Miamı, FL. Central Agency for Jewish Education, 1983.

Atkins, S., with Slosser, B. *Child of Satan: Child of God.* New York: Bantam Books, 1978.

Bugliosi, V., & Gentry, C. *Helter skelter.* New York: Bantam Books, 1974.

Chen, T. E. H. *Thought reform of the Chinese intellectuals.* New York: Oxford University Press for Hong Kong University Press, 1960.

Cinnamon, K., & Farson, D. *Cults and cons: The exploitation of the emotional growth consumer.* Chicago: Nelson-Hall, 1979.

Clark, J. G., Jr., Langone, M. D., Schecter, R. E., & Daly, R. C. B. *Destructive cult conversion: Theory, research and treatment.* Weston, MA: American Family Foundation, 1981.

Delgado, R. Religious totalism: Gentle and ungentle persuasion under the first amendment. *Southern California Law Review*, 1977, *51*, 1–98.

Dellinger, R. W. *Cults and kids: A study of coercion.* Boys Town, NE: Boys Town Center, 1982.

Etemad, B. Extrication from cultism. *Current Psychiatric Therapy*, 1978, *18*, 217–223.

1. A number of well-established parent and ex-member networks and agencies provide information about cults and related group processes: Citizens Freedom Foundation, P. O. Box 86, Hannacroix, NY 12087; the American Family Foundation, P. O. Box 336, Weston, MA 02193; Family Action Information and Rescue, BCM Box 3535, P. O. Box 12, London WC1N 3XX, England; Spiritual Counterfeits Project, P. O. Box 4308, Berkeley, CA 94704; Cult Education Program, International B'nai B'rith, 1640 Rhode Island Avenue, N.W., Washington, DC 20036; and Youth Program Director, Central Agency for Jewish Education, 4200 Biscayne Boulevard, Miami, FL 33137.

Goldberg, L., & Goldberg, W. Group work with former cultists. *National Association of Social Workers*, 1982, *27*, 165–170.

Hearst, P., with Moscow, A. *Every secret thing.* New York: Doubleday, 1982.

Hinkle, L. E., & Wolff, H. G. Communist interrogation of "enemies of the state." *Archives of Neurology and Psychiatry*, 1956, *76*, 115–174.

Lifton, R. J. *Thought reform and the psychology of totalism: A study of "brainwashing" in China.* New York: W. W. Norton, 1961.

Mindszenty, Josef Cardinal. *Memoirs.* New York: Macmillan, 1974.

Ofshe, R. *Second generation thought reform programs.* Address to Citizens' Freedom Foundation, Los Angeles, October 29, 1983.

Reiterman, T., & Jacobs, J. R. *Raven: The Untold story of the Reverend Jim Jones and his people.* New York: E. P. Dutton, 1982.

Rogge, O. J. *Why men confess.* New York: Thomas Nelson & Sons, 1959.

Schein, E. H. *Coercive persuasion.* New York: W. W. Norton, 1961.

SCP Newsletter. An interview with Dr. Margaret Thaler Singer. *Spiritual Counterfeits Newsletter*, 1984, *10*.

Singer, M. T. Coming out of the cults. *Psychology Today*, 1979a, *12*, 72–82.

Singer, M. T. Cults: What are they? Why now? *Forecast for Home Economics*, 1979b, *9*.

Singer, M. T. *Psychotherapy cults.* Address to Citizens' Freedom Foundation, Los Angeles, October 29, 1983.

Temerlin, M. K., & Temerlin, J. W. Psychotherapy cults: An iatrogenic perversion. *Psychotherapy: Theory, Research and Practice*, 1982, *19*, 131–141.

Tipton, S. M. *Getting saved from the sixties.* Berkeley: University of California Press, 1982.

Watkins, P. *My life with Charles Manson.* New York: Bantam Books, 1979.

Webster's third new international unabridged dictionary. Springfield, MA: G. Mc. Merriam, 1966.

West, L. J., & Singer, M. T. Cults, quacks, and nonprofessional psychotherapies. In H. I. Kaplan, A. M. Freedman, & B. J. Sadock (Eds.), *Comprehensive textbook of psychiatry* (Vol. III, 3rd ed.). Baltimore: Williams & Wilkins, 1980.

18

SYSTEMS CONSULTATION WITH AGENCIES DEALING WITH DOMESTIC VIOLENCE

HARLENE ANDERSON
Private Practice
Boston, Massachusetts
Galveston Family Institute
Galveston, Texas

HAROLD GOOLISHIAN
Galveston Family Institute
Galveston, Texas

Consultation with agencies is an intricate dance. When you add the very difficult problems of family violence, the dance becomes even more intricate. The methods and techniques of consultation with agencies working with family violence must be individually tailored to the structure of that agency, to the agency's role and definition in the total network of community services, and to the particular problems defined by the agency and its staff in their work with clients, families, and other agencies.

In general, agencies request consultation from a family therapist or other professional when staff intervention has not succeeded in meeting agency or client goals, in other words, when the client–agency system is "stuck." Successful consultation from a systemic view must avoid the stuckness that led to the request for consultation. Central to success is the consultant's ability to operate in a complex interactive system having input from a multitude of conflicting realities. The consultant must develop a systemic position that avoids collusive "side-taking" in order to maximize information exchange and potential for change. The consultant is, after all, being asked to assist the staff in bringing about these changes that they (the agency and staff) desire.

Consultation is not the process of supervision. It is, rather, the process of assisting agencies and their staff in the struggle to accomplish their work in an effective and efficient manner. It must not involve "taking over" by the consultant in ways that disempower the consultee; it is ordinarily limited to those inputs and activities effective in overcoming impasses and blocks to effective treatment and counseling.

In our view, the practice of consultation parallels the practice of therapy and differs only in the point of application, that is, in who is involved in the direct consultative activity. Just as the task of the therapist is to influence change with a family vis-à-vis its problem, the task of the consultant is to influence change in regard to the problem defined by an agency. Consultation can include addressing intra- and interagency interface problems, agency–board and broader community-related problems, program or subgroup problems within an agency, or work with a single staff member or a team in the management of a particular "stuck case."

This chapter presents examples of our consultation experience with agencies that came to us with problems and the ways in which we as consultants positioned ourselves to be of service to the total treatment system.

KEY ISSUES IN CONSULTATION WITH AGENCIES DEALING WITH DOMESTIC VIOLENCE

Key issues that the systems consultant must recognize in order to achieve a metaview and to facilitate an effective working relationship with those agencies working with family violence include (1) cultural myths, stereotypes, and negative biases; (2) complications of multiple systems; (3) development of resistance in the referral process; (4) dualistic and hierarchical structure of agencies; (5) implicit and explicit messages conveyed by the identity of the agency system; and (6) processes of client and problem identification.

Problems in management of family violence occur within at least three levels of systems: the individual level, the family level, and the societal level. Depending upon the observer's position, these problems traditionally have been viewed as occurring within only one of these levels. On the *individual level*, family violence is considered a symptom that results from a defect in the individual's psychological makeup. When viewed at the *family level*, it has been considered to be representative of pathology of the family organization and structure. On the *societal level*, family violence usually is viewed as pathology associated with a particular socioeconomic class or sex-role learning.

We view the problem of family violence from a framework that includes all three system levels as interrelated, not as separate entities, and believe it must be viewed as a symptom of stressful relationships in, between, and among these three systems. People within each of these systems usually have different views of reality regarding the nature, cause, and remedy of family violence. The domain of family violence becomes even more complicated once it broadens to include agency systems. The same can be said for the entry of a systems consultant with family therapy experience. Both the agency system and the consultant enter with additional views of family violence and what should be done about it, adding more elements to an already complex issue. When people hold different views, each feeling his or her own view is the total reality, struggles will surely ensue. These multiple views may totally block the capacity of one member of the system to communicate with another as they begin to try to negotiate a working relationship and to validate their positions vis-à-vis the problem. This process can maintain and escalate the very problems they are trying to remedy. A tug-of-war can ensue.

Consultants must develop a metaview of these multiple points of view, or they will become just another struggling part of the dysfunctional system in which each subsystem is trying to establish the validity of its partial view and understanding. Without a metaview, the consultant participates in the maintenance or worsening of the interactions around the problems.

Although these key issues are addressed separately in this paper, in reality they are by no means discrete entities. They are interwoven issues.

CULTURAL MYTHS, STEREOTYPES, AND NEGATIVE BIASES

Problems within the realm of family violence are embedded in a myriad of cultural myths, stereotypes, and negative biases. They cross the boundaries of many cultural, political, moral, and economic arenas. It is important for the systems consultant to understand these pervasive perceptions of family violence and their implications for the family and the agency.

In our society, family violence stigmatizes the family and is often associated with minority groups and with chaotic, low socioeconomic families. It is almost always viewed from moralistic points of view. Many of the labels used by agencies and other "helpers" to describe those involved in family violence are pejorative and gender biased.[1] Participants in family violence are commonly described by such labels as "victim" and "victimizer." Women involved in family violence are characteristically defined as victims and stereotyped as lacking self-confidence, fearing abandonment,

1. The term "helpers" refers to all those involved in trying to change an individual family member or the family and can include, among others, extended family, friends, neighbors, physicians, school personnel, ministers, and community agency staff.

and needing to be subservient and exploited. They are often blamed for provoking the abuse, for "asking for it"; they are thought to create their own victimization. Men are usually stereotyped as victimizers who lack self-control, who need to dominate, and who lack respect for women. Both the women and the men are frequently described as unmotivated and resistant to treatment.

Agencies reflect these same cultural myths, biases, and stereotypes vis-à-vis policies, regulations, funding sources, and the attitudes and belief systems of individual staff members. In viewing family violence as a disease or symptom of an individual family member or of the family, agencies fail to recognize it as a macrosystemic as well as microsystemic problem. Clinical classifications, such as child abuse, battered wife, and family violence, suggest overly simplified models of etiology (Daniel, Hampton, & Newberger, 1983). The complicated nature of the problem is obscured by this nosological simplicity; and, in turn, issues such as poverty and social isolation and their relationship to stressful family relationships are masked (Daniel *et al.*, 1983).

Stereotypes also have a constraining influence on the agency staff's ability to manage and treat families involved in family violence. The majority of families these agencies work with are from a multiproblem, low-income, socially disorganized strata of the population. In contrast, the staff usually reflect value-laden, middle-class views. Thus, staff members who stereotype individuals and families according to their own socioeconomic class and fail to see the uniqueness of each situation must be made aware of these cultural myths, stereotypes, and negative biases, and the ways in which they influence and hinder the agency's capacity and ability to work with the problems of family violence.

The unattractive couple: A case example. A therapist requested consultation with a case that was a court-ordered referral for family therapy. The referral was part of the conditions of a probated sentence for a husband who had abused his wife and children. The therapist interviewed the man, his wife, and their three children once. In her description of the interview, she portrayed the man as extremely upset at being there, to the point of becoming belligerent at times. The wife was passive and the children's behavior was chaotic. The therapist particularly focused on the family's physical appearance. The husband was quite vividly described as seedy, weighing at least 300 pounds, and wearing shirtless overalls that revealed rolls of fat. The wife was described as missing her front teeth and looking as though she needed to be laundered from head to toe. From the therapist's presentation of the case it was apparent that she felt disgusted and intimidated by this family, particularly by the husband. She felt in a bind; although she saw the family, and especially the husband as totally untreatable, she had to see them because of the nature of the referral.

We were aware that the therapist's stereotype of this family as undesirable and untreatable was not only handicapping her work with them, but also making an already difficult situation worse. Although the consultation could have many dimensions as a first step, it would be important for us to avoid viewing the case from any position that would continue to stereotype the family. Stereotyping would only handicap and immobilize us just as it did the therapist.

In our consultation, we avoided focusing on the descriptive characteristics of the family and the content of the interview. Instead, we focused on the context of the referral and the therapy interview. We felt that an understanding of the context of the husband's "resistant position" would help the therapist alter her view of both the husband's and the family's behavior, thus freeing her from her own "resistant position."

As a result of the consultation, the therapist was able to view the husband's position as not totally reflective of inherent personality characteristics, and also as a fairly predictable response for a man who felt unfairly treated by the legal system, suspicious of a therapist he viewed as working for the courts, and fearful of losing his wife and children. The therapist later reported that she not only found herself in less of a struggle with this family, but also felt she was even beginning to like the husband.

COMPLICATIONS OF MULTIPLE SYSTEMS

It is vital for the family therapy consultant to understand the importance of those people outside the immediate family who are intensely involved in the family's problems (Goolishian & Anderson, 1981; Imber Coppersmith, 1983), particularly the influence these multiple relationships can have on the family as they consult with agencies around the issues of assessment and treatment. The family therapy consultant must help the agency to become aware of this issue while at the same time understanding that the agency itself may also be an invested member of the multiple systems.

When identified clients, whether an individual family member (child or adult) or a whole family, seek help from outside their own systems, they usually enter a multiagency system. Immediately they can become clients of two or more agency systems and find, more often than not, that each agency's view of the problem and goal is different from, and perhaps contradictory to, the other agencies' views. For example, the family as a unit can simultaneously become a client of a particular legal system, a child welfare system, and a women's shelter system through just one telephone call to the police or a crisis hotline. To complicate the situation even more, it is not unusual for the individual or the family to have one or more staff members (or program units) of each agency working with them, depending upon the agency's mission and the intricacy of its internal organization. Communication and cooperation between the participating agencies are often inadequate or even nonexistent, leading to a situation similar to the classic story of the blind men who try to describe the elephant according to what part of the elephant they are feeling. It is also not unusual for individual members of a family to be a client of different agencies. For example, it would not be atypical for the man to be the primary client in a legal system, the woman in a women's shelter system, and the child in a child welfare system. The result at the agency level and the interagency level is a fragmentation of services and, often, competition.

This complicated, inclusive ecosystem may seem to contradict the common belief that families involved in family violence tend to be isolated. What is important is that families are no longer isolated systems by the time they reach the attention of the courts and community agencies. Any attempts of the family members to isolate themselves because of the sensitive and embarrassing nature of the problem are interrupted by those people in the larger system who are trying to help. By the time a family therapist is approached to serve as a consultant, the domain of the problems he or she confronts can include several of these helpers, including the family-violence agency, program units within it, and its staff members. All have the same goal in mind: resolution of the problem and achievement of peace. However, each has a different view of the problem and different means of reaching the goal. The consultant must understand the importance of the total system context in which problems evolve, including the power of differing views and the difficulties that can occur when they meet, and remember that these differing views in and of themselves can maintain and escalate a family's problems (Auerswald, 1968; Hoffman & Long, 1969).

A devil of a case: A case example. We were asked to consult with a family therapy team at a child guidance agency. The team was in a struggle with a referral source around the issue of who in the family should be treated and how.

A church counselor had referred the family out of concern that the mother was disciplining her three preschool children to the point of physical abuse. She understood the problem as the mother's response to being "left alone" to care for the children at home while her husband worked two jobs, which kept him unavailable for any support other than financial. Her proposed "solution" was for the team to support the wife in convincing the husband to give up his second job and spend more time at home with her and the children. The counselor, having herself failed in efforts to do this, hoped that the team would be better able to achieve this result.

After an initial appointment was scheduled, but before the family was seen, the team received another referral on the same family from a caseworker at a children's protective service. This worker informed the team that the mother had been reported by a neighbor for child abuse. The mother had told this neighbor that the children were out of control because "the devil was in them" and God had told her that she would need to "beat the devil out of them." The caseworker tried to reason with the mother, to explain that she was under severe stress and that God was actually not saying these things to her. The more the caseworker tried to reason with her, the more the mother "talked crazy about God and the devil," verifying the caseworker's belief that the woman was indeed "crazy." The caseworker, knowing that the church counselor had been counseling the mother, was also convinced that the counselor, in her view not a legitimate mental health professional, was probably making the woman crazier because the counselor herself was associated with the church and was negligent in not having reported the child abuse. The worker related that she had strongly recommended to the mother that she should be counseled only by the family therapy team because they were experts in child-abusing families. On the day of the appointment, the caseworker again called the team and reiterated her impression of the mother and of the need for intensive work with the family. She further stated that if the mother did not stop the "crazy talk about the children, the devil, and God," she would have to remove the children from the home for their own protection while the mother and the family received therapy.

When the therapy team initially saw the family, they learned that the husband believed that he was doing the best he could by holding down two jobs in order to financially support his family. He saw his wife as being overly involved in church activities to the point of neglecting him, the children, and the house. The wife expressed concern about her children's behavior and stuck to her belief about the influence of the devil and the guidance of God.

The team's view of the family's present problem was that the church counselor and the caseworker were interfering, thereby escalating the parents' stress and blocking the team's joining moves. Team members had fruitlessly tried to convince both women to withdraw from the case and allow the team to handle the family alone. As the referrers had hoped the team would be more powerful than they at achieving the referrers' goals for the family, so did the team want us, as consultants, to use our power and authority to achieve the team's goals: disengaging the referrers from the family.

The consultants suggested to the team that perhaps it was unrealistic to imagine that the two referrers, who were so obviously invested in this family, would not continue to be involved. Whatever might be best for the family, it was abundantly evident that the team's efforts to decrease the referrers' involvement had consistently resulted in increased involvement. Such efforts could only result in escalating struggles between helpers, not more effective help for the family. A more effective harmonious result could be achieved by the team's respecting and emphasizing the importance of the referrers' roles with this very difficult family.

We recommended that the team schedule a meeting with the referrers in which the importance of their input would be emphasized, particularly the ways in which each of their differing positions in relation to the family offered invaluable data for designing an optimal treatment plan. In addition, it would be important for the team to recognize the caseworker's job of preventing child abuse and realize her helpful intentions. The team needed to both support the caseworker's concerns about the children and to address the religious issue in a manner that did not violate either the church counselor's or the caseworker's belief system.

As a result of the consultation, the team moved toward a nonpartisan stance. By supporting each referrer's concerns, they were viewed by both the church counselor and the caseworker as being supportive of their respective goals for the family. They were not viewed as a controlling agent to be struggled against but, rather, as a helping agent with which to cooperate. The team's new position allowed the referrers to see the team as understanding the serious and delicate nature of the family's problems. Their maneuverability with the referrers, and hence with the family, was increased. The team felt more in control by having less control. They continued working effectively with both the family and the referrers.

DEVELOPMENT OF RESISTANCE IN THE REFERRAL PROCESS

The intensely emotional nature of family violence and the multiple agencies that can quickly become involved make a ripe context for the development of resistance to treatment. Likewise, when an agency requests consultation for these difficult cases, resistance to the consultation commonly appears even during the referral process. The management of resistance in both the agency–family system, and the agency–consultant system, can become an acute problem. While the traditional view of resistance is that reluctance to change is a characteristic of any client system (individual or family), we find it more useful to view resistance as an interactional phenomenon occurring in the relationship between the family, agency, and referring persons. The most frequent form of resistance is a covert struggle over whose understanding of the problem and whose solution will prevail. In other words, when a treatment system is stuck and a client system is being called "resistant" by the treating system, there is probably a violation or challenge to the basic premises of both groups. For example, the agency worker's use of pejorative labels and problem definitions that are contrary to the family's views may insult and violate the family's belief system. The consequence is that the family appears to the worker and the agency to be resistant, unmotivated, and possibly denying that it even has a problem. This behavior on the part of the family challenges the agency worker's beliefs about what would constitute a positive change. What appear to be simply polarized positions are, in fact, recursive feedbacks that can only be destructive to the therapeutic relationship.

While violent families may have made a number of attempts over time to get help, each agency contact is usually initiated during severe crisis and may be induced or influenced by a family member who then becomes the "referring person" (Selvini Palazzoli, Boscolo, Cecchin, & Prata, 1980). Referring persons are often in a struggle with the family at the time of referral. They have usually been involved or overinvolved with the family and its problems over a period of time, and they often initiate the referral at a point when their abilities to help or control the family's problems have been exhausted (Clark, Zalis, & Sacco, 1983).

It is often during the referral process that preexisting labels and new diagnostic labels begin to solidify and stick, becoming roadblocks to treatment. For example, the most common definitions of the problems of family violence usually first appear as dualistic labels such as battered–batterer and victimized–victimizer. These labels attribute motivations to family members and convey pejorative, negative connotations.

Two of the most significant connotations are blame and guilt. For example, in abusive marital relationships, the man and the woman can be simultaneously blamed for problems of family violence, though for different reasons. Attributing the problem to the man and labeling him as victimizing puts him on the defensive. He then sees these well-meaning people, the referring person and the members of an agency, as not only unhelpful but as actually unduly influencing his wife and interfering with his family. Criticizing the woman for her refusal to leave or for her inability to grow beyond her childhood dependencies is equally resistance engendering. As with the man, this may lead to a major reluctance to join in the treatment effort. This reluctance to engage and continue in treatment can be exacerbated as the referral process, the labeling process, and the diagnostic process become homeostatic mechanisms for "no change" in the family system (Hoffman, 1980; Selvini Palazzoli *et al.*, 1980). Thus, the family system and the enlarged treatment–family system (which can now include a matrix of agencies) collusively participate in maintaining and often excalating the very problems they are trying to alleviate: psychological and physical abuse, lack of motivation to change, and resistance to treatment.

Including the man's point of view: A case example. We were asked by the directors of a women's shelter and crisis counseling program to consult with their agency around difficulties they were experiencing with their staff and various program components. One of their concerns was that a large number of women left the shelter and returned to an unchanged, abusive relationship only to seek help from the shelter again at a later date. In addition, they were concerned with threats made to the women and often the shelter itself by men associated with the women clients. On one such occasion, a man actually drove a truck through the front door of the shelter. Their directors saw the cause of this problem as possibly related to the overwhelmingly difficult problems their clients presented. As the shelter had become more prominent in the community, their client referrals had increased and they had begun accepting only the most severe cases of battered women.

As a result of the theoretical position of our own system and previous experience in consulting with community agencies, we felt it would be important to move in the direction of broadening the treatment system to include the men. We wanted to influence the shelter to develop an understanding and awareness of the systemic context of family violence and to redesign their program services in a manner that would take this into account. Since shelters by their very nature are designed to be protectors and advocates for women involved in abusive relationships, their efforts are targeted toward women, not men. Our priority in the consultation process was to avoid behaving in a way that violated the integrity or belief system of the shelter and its staff. We were also aware that the consultation must be consistent with the shelter's definition of the "presenting problem."

During the consultation process, we were able to develop with the shelter staff a consensus about the necessity of involving the men, at least to some degree. In other words, the message to the shelter was that involving the men in a cooperative, or at least a less adversarial, position with the shelter would minimize the chances of the men sabotaging the shelter's efforts to help the women. We suggested that perhaps groups for the men would be an initial step in this direction. It was important that the men be invited to the groups in a way that would communicate to them that their views of the problems were not only important but necessary. It was our hope that, with the men's involvement, the shelter would be in a better position to understand the interactional aspects of family violence and the idiosyncratic nature of each couple's cycle of violence.

Initially, the shelter staff felt that they did not have enough personnel to conduct the group meetings. They also did not want the group meetings to be held at the shelter because of their philosophy of not disclosing its location. It was mutually agreed to have the groups led by therapists on our faculty who would have the advantage of not having already alienated the men during the initial referral of the woman to the shelter. We realized, however, that the therapists could not avoid being seen as representing the shelter and aligning with the wife. The therapists needed to be sensitive to the men's mistrust of the system; therefore, the manner in which the men were to be invited would be crucial.

The groups were led by male therapists who simply invited the men to tell their sides of the obviously complicated situation; they were not being invited in for therapy. The modest goal of the therapists was to join and engage with the men in a manner that would permit the men to feel that their views were understood and that they were not totally to blame for the problems. They hoped that this approach would help defuse any struggles with the shelter. The group meetings did lessen the men's resistance, and a majority of the men asked to be seen in therapy with their mates. The therapists began seeing the couples. This approach is consistent with the systemic view that seeing both the men and women in therapy would lead to a better understanding of the interactional issues of the violence. In addition, we realized that the influence for change in the agency would have been minimized if the couples were seen simply on a referral basis.

The shelter staff needed to be included in the treatment context; therefore, the therapists needed to broaden their role to include consulting with the staff around each case. The therapists would need to engage with each system (staff and client) so as to avoid aligning with one against the other. This neutral position would decrease the chances of creating resistance in any part of the treatment context and, thus, increase the chances of a more successful outcome of the therapy, the case consultation, and the broader agency consultation. To achieve this end, the shelter staff were invited to observe the therapy sessions with the couples from behind a one-way mirror, and to spend time with the therapists before and after the therapy sessions in order to discuss the course of therapy. The therapists also related these consultation cases to the staff's work with other women at the shelter.

The consultation had several positive results. We were able to work with the directors, and the therapists were able to work with the clients. Each group could consult with their representative staff members in a manner that did not violate the integrity or belief system of the agency, its staff members, its clients, or the larger agency–staff–client system. As a result of the staff's involvement in the clinical work, they began to view family violence as an interactional phenomenon. The shelter increased the frequency of involving men in groups, and couples in therapy, and decreased its almost automatic position of advising separation. This helped to interrupt the cycle of women leaving and then returning to the shelter.

This case example illustrates how resistance can develop in the early stages of the consultation process. It is important that the systems consultant avoid making premature judgments that challenge or violate the belief system of the agency. Such judgments limit the consultant's options for effective interventions. The consultant's awareness of the agency's belief system and its views of family violence and a willingness to work with these views in mind will help minimize the likelihood that resistance will develop.

DUALISTIC AND HIERARCHICAL STRUCTURE OF AGENCIES

Gregory Bateson proposed that the mental health field traditionally has viewed human dilemmas from hierarchical and dualistic positions, drawing arbitrary boundaries between itself and those it tries to help (Keeney, 1983). This position implies that the therapist is separate from the clients and their problems, and follows a classical medical model in the sense of diagnostic procedures, nomenclature, and treatment. In other words, therapists do things to people. In contrast to this view, an ecological systems framework includes the therapist, the broader treatment system, the client, and the context of the client's problems as interrelated entities with reciprocal influences (Auerswald, 1968, 1973; Hoffman & Long, 1969; Keeney, 1983).

These traditional, dualistic, and hierarchical categories are evident in the structure of agencies and the services they provide. The service that agencies are designed to provide falls into two main categories: treatment and social control. These categories are considered to be dualistic in the sense that they are at opposite ends of a continuum. On one end there are those services for problems identified as needing treatment, and on the other end, there are those services for problems identified as needing social control. Agencies are often called upon to respond to a family's problems by providing both treatment and social control: (1) supporting, protecting, or counseling; and (2) controlling or seeking assistance in controlling particular behaviors. These services are contradictory and often conflicting. This situation is created when an agency, by the nature of its mission, finds itself in an alliance with one member or part of a family system against another. For example, when a child protective service protects the child from the parents, it is in fact aligning with the child against the parents. When a women's shelter shelters the woman from the man, it is aligning with her against the man. Court systems align with society to protect family members from those whose behavior has been determined to need social control. The agency, by aligning itself with one faction of the family against another, participates in already existent family problems and also creates new ones. Family members now not only have each other to deal with, but they are also at the mercy of the agency whose mission is to help and often simultaneously control them.

There are further implications for the agency and its staff that are created by this inherent and hierarchical structure. Staff members within the agency (e.g., a women's shelter counselor, a children's protective service worker, a juvenile probation officer) often wear two hats: "helper" and "law enforcer." As helpers, their role is to protect, support, counsel, and advocate. As law enforcers, their role is to investigate, monitor, and control. For example, a caseworker in a child protective service may have the role of protecting and counseling a child who has been neglected and abused. At the same time, he or she may have the role of investigating and monitoring the parents. These dualistic roles are frustrating, making the job difficult and leading to burnout.

Consultants must be aware of these dichotomies and the problems they can cause within an agency and between an agency and its clients. They must not place themselves in a dualistic or hierarchical position as they consult with the agency or its clients; to do so would only aggravate the very problems they have been hired to remedy.

IMPLICIT AND EXPLICIT MESSAGES IN THE AGENCY IDENTITY

The public identity and perception of an agency, including its name, are influential in the treatment process with families and in the consultation process with agencies because they convey implicit and explicit messages about its philosophy, tasks, and goals to the public, its clients, other community agencies, and the systems consultant. The agency may be viewed as one that is helpful and can be trusted or it may be viewed as one that is intrusive and has law enforcement powers. Most likely, the agency, the public, the clients, the other community agencies, and the consultant will view the agency through different-colored glasses. In addition, some agencies may not be viewed as having the prestige of a private clinic. Consequently, the staff members, regardless of their credentials and competencies, are not seen as having the prestige of persons associated with a private clinic or of private practitioners. Therefore, they become disillusioned as they try to work with the problems of family violence, and apathetic in the struggle with these difficult, demanding clients who are viewed as unmotivated and low on personal resources (Clark *et al.*, 1983).

The understanding wife: A case example. While consulting with a community agency, we interviewed a woman the agency was counseling. The 39-year-old woman was in a long-time, physically abusive, marital relationship. She was described by the agency as a highly resistant person who continued to stay in the relationship despite the agency's advice to terminate it and get on with her life. During the interview, it became apparent that she was very protective of her husband and was frustrated in her attempts to get her therapist to understand why she stayed in the relationship. At the end of the interview, we asked the woman if she had any advice she could give the agency that would help them in working with other cases similar to hers. She replied, "Yes, it would be helpful if you didn't have such an uppity attitude. And you shouldn't blame the husband." She related these suggestions to her own situation: "Even though my husband beats me, he does it because of things that happened to him when he was a boy. If you had been more sympathetic toward him he would have come in. You know people, know when they need help. Why make it so difficult for them to get it?"

We talked with the staff members about the woman's view of the agency in a way that led them to understand that trying to influence the woman to leave her husband was viewed by her as working against her. In future therapy sessions, the therapist was able to begin joining the woman in her quandary about leaving her husband, which resulted in the woman feeling the therapists were working with her, not against her. During a follow-up two months later, we learned that the woman had a part-time job, was thinking of enrolling in a community college, and was not feeling pressured either to stay with her husband or leave him.

It is important for systems consultants to be aware of how, and by whom, an agency is viewed. They must recognize and understand these different views of the agency and the implications for treatment and consultation. They must consult with the agency in a manner that helps the agency to view itself as working with its clients and not against them. In addition, consultants must be aware of how they themselves are perceived by the agencies; they should place themselves in a position in which the agency can view them as working with it, not against it.

PROCESSES OF CLIENT AND PROBLEM IDENTIFICATION

The processes of client identification and problem identification influence the treatment and management plans for the client and the family. These processes also crucially determine how successful an agency will be in influencing change through its treatment and management plans. Traditionally, agencies are designed to accept individual family members as the designated client. It is the exception to the rule for an agency to view more than one member of a family or the whole family as the client. The symptom bearer in the family is usually defined and presented as the problem and, thus, is the major target of treatment. Treatment plans for the client, and often for the family itself, are usually based on an assessment of the behavior of the one family member who has been identified as the client, without considering the family system and the broader ecological system. This view oversimplifies typologies of individuals, couples, and families, creates categories of problems that limit the agency's ability to work with families, and minimizes the agency's effectiveness.

Keeney (1983) cautions against making assessments and inferences about dyadic interactions and relationship systems from information based only on observing or knowing the individual system. He says it is a mistake to use information from one level of a system to make inferences about another level or unit of a system. When individual, dyadic, and family system levels are confused, assessment of the problem becomes confused and information necessary for an accurate assessment of the family's problems is thereby limited.

For example, in a women's crisis center, the treatment and management plans for a woman involved in an abusive relationship may be based on inferences and understandings about individual and family-wide relationships derived from observations of only the woman. Most women's crisis centers do not seek contact or work with the man involved in the relationship (Walker, 1979). Therefore, the assessment of the problem and the decisions regarding plans for intervening in the woman's life, the marital relationship, and the family, are based on observations and information from an individual relationship system. The more limited the view an agency has of the system relevant to the presenting problem, the more limited its range of alternatives for working with the problem will be. In addition, the probability increases that the limited range of alternatives may not include relevant solutions to the problem or family.

Therefore, it is important that, in working with agencies, the systems consultant be aware of the system level from which the agency ordinarily views its clients. In addition, the consultant must work with the agency in ways that will help the agency understand the advantages of viewing problems from multiple system levels.

SUMMARY

There are often impasses between an agency and its clients that are the results of differences in belief systems and views of reality. In addition, there are various understandings and explanations of the nature, cause, and remedy of the problems. The implications of these multiple views are far-reaching and relevant to the process of systems consultation. A key to a successful consultation is to consult with the agency in the language of its belief system. At the same time, the consultant must encourage the agency to develop a sensitivity to, and an understanding of, the family's language and reality, without violating the integrity of either the family or the agency. The consultant needs to maintain a metaview of the agency, its clients, and the agency–client interface. That is, the consultant needs to know and understand the belief systems, frames of reference, and languages idiosyncratic to each system. Having a working knowledge of the issues presented in this chapter will enable them to achieve a creative and fruitful consultation.

Although this chapter has focused on consultation with agencies with clinical care problems, it has been our experience that the same concepts and key issues are applicable in consultation with agencies with organizational problems. Only the players and the context of the problems are different.

REFERENCES

Auerswald, E. H. Interdisciplinary versus ecological approach. *Family Process*, 1968, *7*, 202–215.

Auerswald, E. H. Families, change, and the ecological perspective. In A. Ferber, M. Mendelsohn, & A. Napier (Eds.), *The book of family therapy*. Boston: Houghton Mifflin, 1973.

Clark, T., Zalis, T., & Sacco, F. C. *Outreach family therapy*. New York: Aronson, 1983.

Daniel, J. L., Hampton, R. L., & Newberger, E. H. Child abuse in black families. *American Journal of Orthopsychiatry*, 1983, *53*, 645–653.

Goolishian, H., & Anderson, H. Including non-blood related persons in family therapy. In A. Gurman (Ed.), *Questions and answers in the practice of family therapy*. New York: Brunner/Mazel, 1981.

Hoffman, L. *Resistance revisited workshop*. Galveston Family Institute, Galveston, TX, 1980.

Hoffman, L., & Long, L. A systems dilemma. *Family Process*, 1969, *8*, 211–234.

Imber Coppersmith, E. The family and public service systems: An assessment model. In B. Keeney (Ed.), *Diagnosis and assessment in family therapy*. Baltimore: Aspen Publications, 1983.

Keeney, B. P. *Aesthetics of change*. New York: Guilford, 1983.

Keeney, B. P. Ecological assessment. In J. C. Hansen & B. P. Keeney (Eds.), *Diagnosis and assessment in family therapy*. Rockville, MD: Aspen Systems Corp., 1983.

Selvini Palazzoli, M., Boscolo, L., Cecchin, G., & Prata, G. The problem of the referring person. *Journal of Marital and Family Therapy*, 1980, *6*, 3–9.

Walker, L. E. *The battered woman*. New York: Harper & Row, 1979.

19

AT THE CENTER OF THE CYCLONE
Family Therapists as Consultants with Family and Divorce Courts

ADELE R. WYNNE
Private Practice
Pittsford, New York

LYMAN C. WYNNE
University of Rochester School of Medicine and Dentistry
Rochester, New York

In the last two decades, as the divorce rate has mounted, courts across the country have been flooded with ever-increasing numbers of difficult decisions regarding family issues. As more options for divorce, custody, and visitation settlements have been championed and legitimized, the complexity as well as the number of court decisions regarding families has escalated. With increasing frequency, child and family clinicians have been called in as consultants to aid judges in resolving these complex cases. In addition, the courts have embraced, even created, new avenues and processes for out-of-court settlements that reduce the economic and emotional cost of contested trials. We believe that the need and opportunity will continue to grow in coming years for consultative and therapeutic contributions by family clinicians working with family court systems.

HISTORICAL PERSPECTIVE

Over the years, drastic changes have taken place in value orientations about the related issues of divorce settlements and child custody and visitation decisions: Whose rights and interests are primary after marital dissolution? How can custody and visitation disputes best be resolved? Gone are the days of simple consensus about whose rights and interests are primary—father, mother, child, or family. Also, since the 1960s, the procedures for no-fault settlements, joint custody, and a variety of counseling and mediation programs, have rapidly proliferated.

THE RIGHTS OF FATHERS

Under Roman law and English common law, sole custody of children was automatically granted to the father, who was regarded as the children's "natural guardian" (Myricks, 1977). Not until the 19th century did the father's absolute right to custody begin to evolve into the idea of his rights balanced by his responsibilities. For example, a New Hampshire judicial opinion stated in 1860:

> It is a well-settled doctrine of the common law, that the father is entitled to the custody of his minor children, as against the mother and everybody else; that he is bound for their maintenance and nurture, and has the corresponding right to their obedience and their services. (Derdeyn, 1976, p. 1370)

THE "TENDER YEARS PRESUMPTION"

Very gradually and inconsistently in the late 19th century, the mother's rights began to be upheld under the Doctrine of Tender Years:

> An infant of tender years is generally left with the mother (if no objection to her is shown to exist) even when the father is without blame, merely because of his inability to bestow upon it that tender care which nature requires, and which it is the peculiar province of a mother to supply. (Kaslow, 1979–1980, p. 733)

"THE BEST INTERESTS OF THE CHILD"

The welfare of the third member of the family triad, the child, was first given explicit attention in a custody case by a Kansas judge in 1881 (Kaslow, 1979–1980). This view was strongly affirmed in 1925 in a landmark decision by Justice Benjamin Cardozo:

> [The judge] does not proceed upon the theory that the petitioner, whether father or mother, has a cause of action against the other or indeed against anyone. He acts as *parens patriae* to do what is best for the interest of the child. (*Finlay v. Finlay*, 1925)

In some jurisdictions since the early 1960s, the courts have sought to safeguard the child's best interests by appointing an attorney as *guardian ad litem* to act as the child's advocate in custody and visitation adjudications. By and large, despite widespread statutory acceptance of the best-interests principle, no child-based criteria have been agreed upon. Instead, until the 1970s, the rule was quite automatically interpreted, in accord with the tender years presumption, to mean that custody should be awarded to the mother except when she was found to be the "guilty" party in the divorce suit. For example, an 1873 legal text stated:

> [The] courts give the custody to the innocent party; because, with such party, the children will be more likely to be cared for properly. (Derdeyn, 1976, p. 1372)

What now seems most striking about divorce, custody, and visitation practice until about 1970 is the emphasis on recognizing the rights and interests of individual family members in accord with arbitrary, adversarial formulas. Viewed from the standpoint of family systems theory, the absence of the comprehensive, integrative framework of systems theory is apparent. Three recent legal changes have markedly altered the adversarial quality of family law: no-fault divorce, joint custody, and the establishment of family conciliation services as arms of the court system.

NO-FAULT SETTLEMENTS

Beginning with the no-fault divorce law that went into effect in California in 1970 (Shipman, 1977), similar laws have been rapidly enacted in the United States, extending to 48 of the 50 states by 1983. This option has made divorce increasingly a matter of negotiation rather than litigation. However, because some state laws allow fault to be used as a basis for custody determinations even when there are no-fault divorce procedures, the adversarial nature of custody adjudications has often continued with little change (Derdeyn, 1976; Kaslow, 1979–1980).

JOINT CUSTODY

Still more recently, the advent of joint-custody laws has opened up additional opportunities—and complications—for negotiation. Although scattered court decisions awarding joint custody were made as long ago as 1948 (Nehls & Morgenbesser, 1980), only six states had joint-custody laws before 1980. Subsequently, such laws have increased very rapidly and have taken a variety of forms, including joint custody as the preferred and mandated choice in some states (Derdeyn & Scott, 1984).

This trend has been at odds with the widely publicized proposal by Goldstein, Freud, and Solnit (1973) who drew upon psychoanalytic theory to argue for maintaining continuity of relationship between the child and one "psychological parent" (not necessarily the biological parent). Their proposal specified that the parent with sole custody would also unilaterally determine the noncustodial parent's visitation rights. However, many courts have rejected this concept as a "specious notion" (Kaslow, 1979–1980) and have strongly moved toward joint custody, even when not requested by the divorcing couple (Jacobs, 1982; Roman & Haddad, 1978).

COURT-CONNECTED COUNSELING PROGRAMS

The use of marriage counselors in the divorce process was introduced in the United States in 1933, when the divorce courts in Milwaukee and Cincinnati each established a Department of Family Conciliation (Shipman, 1977). Counseling programs have taken on new importance since the advent of no-fault divorce laws. Most states have now established within the court system family-service arms staffed by mental health professionals. Originally responsible for pretrial evaluation of parenting capabilities, the scope and mission of these services have expanded to assist conflicted couples in exploring the possibility of reconciliation or, alternatively, of negotiating divorce, custody, and visitation terms without a court-contested trial. It is now widely agreed, even by many divorce lawyers, that court-ordered settlements and a bitter adversarial process are inappropriate for most marital disputes, which are basically "people problems, not legal problems" (Steinberg, 1980).

The legal mandate and the actual functioning of these family-service arms still vary widely throughout the United States and Canada. In some jurisdictions, all litigating couples are ordered by the court to go through the family-service unit. These units have a variety of names, such as the "Conciliation Courts" of California (Elkin, 1973). Especially since 1981, these new arrangements for collaborative spousal settlements have dramatically reduced the number of cases contested in court trials in California and some other states (Francke, 1983). Also, when each party has a voice in the initial, negotiated settlement, the frequency of postdivorce appearances in court has been reduced (Ilfeld, Ilfeld, & Alexander, 1982).

Staff members of these court family-service units are able to offer direct, but usually time-limited help in assessing and resolving many divorce-related conflicts. In those cases that prove to be intransigent, too time-consuming, or involving questions of mental competency, the staff request consultation from a variety of mental health specialists. For individual psychological testing or a mental status evaluation, a psychologist with a PhD or a psychiatrist may be called in. As the issues raised by divorce have moved beyond questions of individual parental competency, family specialists have increasingly been called in as consultants, mediators, or therapists. In addition, lawyers and couples with conflicts sometimes use the court family services as a referral source when they want assistance in resolving problems out of court.

CHILD CUSTODY EVALUATIONS

As a continuation of the adversarial procedures of the past, consultation often is still sought, and provided, for one family member. Probably the most common route by which psychiatrists are contacted to consult in custody cases is by referral from an individual parent's attorney (American Psychiatric Association, 1982). Accepting such referrals "stacks the deck" against working with the family as a system and, with multiple consultants involved, presents the court with a "morass of parent-oriented conflicting testimony" (Derdeyn, 1975). Clinicians, it now seems agreed, can better serve children and families if they consult not for one of the competing adults, but only for the court or its family-service arm.

DIVORCE MEDIATION

A major new vehicle for negotiating divorce settlements with the voluntary participation of both conflicting spouses is a formalized divorce mediation (Coogler, 1978; Haynes, 1978). Mediation is not adjudicatory; it is "a cooperative process by which the parties agree to use the services of a neutral third person whose function is to help them resolve, in a noncompetitive manner, the issues which divide them" (Kaslow, 1979–1980, p. 727). In some jurisdictions, the court family-service staff suggests that divorcing couples work with outside divorce mediators, but, at present, couples themselves more often seek out mediators to avoid expensive and sometimes embarrassing court battles. Structured mediation is conducted in accord with rules that the parties contractually agree to follow in advance (Coogler, 1978). Although "mediation" takes many forms, it has been most useful in the negotiation of "nuts and bolts" issues such as property distribution and support payments. Most mediators work with couples who have already decided upon divorce (Coogler, Weber, & McKenry, 1979).

Thus, three kinds of mental health services to the divorce and family courts now have become available: court-connected counseling and assessment programs, psychiatric and psychologic evaluations of the individual family members by outside consultants, and resolution of "practical" issues through contractual negotations with specially trained divorce mediators.

FAMILY THERAPISTS AS COURT CONSULTANTS

Supplementing these three kinds of mental health services to the courts, systems-oriented family therapists can fulfill a distinctive, valuable function in working with divorce problems. When family therapists are court consultants and proceedings have already begun, they, unlike divorce mediators, do not assume that the decision to divorce is necessarily immutable. Whitaker and Miller (1969) have cogently shown that therapy with couples should be tried in order to clarify whether reconciliation is possible and desirable even after one or both members of the couple have "decided" on divorce. Later, after legal action has definitely taken place, the couple and their children often remain caught up in unresolved emotional tangles. The difficulties of coparenting after divorce usually require new problem-solving skills. In assisting the court family service staff with this broad range of problems within a consultative framework, we have been able to use family therapy skills selectively, and often surprisingly successfully, in brief therapy. The leverage provided by consultative collaboration with the court or its family-service arm has facilitated our therapeutic efforts.

For several years we have been consultants to the family-service unit of the court system in Rochester, New York.[1] This unit does not deal with issues of support payments or division of property, which are handled by outside mediators or lawyers. Rather, the unit is committed to broader fact-

1. The Rochester court family-service unit, headed by Jeanette Minkoff, PhD, is officially identified as the "Adult Intake and Special Investigations Unit of the Monroe County Probation Department." The 11 staff members of this unit have been mandated since 1967 to serve as consultants to both the 5 Family Court judges (who deal with nondivorce family issues such as child abuse) and the 18 Supreme Court justices of the New York Seventh Judicial District (who deal with divorce and custody decisions). Historically, this unit was established under the jurisdiction of the Probation Department because this was already a service arm of the courts for casework investigations. Despite its special name and administrative location, this unit in Rochester functions much like Conciliation Courts in California and similar programs elsewhere. Although this family service unit is an official consulting arm within the court system, it is able to exercise considerable discretion in deciding what data are appropriate to incorporate in their reports and recommendations to the courts. Thus, our consultation to this family-service unit is nested within the larger consultative system set up by the courts.

finding and assessment in order to facilitate reconciliation when possible, and, if not, to negotiate settlements. Family therapists and other mental health professionals are called as consultants whenever the resourcefulness of the caseworker, or the allocated time for each case, proves to be inadequate for the task. In most cases, the judges rely on the recommendations of the unit staff in deciding whether to request specialist consultation.

BRIEF THERAPY WITHIN A CONSULTATIVE FRAMEWORK

As consultants to this family-service unit, we have been impressed with the diversity of problems encountered and the variety of ways in which a family therapist, functioning as a consultant, can interface with this legal system. The following case illustrates incorporation of a brief therapeutic intervention within the context of consultation to the court. The judge had ordered that an evaluation and recommendation be made by the court family-service unit. The unit staff started this process but then concluded that the potentially explosive quality of the problem called for consultation with an outside family therapist.

A Grieving Father and a Fearful Son: A Case Example

In this case, a noncustodial father (George) had initiated court action by asking for redress of denial of his visitation rights with his 12-year-old son, Patrick. Generally, the courts are reluctant to deny visitation by a noncustodial parent unless harm to the child is very likely. George and his former wife, Joan, had separated 7 years previously, following violent quarrels between them. Although Joan had obtained a court injunction prohibiting George from entering the family home, he had twice attempted to do so with the intention, according to Joan, of "kidnapping" Patrick. After being given two large fines for these attempts at entry, George stopped trying to assert his "right to be in my own home."

At the time of the subsequent divorce, George was given 3-hour visitation rights on Sundays but, following an altercation between the parents during one of these visits, during which the father allegedly threatened violence, Patrick tearfully called his father to say that he did not want to see him anymore. George respected Patrick's wish but despaired over the alienation from his son. Two years later Joan married Richard, a professional man with a considerably better social position than George, who was a bricklayer. Joan and Richard moved to another part of the city and got an unlisted telephone number in order to prevent George from locating them.

Thus, at the time the court family-service unit had asked us to do a consultation, George had not been able to contact his son for over 4 years.

We were told by the court family-service unit that Patrick recently had recovered from his "nervous" condition (that included a number of psychophysiologic symptoms) but that he remained in dread of his biological father. Although Joan still believed George to be unpredictably explosive and abusive, George maintained that her views were unreasonable. He said, "I am being blocked from even giving birthday and Christmas presents to my son. I want to see Patrick so that I can show him how much I care for him."

Our first consultative session was with Joan, Richard, and Patrick, interviewing them together as a family and then separately. Patrick hesitantly revealed his continuing fear but also fascination with his biological father. He recalled him as being "crazy," and described his impression of wild scenes in his early childhood, with the police and his father both displaying guns. During the past year he had become comfortable with his stepfather, a calm and self-confident man, and had ceased to have bad dreams and vomiting. He no longer needed to sleep with his mother. His grades in school had improved and Little League baseball was a big part of his life.

Our second session was with George, who seemed surprisingly mild mannered and sincerely interested in reestablishing a relationship with his son. At the conclusion of a wide-ranging evaluation of the father's past and current functioning and of his understanding of his son's emotional state, we said that Patrick still feared him but that we believed a meeting would be reassuring to Patrick and would give him a chance to see his father as a more humane person than he remembered him to be. Also, we said that Patrick's fears about being kidnapped needed to be allayed. George conceded that he would be relieved and satisfied at this time if he could only see Patrick again and let him know how much he loved him.

In a third session, this time with Joan and Richard, we explored the possibility of a meeting between Patrick and his father in the neutral atmosphere of our office, with the limited goal of reducing Patrick's apprehensions and misunderstandings. We promised that the meeting would not be a prologue to a new court battle about visitation rights. Joan was apprehensive about such a meeting but agreed to its taking place if Richard were in an adjoining room "in case Patrick needed help."

The meeting between father and son began with great tension and caution between them, but unfolded with surprising smoothness. George carefully and quietly drew Patrick out. At first Patrick was tight and terse in his responses; slowly he engaged more positively with his father as they discovered unsuspected mutual skills and interests such as playing baseball.

Patrick finally asked his father about his hobbies and his grandmother. There was a moment of high drama when George offered, and Patrick hesitantly accepted, a box of Christmas presents (this was August) that George and the grandmother had sent the previous Christmas "to show our love." The box had been returned unopened.

Before leaving with Patrick, Richard entered the room and engaged George in a most cordial conversation. We closed the case by summarizing for George how important it was to let his son decide, in his own time, when he was ready to make more contact. We reported what Patrick had told us: "I would like to get to know my father better when I am older, like when I'm 16." George was extraordinarily pleased to see for himself that his son was doing well and was growing less fearful of him. He agreed to forgo demands for visitation rights at this time.

We recommended to the court that restrictions on the relationship between father and son probably could be eased as Patrick grew older, especially if there were indications that the adults were supportive of Patrick's making his own decisions. Further follow-up was thus turned back to the court family-service unit. Our consultative contact was concluded within a few weeks after a total of four sessions.

It was our impression that it was indeed possible to have a brief intervention that could be both therapeutic and preventive within the consultative framework. Prior to our meeting, George had planned to carry his visitation requests into a court battle in which the son would have had to appear, and the grievances and emotional turmoil of the earlier years would have been painfully put on display. It seemed to us that either forced visitations or, alternatively, no contact whatsoever, would be developmentally damaging to Patrick and a serious strain for the adults as well. All of the adults expressed their appreciation for our help in mitigating the intense feelings that they had long been harboring.

REVISION OF JOINT CUSTODY AGREEMENTS

Under joint custody, both parents share responsibility for making major decisions that affect the children. Optimally, joint custody permits more appropriate flexibility because the legal system does not have to be involved when changes are warranted, such as the scheduling of residence with each parent. Because parents who divorce are usually unskilled at cooperating, joint custody does not always proceed smoothly. When conflicts arise that cannot be resolved, some parents who have joint custody may choose to use a family therapist instead of calling in their lawyers. Having become familiar with the court family services in obtaining their divorce, they may contact these services to obtain the names of family therapists for help in negotiating their impasses.

The Ping-Pong Sharing of Children in Joint Custody: A Case Example

The following case was referred to us by the court family-service staff after the mother had asked them for assistance. She and her former husband could not resolve a dispute about changing their self-imposed arrangements for joint custody of their children, and they wished to avoid a court hearing. The husband did not want counseling from the staff, but he agreed to a single meeting with us after the staff reassured him that we were "objective," outside consultants. The mother, Elsie, proposed a change in the living arrangement for their children, a boy 12 and a girl 9. Elsie proposed that each parent have the children for a week at a time, while the husband, Stephen, strongly preferred the present schedule, namely, that the children sleep in each residence alternate weeknights and alternate weekends. He liked having them with Elsie two weeknights because it gave him "recreational time" for himself. Elsie found the present arrangement unsettling for the children and for herself because it meant that the parents had to chauffeur them 10 miles each way almost daily, and she perceived that both of the children were beginning to show eating and sleeping disturbances. Stephen presented himself as being "in control" financially and psychologically and wanting to retain this position.

We used the first session to establish a relationship with both parents. A consensus emerged that it would be helpful for us to see the children in each home environment. While one of us (L.C.W.) was out of the country for 2 weeks, the other (A.R.W.) made a visit to each home. (Flexibility of scheduling is one of the many advantages of co-consultants.) Stephen and his new wife lived in the pleasant, longtime family home in the suburbs. About 4 months previously, Elsie had bought an old, rundown house in urban Rochester. The house was slowly being rehabilitated by her, but she was barely making ends meet. She had almost no extra money to spend on socialization with other adults. Her financial woes were part of her dilemma, and it was important that she include them in the picture even though they were not part of our initial agenda with the couple.

The children were lively, open, and looked healthy and well-adjusted despite being shifted almost daily from home to home. They said that they liked seeing both mother and father "all the time," and that they had made a few friends in their mother's new Rochester neighborhood. However, Elsie was concerned that they watched television too much when they were with her and she was trying to limit this activity. Stephen later reported that the children seldom watched television while with him: "They do other things which are better for them." Living near longtime friends indeed gave the children more opportunities for peer relationships. Elsie recognized this advantage for them at this stage of their development.

After the two home visits, we met only once more with Stephen and Elsie to explore a more stable residential arrangement. We said that although the children seemed to be doing fairly well under the present schedule, their need for a more consistent home base would become still more apparent as they became older and more involved with peers and after-school activities. We suggested that the suburban home might be the logical weekday base since Elsie lived outside their school district. Stephen agreed to this idea with the provision that he have at least one evening during the week to do his own "recreational" projects at his firm's laboratory. Elsie was more than willing to take the children for supper on Wednesday evening and return them to Stephen before their bedtime. Each parent would continue to have the children on alternate weekends.

With the resolution of the specific presenting problem, we left it that we would not see them again unless they had other problems with which they needed help. We believed that Elsie would have liked to address other areas left unresolved by the divorce, but Stephen was resistant to exploring more issues than he "had bargained for."

At the conclusion of the brief therapy that took place within this consultation, this couple was still enmeshed with each other. Both were struggling for control in many areas. A redeeming factor was that they both had a strong concern for the welfare of their children. The new arrangement for joint residence differed from what either parent had proposed. Both were willing to accept a plan that would be better for the children in that it gave them more continuity in a home base. As Kaslow (1979–1980) has pointed out: "The essence of joint custody lies not in the parents' equal division of the children's time, but in their joint responsibility" for their children's lives (p. 738).

In this case we were not court consultants by virtue of an order given to the couple by a judge. Rather, we were consultants with the family-service arm of the court with the couple's voluntary agreement. Therefore, we discussed with the couple, both in the initial and the concluding meeting, our relationship with the family-service staff. We stated that we wanted the thinking in our meetings with the couple, and the problem resolution we had reached, to be known to the service-unit staff in the eventuality that the couple might ask for legal assistance or redress in the future. The couple was pleased that the staff would learn of "our success in resolution."

RECURRING NONCOMPLIANCE WITH COURT ORDERS

The dysfunction inherent in a family system leading to separation or divorce may long endure after the divorce decree is finalized. Even when one or both of the divorced couple remarry, unresolved conflicts and continuing enmeshment with the former spouse may continue to take the form of bitter disputes over custody and visitation rights. A common pattern is for fathers to stop child support payments and mothers to deny visitation rights. Such retaliatory actions are in explicit violation of court orders. When such noncompliance with court decrees persists, the legal system alone is ineffective. We believe that this is a useful time to call in family therapists as consultants.

An Attorney–Therapist Affair: A Case Example

The following case illustrates how a divorced but still emotionally enmeshed couple can circumvent resolution of their problems by repeated litigation over visitation rights. It also exemplifies how our functioning as family consultants interfaced with three components of the legal system: the attorneys (one for each parent and one for the children as *guardian ad litem*), the judge, and the court family-service unit. In order to interrupt this cyclical pattern, it was necessary for us to collaborate not only with the family but also with the entire legal system. Joseph L. Steinberg (1980), a divorce lawyer, has persuasively described the need for interdisciplinary teamwork between attorneys and family therapists in "marriages or, at the least, an affair" (p. 259). We will present this case in detail because it illustrates a number of ways in which the family consultant and the court can become supportive allies, helping the couple to end a cycle of repetitive court decrees and noncompliance.

The Grasso family consists of divorced parents, Roberto and Eileen, a daughter Betsy (age 12), and two sons, Carl (age 9), and Matt (age 7). The Grasso parents reported that they had enjoyed a lively, close family life when the children were of preschool age. Eventually, however, Roberto's authoritarian concern with behavioral rules clashed with Eileen's extreme sensitivity and responsiveness to the feeling states of the children. On several occasions, Roberto had hit his wife when she undercut his orders to the children. Four years previously, they had agreed that Roberto should move out, with the understanding that the children might visit him often. After a year of disagreement about these visits, there was an especially heated altercation when Roberto wanted to begin taking 4-year-old Matt to his apartment for overnight visits. Eileen thought Matt was too young. From that point on, Eileen allowed Roberto to see the children only in the family home. Two years later, they were legally separated. Roberto reluctantly conceded sole custody to Eileen but with the stipulation that he be given extensive and explicit visitation rights.

Despite the court order specifying Roberto's visitation rights, the children refused to go out with their father. Eileen insisted that he visit them in the home where she could "protect the kids" from their father. More surprisingly, the parents would sleep together whenever Roberto came to "see the children," and they continued to do so even after the divorce decree was finalized a year later.

After several unsuccessful, traumatic attempts to pressure the children to spend time with him at his home, Roberto took Eileen to court where she was cited for contempt for repeatedly ignoring visitation guidelines. The judge then ordered 8 months of "family counseling." Roberto went to one meeting with a female therapist and then angrily bowed out. Eileen and the children continued seeing this therapist while Roberto sought out a male psychologist for himself. After the 8 months of court-ordered therapy, Roberto went to collect his children for a visit. More adamantly than ever, the children again refused to go with him, and there was a tempestuous scene at the front door. Roberto asked his attorney for a stronger court order.

Roberto's attorney realized that further court decrees would not alter the children's resistance. He called the court family-service unit for help and was advised to join with Eileen's attorney in persuading both parents to contact us for therapy. Roberto's attorney then made the referral, but warned us about an imminent hearing before a new Family Court judge (known for his staunch support of the rights of fathers). This judge agreed to postpone the hearing until he received a consultant's report from us. Hence, through collaborative discussion with both attorneys and with the family-service staff, we became consultants with the court and, within that framework, we had the option of becoming therapists with the family if we decided that this was appropriate.

When Roberto and Eileen called us for an appointment, we requested an initial consultation with the whole family. We said that we would then try to reach agreement with them about how to proceed. We explained that we worked as co-consultants. The fact of our being a man-and-woman team turned out to be of great importance to this couple, as it has been with most embattled couples we have seen. Roberto believed that the female therapist whom they previously had seen had sided with Eileen against him; they both welcomed the presumably "balanced" viewpoint that we could provide as a team.

The first session included both parents and their three children. Betsy was at first sullen and then bitterly articulate: "I hate my father. He can't change. I wish he were dead." Her younger brothers expressed similar feelings, but seemed to be following her lead. In addition to their anger, we sensed that they were truly afraid of being alone with their father. The next day Eileen called and insisted that we not include the children in our sessions: "It is too hard on them. Betsy couldn't sleep and was in tears."

In the second session, without the children, the parents agreed that the children's fear of their father's temper was a mutual concern. Roberto saw their fear as stirred up by Eileen; Eileen worried that Betsy was growing up hating all men. We inquired under what circumstances Roberto and the children could meet without Eileen being present. She could think of no possible circumstances.

Working toward the smallest possible change to which both could agree, Eileen at last suggested that she and the two younger children might go with Roberto for hamburgers at the children's favorite fast-food restaurant. When this outing had gone smoothly, we pushed them to agree on a next step: Roberto took Carl and Matt to the same restaurant for a half hour outing with Eileen's sister acting as chaperone.

Minute changes were thus maneuvered into these visitations, although Roberto kept complaining that the changes were too little. Our expectation was that they agree upon *some* change and then try it out as an "experiment." A turning point came after Eileen began taking all the children to Roberto's soccer games on weekends and Roberto insisted that she stop coming with them. The next weekend, the two youngest children went to the game without their mother and without intransigent Betsy.

The parents' continuing sexual relationship and the unabated hostility of Betsy concerned us. At 12, she was upset when she saw her parents in the same bed and often denounced their immorality. "Dad should stop coming to the house. He's a beast!" Eileen was irately jealous of Roberto's girlfriends and continually begged him to give them up. We challenged the couple's stated interest in getting on with their separate lives as long as they continued to sleep together. We pointed out that this was offensive and confusing for prepubescent Betsy who was struggling to find a moral code for herself. Their efforts at sexual abstinence were feeble and shortlived, and we were repeatedly frustrated in our efforts. Both parents colluded in refusing to decouple, although Roberto would sometimes complain that "this woman will not leave me alone" and Eileen periodically claimed that he "used" her. Faced with their insistence on remaining bed partners, our goals were reformulated to focus on stabilizing the family system so that the couple could work together more harmoniously in their functions as coparents.

Roberto was now making current child support payments, but Eileen threatened court action to obtain unpaid back payments. Roberto asserted that he was too much in debt from all the legal fees, and Eileen finally backed off. Both parents were creatively facilitating the amount of time the two younger children spent with their father. We sensed that both parents thought things were going well even though the children had spent no overnights with their father (a stipulation in the visitation agreement).

Abruptly, after 2 months of weekly meetings, Roberto announced that he was going ahead with the delayed hearing before the Family Court judge who had a reputation for supporting the rights of fathers. We were subpoenaed to testify in court a week later. Dismayed, we believed that a trial involving renewed threats of jail for Eileen and court testimony by the children would destroy the slowly evolving rapport between Roberto and the children.

We immediately contacted Roberto's attorney, who said, "The judge wants this visitation dispute settled at once or he will settle it in court. Of course, he thinks it would be better if they could resolve it out of court. He hopes you can work out a written agreement between the parents that can be incorporated as a stipulation in a new court order by him."

We told the attorney that we would work on a written, step-by-step schedule that could lead to compliance with the father's extensive, court-ordered visitation rights within 4 months. Such a plan was the only basis on which we would work with the family. The attorney thought that the judge might go along with such a "transition period," if that were our proposed solution. We were asked to meet in 3 days with the judge in his chambers, together with both parents, their attorneys, and the children's court-appointed attorney to discuss the visitation question.

We immediately met with both parents and used the judge's deadline as leverage to obtain agreement with them that their own, and the children's, best interests lay in progressing with the gradual changes that had already been taking place in the visitation arrangements prior to Roberto's resorting again to court action. Working with the couple intensively, we wrote out a detailed plan that was a compromise between the parental preferences, but was a schedule that the couple agreed we should present to the judge.

From our discussion with the attorneys, we were concerned that the judge would require immediate and precise compliance with the stipulations of the last visitation order. This expectation, we believed, would only result in further noncompliance. Hence, we concluded our statement as follows:

> We concur with the Court that basic structure is necessary as the foundation for the growth of a good parent–child relationship. However, the *quality* of the time together is also important in achieving stabilized compliance without the use of force. We would welcome the support of the Court toward reaching the goal of improved "quality *and* quantity" of the time the children spend with their father.

Within the framework described above, we are willing to continue to work with the parents (and with the children when appropriate) if the Court, the attorneys, and both the parents all agree to the 4-month goal described above, and to the principle of progressive change in definite stages.

At the hearing in the judge's chambers, after carefully reading the new schedule and statement, he announced: "This is the only way to go when there has been so much distrust." He then drew up a court order in which our schedule and statement were officially included. By working collaboratively, a trial was thus avoided that would have been costly, emotionally disturbing, and counterproductive for all five family members.

During the summer months, Roberto became more committed to the concept of slow transitions. He was seeing enough of the children so that he was quite unconcerned that the overnight visits to his home had not been fully implemented by the end of the 4-month period when we terminated our work with the family. Eileen was working part of the day in Roberto's office, helping him get his financial affairs in order again. Betsy was still distancing herself whenever her father spent a day (or night) at the family home. She no longer retreated to her room and was usually polite to him, but she refused to accompany him away from home. Roberto accepted our explanations that Betsy, as a 12-year-old, needed to sort out her own identity and values. Most important, everyone's emotional volatility had abated as had the constant threat of recourse to the courts. We ended our consultation to the court with a report to the judge stating that limited but not optimal goals had been achieved and that we would be available for further consultation if needed.

THE RELATIONSHIP OF "CONSULTANT" AND "THERAPIST" ROLES

Ordinarily, we have found that a clear referral or mandate from the court gives us increased leverage for effective therapeutic interventions. Under these circumstances, we explain to the couple that, because we are court consultants, we shall be reporting to the court, but that we shall first discuss the report with the couple. In this way, we are able to function therapeutically with the couple or family within a consultative framework. However, we do not label our clinical work "therapy" unless the couple introduces this concept and identifies a problem that they cannot resolve alone. For many persons (but not for us), the concept of "therapy" is associated with an expectation of long-term dependency for treatment of an illness. Because "therapy" so frequently has negative and debatable connotations, we simply tell couples and families that our approach involves short-term, collaborative meetings to achieve resolution in a specific, problematic area.

The distinction between our consultative relationship with the court and our therapeutic relationship with the family has, most importantly, posed no difficulties for the court family-service unit, which specifically encourages this dual relationship. It welcomes the "bonus" of therapeutic resolution, but regards our assessment of the family situation as of primary value if further legal action is necessary. Considering the intensity and duration of the alienation and turmoil in these families, the proportion of our referrals that have achieved problem resolution without coming to trial has been surprising and gratifying to us. It has been helpful that the court has respected our judgment in setting a realistic time frame for our work with each family, perhaps because we have made known to the unit staff that we use a brief, problem-solving approach.

In instances in which the referral is made before court action has taken place, as with couples who wish to avoid an adversarial battle (see our second case example), we are not formal consultants with the court. We then engage the couple or family in *direct* consultation before deciding whether "therapy" will be needed. Usually three to six "consultation" sessions are all that are needed for focused problem resolution in which we expect the couple to take explicit responsibility for identifying the problems that they want to work on. By making clear that we shall not go on and on in a vaguely defined therapeutic relationship, we find that our impact is both more focused and more effective.

REPORTING TO THE COURT

The keystone of our formal consultative role with the court family-service system is the report that we file about our observations and recommendations. When psychiatric consultation is provided to the legal system, the issue of confidentiality is usually handled differently than is customary in other clinical relationships. For example, the American Psychiatric Association Task Force on Clinical Assessment in Child Custody (1982) recommends: "The psychiatric consultant must actively dispel the expectation that confidences will be kept, and some require adults to sign a statement permitting the psychiatrist to share findings with the court and with the other parent and lawyer" (p. 17). As described in our work with the Grasso family, our approach is different. We discuss with the parents our planned recommendations to the court and what background data will be included to make these recommendations understandable to the court. We explain that in our report we will try to present a balanced view of the needs of each family member and of the family as a whole. Often, this sharing of our proposed report with the couple uncovers points of ambiguity and delineates residual, unsolved problems.

At the discretion of the service-unit staff, our written statement, in whole or in part, is incorporated into the staff's more comprehensive report to the judge. This report is filed in the judge's chambers, where it can be reviewed by the contesting attorneys before further judicial action is taken. The attorneys may choose to relay its contents to their clients, a possibility that makes collaborative discussion of our recommendations with the couple especially desirable.

Whenever our consultative assessment of the mental status of a family member is pertinent but possibly inflammatory, this information is shared with the family-service unit director in a separate letter. This information may be used to help the mental health professionals of the service unit understand our views when they prepare their overall recommendation to the judge, but the details of such information remains confidential with the staff if we so request. In effect, we are making a distinction between our mental health consultative role and our legal consultative function. This distinction is crucial because it helps us maintain and protect our therapeutic relationship with the couple or family within the context of the consultation with the judicial system.

TESTIFYING IN COURT

A common worry of mental health professionals about contact with the legal system is that they may be required to testify in court. This possibility has not turned out to be a problem in our work as family consultants. Technically, consultants can be called to testify, but at least two factors are now making this an infrequent occurrence. First, the number of trials involving family disputes has diminished as out-of-court settlements have greatly increased with new conciliation procedures. In San Francisco, a judge previously had 15 custody disputes a day on his calendar, but with the establishment of a conciliation court, only 3 cases were heard during all of 1981 (Francke, 1983).

Second, when court testimony is needed, the court family-service unit in Rochester (and in similar units elsewhere) serves as a buffer between the judge and the consultant from the community. If testimony is needed, the judge relies on the unit staff, which then incorporates our opinions into its recommendations to the judge. Even so, the unit staff was called to testify in court in only 19 out of 320 cases they handled in the past year; outside consultants were subpoenaed only rarely. (The Grasso case is the only instance in which it has been necessary for us to meet personally with the judge.) Thus, the reluctance of many mental health professionals to work with the legal system because they might have to testify in court is becoming less and less justified. For those who work in jurisdictions where court testimony is an issue, helpful suggestions have been provided by Goldzband (1982) and by the American Psychiatric Association Task Force (1982).

CONCLUDING COMMENTS

In our role as consultants to divorce and family courts, we have worked with cases involving a diversity of custody fights, intergenerational and spousal visitation disputes, and residency problems under joint custody. Especially challenging (and rewarding) are those cases in which the children refuse to visit with their noncustodial parent. In our work with these families, we have been effective in establishing mutually acceptable visitation plans. The strategies and details may differ but, conceptually, these cases are similar in their need for restructuring of the "pre-divorce family system."

In recent years, the legal system is recognizing the help of family therapists as consultants in cases with deeply entrenched, systemic conflicts. Reciprocally, as family therapists, we have begun to appreciate how the consultative framework provided by the legal system may function to support us in therapeutic interventions. Together, legal and mental health teams may achieve more than either could alone.

REFERENCES

American Psychiatric Association. *Child custody consultation: Report of the Task Force on Clinical Assessment in Child Custody*. Washington, DC: American Psychiatric Association Press, 1982.

Coogler, O. J. *Structured mediation in divorce settlement*. Lexington, MA: Lexington Books, 1978.

Coogler, O. J., Weber, R. E., & McKenry, P. C. Divorce mediation: A means of facilitating divorce and adjustment. *Family Coordinator*, 1979, *28*, 255–259.

Derdeyn, A. P. Child custody consultation. *American Journal of Orthopsychiatry*, 1975, *45*, 791–801.

Derdeyn, A. P. Child custody contests in historical perspective. *American Journal of Psychiatry*, 1976, *133*, 1369–1376.

Derdeyn, A. P., & Scott, E. Joint custody: A critical analysis and appraisal. *American Journal of Orthopsychiatry*, 1984, *54*, 199–209.

Elkin, M. Conciliation courts: The reintegration of disintegrating families. *Family Coordinator*, 1973, *22*, 63–71.

Finlay v. Finlay, 148 N.E. 624 (N.Y. 1925).
Francke, L. B. *Growing up divorced.* New York: Simon & Schuster, 1983.
Goldstein, J., Freud, A., & Solnit, A. J. *Beyond the best interests of the child.* New York: Free Press, 1973.
Goldzband, M. G. *Consulting in child custody: An introduction to the ugliest litigation for mental health professionals.* Lexington, MA: D. C. Heath, 1982.
Haynes, J. M. Divorce mediator: A new role. *Social Work*, 1978, *23*, 5–9.
Ilfeld, F. W., Ilfeld, H. Z., & Alexander, J. R. Does joint custody work? A first look at outcome data of relitigation. *American Journal of Psychiatry*, 1982, *139*, 62–66.
Jacobs, J. W. The effect of divorce on fathers: An overview of the literature. *American Journal of Psychiatry*, 1982, *139*, 1235–1241.
Kaslow, F. W. Stages of divorce: A psychological perspective. *Villanova Law Review*, 1979–1980, *25*, 718–751.
Myricks, N. The Equal Rights Amendment: Its potential impact on family life. *Family Coordinator*, 1977, *26*, 321–324.
Nehls, N., & Morgenbesser, M. Joint custody: An exploration of the issues. *Family Process*, 1980, *19*, 117–125.
Roman, M., & Haddad, W. *The disposable parent: The case for joint custody.* New York: Holt, Rienhart, & Winston, 1978.
Shipman, G. In my opinion: The role of counseling in the reform of marriage and divorce procedures. *Family Coordinator*, 1977, *26*, 395–407.
Steinberg, J. L. Toward an interdisciplinary commitment: A divorce lawyer proposes attorney–therapist marriages or, at the least, an affair. *Journal of Marital and Family Therapy*, 1980, *6*, 259–268.
Whitaker, C. A., & Miller, M. H. A re-evaluation of "psychiatric help" when divorce impends. *American Journal of Psychiatry*, 1969, *126*, 611–618.

20

CONSULTATION WITH THE CLERGY
A Systems Approach

TIMOTHY T. WEBER[1]
Colorado Center for Psychology
Colorado Springs, Colorado

JOHN CHARLES WYNN[1]
Colgate–Rochester Divinity School
Rochester, New York

The clergy historically have been a significant force in influencing social behavior and shaping the lives of countless individuals and their families.[2] As a contemporary example of this influence, it has been documented that people in trouble will turn to the clergy first and more often than to other members of the helping professions (Fairchild, 1980; Wynn, 1982). Moreover, for many people the clergy and their congregations have functioned as an extension of, and, in some cases, a trusted substitute for, the family in providing steady nurturance, education, advice, guiding mythologies, and rituals to assist with moving through transitions across the life span. Because the clergy are intensely involved with families, they may be eager to collaborate with the consulting family therapist. This chapter will examine issues in such consultation from a systems perspective.

A PROFILE OF THE CLERGY AND THEIR CHURCHES[3]

Clergy and churches vary widely in style and habits, each context being unique. However, this general profile of the clergy and the church context,

1. In addition to working as family therapists and teachers of family therapy, both authors are graduates of theological seminaries and have served as professionals within a variety of congregations.
2. We will use the term "clergy" to refer collectively to leaders of religious organizations (e.g., priests, rabbis, pastors, or ministers).
3. By and large, the principles and problems discussed in this chapter apply to both churches and synagogues. For simplicity of exposition, we will use the term "church" except where a synagogue is explicitly mentioned.

while oversimplified, may help orient the consultant to some of the salient issues in consulting with the clergy.

THE CLERGY

Those who work with the clergy know them to be a profession of generalists who serve as theologians, preachers, teachers, administrators, and counselors. These widespread duties can leave them with feelings of inadequacy in many of their tasks. Because they work with people all week long, they generally become adept in human relations. And yet they may feel inferior to consultants who have expertise in psychotherapy. If consultants are sensitive to this situation, they will be able to accept clergy as colleagues in the helping professions, recognizing their competencies and avoiding the risk of making them feel more inadequate in this encounter.

Recently, many more members of the clergy have become open to collaborating with consultants from the helping professions. Training in theological seminaries has included courses in counseling and clinical experience in pastoral care, a development that has made the clergy more receptive to behavioral sciences and mental health education than ever before. Their own numerous journals (e.g., *Pastoral Psychology*, *Religion and Health*), their professional associations (e.g., American Association of Pastoral Counselors), and their participation in therapy organizations (about 16% of the membership of The American Association for Marriage and Family Therapy is trained as clergy), are indications of a greater interest and sophistication in the field of therapy. Once wary of psychology and suspicious of psychotherapy (McWhirter, 1968), the clergy have begun to shift to a cross-disciplinary cooperation with representatives of the mental health field.

Still, their willingness to collaborate with consultants may be affected by their relative isolation. Members of the clergy, both by education and work, tend to be isolated, sometimes standing far apart from their own colleagues in ministry as well as from their congregations, despite their many social responsibilities. Such a position may make it difficult for some to request help when they need it. Overworked in their congregations, competitive with peers and other professionals, often unclear about the exact criteria for "successful ministry," many may endure chronic, low-grade depression.

Perhaps because of this emotional isolation, many members of the clergy tend to become overly involved with individuals in their congregations. In addition, their training conditions them to be helpful. Sometimes overinvolvement is the result of their seeking support and gratification from their work. It may also stem from a need to prove their competency and their dedication to their faith. Their ambiguous job descriptions may propel them to do more and more in an effort to satisfy their parishioners. Because many people jokingly describe the clergy as "working only on Sunday," clergymen or women may overwork to prove that "I am really needed in this place." For whatever reason, an overfunctioning leader can elicit an underfunctioning system in the church, thereby increasing the demands on the professional staff and eliciting diffuse complaints from the underutilized membership. Not a few members of the clergy under similar circumstances have felt burned out and have either dropped out of the profession or have continued as people who feel "trapped in ministry," believing there are no other vocations open to them.

THE CHURCH

The clergy cannot be understood apart from the tradition of religious organizations in which they work. The term "church" evokes a composite picture of plurality and diversity. It denotes many different denominations and sects with their own unique, ethnic heritages, values, traditions, and beliefs that often span the centuries. Churches may differ markedly in their values regarding such issues as divorce, birth control, mental health programs, tolerance for diverse beliefs, and social outreach. The belief systems and language of the clergy and their churches will influence their response to interventions. Therefore, it is important for the consultant to understand something of the specific historical background of the consultee's church. For example, one Jewish consultant with whom we are acquainted has frequently consulted with Christian clergy and has done so very effectively. Her approach from the beginning is to admit that by heritage she has little understanding of their theology and will require some coaching in order to appreciate the problems with which they will be working. As clergy cannot resist explaining their traditions to inquirers, this introduction invariably opens the way to an easy working relationship.

Religious systems, of course, have much in common with secular systems. However, they also have their unique characteristics. Four in particular are relevant to the consultant: (1) the decline of religious influence, (2) the voluntary nature of North American religion, (3) conflict patterns of religious groups, and (4) the service record of churches.

1. Many of the mainline churches of North America have either gone into decline during the 1970s and 1980s or else failed to maintain membership levels commensurate with the growth of the national population. The leadership of religious groups has shown concern over this perceived loss of

influence and the decrease in prestige and numbers. Some of the most attractive courses in seminaries have been those dealing with techniques to enhance church growth. It is a time of notable change and widespread uncertainty in religious institutions, but it is also a time of openness to new models of ministry and to consultation. The crisis status of many churches signals not only danger but also opportunity to experiment with new models of ministry.

2. That a church is a voluntary organization leads to rather natural but vexing results for clergy. Persons may enter and leave membership almost at will. Loyalty to the institution and its tenets remains largely an idiosyncratic matter, with members choosing whether to be active or inactive, faithful or indifferent. It follows that an organization whose power may be in decline and whose constituency cannot be expected to show unanimous support may likely be a system undergoing discontent and in some need of restructuring.

3. Conflict management and conflict resolution loom large in what is dubbed church polity (governance) because the systems we are describing necessarily produce inner conflict as an inevitable by-product of their complicated lives. But the conflicts tend to be covert and, thus, more hazardous than in organizations where conflict is more overt. Given the ideal that they ought to live at peace with one another, but being unable to do so all the time, church folk will often try to deny or submerge conflict. Believing that they are not like other groups who fight with each other, church members may insist that they must think positively and "love one another." Thus, the submerged conflict can increase the discontent already mentioned and complicate the problems of church organization.

4. It is the theme of servanthood, if anything, that characterizes the churches in their social behavior. The ideal of a servant group, ministering to the needy and bereft, is Biblically based and the subject of thousands of sermons. Believing themselves to be a servant organization, churches can err in two rather typical ways: by turning inward and developing a thick membrane between themselves and the rest of the world, or by minding almost everyone else's business and neglecting their own internal needs. In either direction lies the possibility of guilt, a problem to which religious people are by nature and training particularly susceptible.

There remains one factor that the consultant should keep in mind: The church is really a family in which there are many smaller families. Historically, the Judaeo-Christian tradition has been imbued with the ideal that their religious units comprise an extended family. This ideal is hallowed by the Scriptures and preached from pulpits. It is no small wonder, therefore, that a good portion of church members believe this ideal and may use the church as a buttress or substitute for their own family. Yet, owing to the voluntary nature of commitment alluded to above, that wish for nurturance and support may be frustrated and many persons can be disappointed by unrealistic expectations. As a surrogate family, the religious group can evoke intense loyalty, incite harsh emotional conflicts, and increase dependency. On the positive side, the church can also stand by people with family-like rituals at times of birth and baptism, puberty and confirmation, marriage and wedding, separation and divorce, death and funeral rites. Thus, through its liturgy the church can foster family solidarity and bring meaning to life's transitions.

ENTERING CONSULTATION: ROLES, AVENUES, AND ISSUES

THE CONSULTATION ROLE

Consultants with the clergy provide expert advice on the diagnosis and management of work-related problems from a systems perspective; the consultee provides the consultant with an orientation to the specific problem and the surrounding context. Thus, the process between the consultant and the consultee is one of mutuality and collaboration. It is not mandatory that the consultant's advice be followed, as it would be in a supervisory relationship. Rather, the advice is made available and is often reshaped in the mutual dialogues between the consultant and the clergyman or woman.

In contrast to direct service, in which the provider (teacher, therapist, leader) addresses the problem directly, consultants address the problem *indirectly* through the clergy, who maintain ongoing, primary responsibility for managing the problem. As an extension of the consultation, the consultant may deliver services such as teaching, training, supervision, or therapy. For example, one of the authors once taught a 10-week seminar on "Marital Therapy in Pastoral Care" after several participants independently asked for a more didactic segment on pastoral counseling with couples. In this instance, teaching was an adjunct to consultation, a means of giving these members of the clergy information to assist them in managing problems within their congregations.

A clear consultative relationship has the advantage of enabling members of the clergy to use their own resources more effectively, in contrast to a direct service model in which they hand over problems to the family therapist for solving. While the direct-service model may indeed be useful at times, for example, when serious psychiatric or family disturbance is involved, the consulting model does not de-skill a member of the clergy but, rather, supplements his or her confidence and functioning.

ENTRY AVENUES

There are many direct and indirect avenues that lead to consultative relationships with the clergy. A family therapist may be asked to provide specific, time-limited teaching and/or training for either congregational members or clergy. There is often keen interest in programs that address some aspect of single adulthood or marital and family life. For example, some of the workshops and retreats may focus on such issues as parent–child communication, living in a stepfamily, marriage and the extended family, leadership training, and death in the family. This program format may be a convenient opportunity for both teaching family therapists and the clergy to "test the water" without making further commitments for consultation. We have found that these programs often open opportunities for later specific consultations related to issues discussed in the program.

Most consultations, however, begin more directly when an individual member of the clergy requests help in dealing with one of the following three problems: counseling with members of the congregation, internal staff conflicts, and major conflicts between the church leadership and members of the congregation. Providing assistance in one area may uncover problems in the other areas. Ecclesiastical superiors may request a consultant to assist them in dealing with pastoral or organizational problems in the churches under their auspices. However, this kind of invitation is infrequent and is usually directed to those "insider" consultants who already have a trusted role within the church.

Occasionally when the clergy are in an impasse in counseling with parishioners, they refer these clients to a family therapist for continuing, more "high-powered" therapy. If the family therapist automatically accepts the referral without deliberately exploring other options, a difficulty may be experienced as a major problem for both the pastor and his or her clients: *Pastor*: "I failed my clients and had to send them elsewhere." *Clients*: "We must really be bad if our pastor can't help us and thinks we need a shrink." A better solution may be for the family therapist to discuss the case with the pastor and consider the option of a consultation with him or her, with or without the presence of the clients.

"Options at the impasse": A case example. After working with a couple in his congregation for several months, Father Schweizer began to feel discouraged that he had not made significant progress. He had used a number of counseling techniques that he had learned in his clinical training. However, except for a few positive responses by the couple, his arduous labors had produced little positive change and reconciliation. At that point, Father Schweizer referred the couple to a family therapist. After hearing about the case and sensing undertones of discouragement, the family therapist suggested a consultation—first with Father Schweizer and then with Father Schweizer and the couple together. Although Father Schweizer initially suggested coming to the consultant's office with the couple, the family therapist consultant proposed that the consultation be held at the church. This geographical strategy was intended to define more clearly the roles of the consultant and the consultee; the clergy-consultee was to remain in charge of the case (meeting on church "turf" would reinforce this notion), and the consultant was more free to "return" the case to the clergyman after offering his expertise. During the initial meeting, Father Schweizer confessed to a sense of trepidation, "I'm a little nervous. I've never been observed before." The consultant responded, "That makes two of us. We've never worked together before and here I am, supposedly knowing something about these kinds of things!" Both laughed and began a collaborative series of productive consultations with the couple in which Father Schweizer and the consultant learned from one another.

In this case, and in others like it, the goals of the consultation are to assess the impasse in the system and explore how the impasse can be resolved, by instituting a new treatment plan in continued counseling with the couple, by referral to a family therapist, by termination of therapy, and so on.

Members of the clergy, like a great many other professionals, guard their own turf with considerable zeal. Concerned that their members may stray out of reach if referred to other specialists, and worried about the image of their own competency among members if they defer to other professionals, they are very careful about the implications of any referral. Sometimes they may continue to work with members long after a referral has been indicated. Consultation may be useful in helping clergy to clarify their skills and limits, instructing them how to refer in a way that will help the member, and how to continue involvement with the professional to whom the members have been referred. If a referral is indicated, the consultation format allows opportunity for a careful framing of the referral to minimize the negative connotations of "failure" on the part of both clergy and clients. Moreover, the consultation format permits a realistic assessment of the risks and benefits of referral so that expectations are not inappropriately minimized or maximized.

When members of the clergy request consultation, they are usually interested in an informal consultation to help them examine a new perspective of the problem and explore alternatives for dealing with the problem. Often consultations do not evolve beyond this informal phase. As they become more familiar with the consultant, they frequently rely upon these informal, ad hoc consultations for both information and support.

There are two risks associated with informal, individual consultation.

First, because the consultant does not have direct access to the larger system and sees the problem only through the eyes of the consultee, the consultant may unwittingly reinforce a limited view and replicate attempted solutions that already have failed. Second, because of the informal nature of these consultations, members of the clergy may increasingly use these meetings not so much to solve professional problems as to remedy the problems of being emotionally isolated, issues that are endemic to the profession. Relying upon consultation for personal support may be necessary at times. However, repeated use of consultation for this purpose may impair their use of support from within their natural systems, that is, with their spouses and church colleagues.

To minimize the risk of seeing the problem through pastoral eyes, we have often suggested a more formal, "data-gathering" consultation in which members of the system involved with the problem (e.g., clients, congregational leaders, staff members) are included. Expanding the frame of reference and opening the consultation to more information may in itself help members of the clergy to discover new alternatives with minimal suggestions from the consultant. The consultant's primary role in this format is to generate a more complex, interactional view of the problem by using the strategies of circular interviewing (Penn, 1982; Selvini Palazzoli, Boscolo, Cecchin, & Prata, 1980). Often, it is sufficient to guide the consultees toward drawing their own conclusions based on the data rather than to give advice directly or to present a new formulation. This questioning process reinforces the clergy's own competency to draw conclusions and enables him or her to continue counseling from a position of strength.

Strengthening the clergy's support base, initially among colleagues, has been our goal in response to the second risk of encouraging dependence through informal, individual consultation. We have found the members of clergy to be enthusiastic about a group case conference format. Here the consultant contracts with five to seven church leaders to meet regularly over a fixed period (e.g., biweekly for 6 months) in sessions in which they present problem cases by rotation and the consultant utilizes part of the sessions for didactic input. Each presenter is requested to bring along a one- or two-page outline of the case that includes a description of the nuclear and extended family, the presenting problem, important variables within the larger system (e.g., work and school issues), a summary of the sessions, including the primary interventions used thus far, and specific questions that they want to work on. The advantage of this structured presentation is that it focuses attention and minimizes rambling and vague theorizing. The consultant's task is to guide discussion of the case, inviting input from other members of the group.

After several months of following this structured framework, the participants present their own genograms or family trees to the group, giving attention to such issues as emotional cutoffs (Bowen, 1978), sibling position, repeated themes across the generations, critical events, occupational histories, and religious patterns (Guerin & Pendagast, 1976). The importance of understanding and coming to terms with issues rooted in families of origin have become increasingly important in preparation for the ministry and in helping clergymen and women to deal with continuing problems in their work (Anderson & Fitzgerald, 1978). The consultant needs to be aware of the possibility that members of the clergy may at times seek to work on their own family problems through working with the problems of the families within their congregations. Although these group presentations may evoke interesting personal explorations, our central task as consultants is to assist the consultees in the use of genograms and other personal data that may illuminate issues in their professional lives. In some cases, members of the clergy have elected to follow up these consultation sessions with personal therapy.

The following issues have emerged as especially important in helping church leaders to better understand their personal and professional development: (1) patterns of overfunctioning and underfunctioning and expectations of being "the responsible one," (2) overt and covert rules for how conflict is expressed and managed, (3) attitudes toward emotional expression, especially the expression of anger and affection, and (4) how their families of origin influenced vocational choice.

"Sacrifice": A case example. Pastor Lierman had been depressed for several years as he dutifully but methodically went about his work in a small suburban congregation. As he explored the issue of vocational choice during his genogram presentation, he recalled how his father had regretted not having gone into the ministry. His father had always felt "second class" to professional ministers but, nevertheless, had vigorously participated as a lay minister for years, in addition to working full-time as a businessman. Although Pastor Lierman had never talked to his father about choosing the ministry as a vocation, he had felt "obliged" to fulfill his father's dream by entering the ministry. His father had reciprocated by being noticeably proud of his son's choice. Since his father's death, Pastor Lierman had become more disenchanted with the ministry. In preparing his genogram, he realized that he was now in the process of "giving up" the ministry and deciding whether he truly wanted to pursue the ministry as *his* choice rather than simply continuing to enact his father's dreams.

In a group, pastors often discover the benefits of using each other as peer consultants and become more accepting of the vulnerability that goes along with asking for help. This vulnerability is protected by stipulating that what is shared in the group is held strictly confidential.

ENTRY ISSUES

In beginning a consultation with members of the clergy, there are several issues that directly affect the consultant's effectiveness. First, it is important to understand the potential advantages and disadvantages of being either an "insider" consultant (clergy-trained or actively religious within the church) or an "outsider" consultant (having no identifiable affiliation within the church). Traditionally, the clergy have been suspicious of secular psychotherapists and their presumed antireligious bias (McWhirter, 1968). Consequently, clergymen and women have been more inclined to seek assistance from those insiders who share their religious values. Although the clergy increasingly has become more receptive to outsiders, the insider at the entry point has a distinct advantage over the outsider who may initially be regarded with some suspicion.

However, the question of who has the most leverage is more complicated than it appears at first glance. After the outsider has been accepted, it may be easier for the outsider than the insider to bring about change and to continue to have an effective influence. Outside consultants, being different from members of the clergy, may be perceived as less threatening and may be able to offer a more objective and challenging viewpoint. Outsiders may make fewer assumptions about the clergy and their organization than the insiders who already *think* they know what is important to know. Furthermore, by being uninformed, the outsider is more likely to inquire about the clergy's beliefs and practices and the functioning of the church organization. Not only may this "one-down" inquiry empower the clergy and foster a collaborative spirit, but also, in the process of educating the consultant, the individual clergyman or clergywoman may clarify particular beliefs and values held by a specific congregation and the church leadership that may be central to solving the presenting problem. The insider, being too similar to the clergy, runs the risk of bypassing these important steps and may be perceived by the consultees as too competitive or not as expert as the outsider. Regardless of whether the consultant is an insider or outsider, effective consultation with the clergy begins by respecting the clergyman's or woman's expertise and ability to acquaint the consultant with the beliefs and rituals that give substance to his or her life with the parishioners. A consultant earns the right to be a strong leader by beginning as a sensitive follower.

A second issue in beginning a consultation with any member of the clergy is reflected in the mandate: "Go slowly." In any kind of consultation, it is important, particularly in the early stages, for the consultant to accommodate his or her approach to the operating style, language, and beliefs of the consultee before intiating any major interventions. With the clergy it is especially imperative. The clergy operate out of a set of assumptions often confusing to lay people. Being theologians, they are trained to measure contemporary conditions against an Absolute, a habit that will color their thinking about ethics and commitment. Being subject to ecclesiastical discipline, they are answerable to denominational rules that define some of their counseling practices (e.g., the permissible bounds in which they may work with divorced persons toward remarriage). Being liturgists, they live with a set of rites meaningful to them, but often irrelevant not only to the outside world, but also to their members.

Furthermore, although members of the clergy may run the gamut from liberal to conservative, they are nevertheless representatives of long and seasoned traditions within the church and, in their job descriptions, they are called upon (overtly and covertly) to preserve those sacred and not-so-sacred traditions and routines. Churches are inherently conservative organizations in both practice and belief. Those churches that have explicitly identified themselves as being theologically conservative have in recent years attracted more members (Kelley, 1972). Members of the clergy may be called upon to be dynamic, but to keep their jobs they often must walk softly. Traditions within the church that may appear to have little to do with the depth of spirituality (e.g., how committees are organized, who is on the altar guild, which hymnal is used, what time do worship services begin and end) are often inflexible routines that, if changed, may invoke wrath from offended parishioners. This penchant for preservation is reflected in one poster circulating among the churches: "The Seven Last Words of the Church: We've Never Done It That Way Before." In consulting with the clergy, therefore, it is crucial to assess and respect the traditions and routines that shape church life.

Third, in beginning a consultation with the clergy in churches with more than one staff member, it is important to consider who else, besides the initial consultee, should participate and to determine whether and how an extended consultation might take place. Identifying too closely with the one staff member as consultee may evoke resistance in others who may perceive the consultant as taking sides in an ongoing staff conflict. Or the consultee may unwittingly use the consultant to gain advantage over other staff members who may, in response, sabotage the consultant's efforts. Proposing a preliminary, exploratory stage with other members of the system who are in leadership positions is useful in mitigating these potential disasters and gaining a broader base of support.

"The Lone Ranger": A case example. Pastor Erhardt was a copastor in a large congregation that included eight staff members who worked under the supervision of the copastors. Pastor Erhardt had been in the congregation only several months when he experienced what he thought to be increasing discontent and apathy among the staff. His colleague, Pastor Tyson, did not share Pastor Erhardt's view. Instead, he thought that Pastor Erhardt was overreacting to the staff's slow response to

Erhardt's enthusiastic entry into the congregation and his many proposals for new projects. Pastor Erhardt then took it upon himself to contact a consultant with the request: "Our staff members at the church aren't working up to their potential. I think they may benefit from a program that could help us all communicate better." The consultant and Pastor Erhardt then discussed the details of a specific program. Before agreeing to the request, the consultant suggested that he meet with Pastor Erhardt and Pastor Tyson so that he could get more information that would help him design a program that would be of most benefit. The consultant suggested this preliminary step in order to gain a broader base of support from the leaderhsip and avert any potential sabotage by competing leaders. The consultant had hypothesized that Pastor Erhardt's recent entrance into the system had destabilized the organization and that his request for consultation was his unilateral attempt to consolidate his role. In that meeting, the consultant was not only able to gain access to information that significantly modified his initial view of the problem, but he was also able to engage both Pastor Erhardt and Pastor Tyson in a way that mitigated an increasing, covert conflict between the two by identifying them as a "team" with a joint proposal for the staff. This collaboration between the consultant and these clergymen was crucial in giving solid foundation to the program and increasing the consultant's credibility with the other staff members.

THE ASSESSMENT FRAMEWORK

In consulting with members of the clergy, we have been asked to deal with a variety of problems ranging from a stuck counseling case to a major rift between factions in the congregation. The extent of the assessment process depends on the breadth and severity of the specific problem. We have found it useful to consider each problem, regardless of its apparent simplicity or complexity, within a larger systemic framework. The eight subsystems in this framework that may affect (usually covertly) each request for consultation include the following: (1) the individual clergyman or woman, (2) his or her family of origin and nuclear family, (3) the clergy–staff team within the church, (4) individuals and families that constitute the church membership, (5) the church organization (e.g., church council, committees), (6) clergy groups within the community, (7) the surrounding community and its sociopolitical issues that have an effect upon the church, and (8) the regional and national administration under whose auspices the church operates. We have already illustrated how the subtle interaction between these subsystems may generate and escalate what appear to be "simple problems" that are presented for consultation. Likewise, these same subsystems may offer resources for resolving problems and should be considered by the consultant in designing interventions.

"There is more than meets the eye": A case example. In a group case conference, Pastor Christopher reported that he had been counseling a young, attractive, female college student for months and had achieved some successful results. His problem was that he did not know if he should terminate with her. Using the framework discussed above, the consultant questioned him further about his dilemma, and the scope of the problem broadened. He anxiously spoke of other issues complicating his decision. His wife had become increasingly annoyed with the "many hours" he had been spending with this attractive student. She had asked her husband to give some "very good reasons" why this woman needed all the counseling she was getting, but he had denied her request because of "confidentiality," which only further enraged his wife and increased her suspicions. Pastor Christopher not only wanted to terminate counseling with this parishioner because of the successful resolution of the problem, but he also wanted to "keep his home from exploding."

However, the parents of this female parishioner, who were long-standing, prominent members in the congregation, had made it unequivocally clear to Pastor Christopher that they wanted him to continue to see their daughter despite his opinion to the contrary. Worrying about their daughter had fueled their desperation and anger at him for suggesting that their perceptions might not have been as accurate as they imagined. He had complied with their demand to see their daughter, anticipating that they would withdraw their support from the congregation were he to confront them further. Because the congregation he was serving had been floundering during the last several years, Pastor Christopher was afraid to take any risks that would further jeopardize its survival and his own status within the district. This was his first congregation and some district administrators had recently been questioning his leadership ability. He also recalled how the parents of his client had reminded him of his own parents, whom he had never directly confronted because he feared the loss of their approval. In the seminary, he had been enamored with the listening/reflective approach to counseling and had avoided more directive/confrontative approaches that were not "his style."

Group members helped Pastor Christopher to redefine the consulting problem of "when to terminate." Both the problem and potential solutions became clearer when the focus broadened to include the interaction among the following subsystems: the individual clergyman, his family of origin and his nuclear family, the parents of the female client, the church organization, and the regional church administration.

Not every consulting problem will interlock with all eight subsystems. However, assessing these subsystems and how they relate to the problem may illuminate the picture and suggest solutions previously unconsidered. Besides assessing the relevant subsystems, the following questions have been useful to us in crystallizing our inquiry.

1. *At what stage in its organizational life cycle is the congregation?* The congregation may have just begun and may be propelled by the un-

bounded enthusiasm and openness to innovation of a small group of eager parishioners. Another congregation might be in the "settling down" stage following years of chaos and a high turnover in membership, and have a low tolerance for innovation and a thirst for stabilization and order. Many congregations that were once affluent and rich in members have recently experienced declines in membership and a consequent depression because they have not adapted to the reality of changing neighborhoods, the leaving of older, charter members who have not been replaced by younger members, and so on. Other congregations have burgeoned with a rapid influx of members and required new building programs and a larger, more comprehensive staff to meet the growing needs. Some congregations have reached a plateau and remained relatively stable for years, a stage characterized by either satisfaction or boredom.

Each stage of the congregation's life cycle, especially during transition periods when there is a significant exiting or entering of members, presents particular issues for the clergy and influences how they experience themselves and how they deal with problems that arise in their day-to-day ministry. For instance, in the previous case example, Pastor Christopher was hesitant to take a decisive step partly because he feared that he would alienate influential members who were desperately needed in his declining congregation. Had the congregation been at another point in the organizational life cycle, his response might have been entirely different. In other congregations, the joy of expansion may mask the difficulty of readjusting old roles and coping with pressing demands without adequate resources. Although members of the clergy adjust to the vicissitudes of congregational life with reasonable success, we have found that connecting issues in the organizational life cycle with specific consultation problems can often normalize these problems and ease tension by relating them to a broader perspective.

2. *What is the history of previous pastors?* Although many Protestant congregations appear to emphasize the "sameness" of the clergy and their congregations, following the belief in "the priesthood of all believers," this "sameness" is an illusion. In fact, the clergy may be experienced by the members of their congregations as powerful parental figures with attributes of "apartness," "holiness," and "magical power," and be expected to nurture, rebuke, counsel, and guard moral standards. As parent-surrogates, the clergy are the constant receptacles for intensely positive and negative feelings. Negative attitudes are indirectly manifested in constant criticism, attempts to remove the clergy, withdrawal from congregational activities, and general passive resistance. Positive attitudes are seen in displays of fierce loyalty and dedication to proposals by the clergy, with strong personal adherence, open praise for the clergy's work, and consistent attendance in worship (Williamson, 1967). Clergymen and women are not simply leaders

who are assigned to accomplish church tasks but, rather, may be regarded as surrogate parents entrusted with the care of large and complex families.

A congregation has a deep reservoir of strong feelings toward former pastors, and this will influence a successor's life in his or her new congregational family. It is important for the consultant to be sensitive to the congregation's "family of origin" and to understand the historical context in which current problems are often firmly rooted. In trying to establish a ministry in the congregation, a pastor may unwittingly transgress honored rituals and protocols set by predecessors. It may be nearly impossible for a new pastor, regardless of his or her best intentions, to spark commitment from parishioners whose energy has been trapped by nostalgic loyalty. Members may use the new pastor to complete unfinished business with the one who came before, just as stepchildren may be sharply hostile to a stepfather because of the biological father's departure from the family.

"The ghost of cleric past": A case example. A young congregation in a growing suburban neighborhood called a fresh graduate, the Reverend Hilary, from the seminary as its first clergyman. The congregation had high hopes for Hilary, who had indicated a strong commitment to evangelism and church growth. He was slowly gaining the trust of his members in the first months of his ministry when he suddenly resigned one day and quickly moved away from the city. The members were shocked. Weeks later they were even more astonished to learn that he had impregnated a young girl from the youth group. It took a number of months before the congregation was ready to call the Reverend Andrews, an older, more seasoned, minister. Nevertheless, Andrews had countless difficulties establishing leadership in the congregation because of persistent complaints and nagging from the membership. After struggling for 6 years in the congregation, he finally resigned. As a last hope, he had attempted unsuccessfully to work with a passionate faction of angry charter members who had brought a long list of both petty and serious offenses to the district bishop. Although Andrews recognized deficiencies in his leadership ability, the charges leveled against him had seemed largely petty and irrational, but excruciatingly persistent over the year.

One previous consultation, 2 years before Andrews had resigned, had focused on helping him and his congregation to air their differences and temporarily resolve their conflict. However, the consultant failed to attend to the congregation's history, its unfinished business with the Reverend Hilary and the intense feelings of anger and depression that had been pushed underground in the wake of Hilary's sudden departure. These feelings had been transferred to Andrews. Over the years, the embarrassing behavior of Hilary had become a secret, and his departure had been framed as a "mystery" to newcomers. Yet the unresolved feelings had not evaporated but, rather, intensified. Andrews, the second clergyman, paid penance for the sins of Hilary, the first clergyman.

3. *At what stage of his or her professional life cycle is the clergyman or clergywoman?* Orientation to work and awareness of personal strengths and liabilities will vary greatly according to the individual's position in the professional life cycle. Borrowing from Daniel Levinson's examination of adult development, Noyce (1983) has outlined the salient ages or "seasons of a cleric's life" from age 25 through age 50. The first stage, "Getting into the Adult World," involves entering the first parish with immense energy and idealistic expectations and moving on to disillusionment. Commenting on this stage, one clergyman said, "You soon learn that the church has levels of commitment not as intense as your own."

The "Age Thirty Transition" is the second stage; at this point, members of the clergy reevaluate their careers, with the result that many of them leave the ministry about 5 years after leaving the seminary. Those who continue enter the third stage (in their mid- and late-30s) of "Settling Down." This stage involves vigorous work in the church, creative ministry, and career advancement. In their late 30s, clergymen and women enter the fourth stage, "Becoming One's Own Person," discard earlier relationships to mentors, become more independent, and offer a more caring leadership to others.

The fifth stage is the "Midlife Transition," in which members of the clergy may think that earlier accomplishments and outwardly successful careers seem shallow and unfulfilling. Concerns of the heart that have been put aside for too long now become dominant. Career-long fantasies of engineering exciting projects in the church or winning a call to the ideal parish or a top denominational post are now tempered to fit reality better. Choices are made with a greater awareness of death. Some react with sudden changes in life-style, jolting congregational members. Others become more distant because of self-analysis, angering those in the congregation who expect the clergy to be available and highly energetic. Some leave church work altogether, while still others become angry over their career choice but feel helpless to do anything: "I'm too old to make a change now." Individual members of the clergy may either work through this struggle or become bitter toward the people they serve. Likewise, men and women who have spent their lives in other occupations may now enter the ministry for a "fresh start."

The sixth stage is a new period of stability in which the clergyman or woman often grows into a new and relaxed maturity. One stated, "I have been much less idealistic—enjoying and allowing people to be where they are without always trying to change them. Maybe I'm just turning into a gentle, loving old man." Younger clergy may be irritated by this stance, regarding it as lacking in prophetic power and as showing indifference to social justice.

Although these stages are not by any means fixed and invariable, they do provide the consultant with a general orientation to the primary issues that shape how members of the clergy may approach their experiences. Moreover, this framework may help the consultant better understand leadership success and conflict in churches with more than one staff member. For example, a clergyman under 40 might be best paired with a post-midlife pastoral colleague who is more attuned to the "hermit" stage. On the other hand, colleagues at the same stage in the life cycle may spark intense rivalry. Even if they are not in conflict, the congregation's needs may not be satisfied because of the absence of complementarity or diversity of church leaders who are at the same stage of the life cycle.

4. *How are people involved with each other in the system?* People typically are involved with each other on a continuum ranging from being overly close and responsive to one another (enmeshed) to having minimal contact and concern for each other (disengaged). From our experience, it is especially important for the consultant to assess the patterns among the following subsystems:

a. *Clergy and colleagues.* Despite extensive social activity, clergymen and women are often personally isolated and feel very much alone. Is the consultee open to support from his or her colleagues or are there unspoken rules about keeping problems to oneself? Many members of the clergy are so conditioned to their autonomy that they find it very difficult to work with colleagues or staff.

"Too many cooks": A case example. When Father Paul requested help from a consultant, it was because he could not make any progress with a family he had known for years, but had worked with in counseling for only several weeks. This family displayed the multiproblem syndrome of disorganized families—an alcoholic mother, runaway daughter, and a 10-year-old son who was already a school dropout. No sooner would Father Paul make some gain with them than it would be erased by the family's sabotage or some other impediment. The consultant soon learned that the director of religious education in the church was also working with this family, unbeknownst to Father Paul and, worse, the two were working at cross-purposes. Bringing them together in collaboration proved to be the prelude to progress with the family and with a church staff that needed more direct communication.

b. *Church and neighborhood.* A church may be overly involved in its internal life, creating rigid boundaries with the community, or it may be socially active while neglecting the nurturance of its members.

c. *Church and regional administration.* Do the clergy and church experience support or alienation from the regional administration? Is the regional administration overly involved in determining the course of the church's life so that members do not take "ownership" of their church and its mission?

d. *Congregational groups.* Within the church, there are numerous subsystems that are determined by such variables as sex, age, length of membership in the congregation, and theological beliefs. How much contact do the church subsystems have with each other? With which subsystems is the clergy over- and underinvolved? To what extent does the church have a common mission that encompasses the needs of the different subsystems? Are there a variety of missions that remain unintegrated or, worse, unheard and ignored?

e. *Clergy and members.* How involved are the clergy in the personal lives of the members? Do they distance themselves from the personal struggles of the members? Or, more typically, are the clergy so enmeshed in the lives of some members that it is difficult for them to gain perspective? Overinvolvement with members may compensate for disengagement and lack of support from family members and clergy-colleagues. Sometimes it is useful to encourage the clergy to become more structured in their contacts with church members with whom they are enmeshed.

"Too close for comfort": A case example. Rabbi David, who was known to have counseling skills, was approached by a couple for assistance. After he had met with both husband and wife several times, the wife began making unscheduled visits to the synagogue. At first Rabbi David welcomed these visits as opportunities to counsel and to assist the depressed wife. After several weeks, these individual meetings increased to the point that Rabbi David was having difficulty completing his office business. Moreover, the husband, who had initially encouraged his wife to visit Rabbi David, was now becoming angry because his wife was contrasting his apparent lack of concern with Rabbi David's "deep love and support." Consultation was useful in helping Rabbi David distance himself from the wife in a way that was still supportive. Rabbi David and the couple agreed that if the wife needed an individual appointment, she could come at a scheduled time during the week. In all other cases, she was to ask her husband for support.

f. *Clergy family, clergy, and church.* Clergy too often function as symbolic bigamists. They are married to their spouses/family and, bound by vows of deep loyalty, they often act as if they are married to the church family. They are on 24-hour call to both families, and they may not put limits on demands for their services. Balancing time between these two families is tricky business even if the individual has a clear sense that a spouse, not the church, is the real marital partner. Any overinvolvement with one family leads to a reciprocal disengagement from the other. Friedman (1978) has written about some of the causes and consequences of tipping this delicate balance between personal family and congregational family. For example, clergy may stabilize an overly tense relationship at home by entering other intense relationships that draw off pressure. An "affair" with the church can relieve pressure from a difficult marriage. Even if this is not the case, those who for other reasons have overinvolved themselves with the congregational family may experience increasing turmoil at home that will necessitate their presence to "do something about the family problem." Sometimes the disengagement from the family will result in the spouse emotionally disengaging from the marriage.

If a pastor and congregational family have together achieved a working relationship and are in equilibrium, this balance may be disturbed in the opposite direction toward home when the pastor needs to attend to such normal developments as the birth of children, sicknesses, the spouse getting a job, and so on. As in a marriage, the congregational family may respond to the cleric's emotional withdrawing by henpecking and criticism or, more indirectly, by creating problems in the church in the hopes of reinvolving him or her. Many congregational problems may be indirect attempts to reengage the peripheral and distancing clergy–father/mother.

"Competing with God": A case example. Sam Lynn, a young seminarian in the Southwest, had been working for several years in a part-time secular job when he was notified that he had been called to a new mission congregation in a neighboring state. Because his job had been part-time, he and his wife, along with their two young children, had had enjoyable opportunities to cement their family after the difficult seminary years. He and his wife had become very close, and both looked forward to their first call.

Pastor Lynn arrived at the congregation in the late fall and not only was immediately besieged with routine parish demands, but also had little time to adjust to the congregation before he was pushing himself to prepare for the church seasons of Advent and Christmas. At the same time, he spent hours visiting people in the community, late into the night, in hopes of quickly increasing the church membership. Pastor Lynn's wife was unprepared for this abrupt disengagement and quickly became depressed. She felt guilty about complaining because her husband was doing "the Lord's work" and who, after all, could compete with God!

A consultant, engaged by the district administration to assist clergy in adjusting to their first call, worked intensively with Pastor Lynn for several weeks, concentrating on organizational issues, time management, sermon preparation, and personal adjustment. The family subsystem was not seriously addressed in the consultation, and Pastor Lynn's wife was only involved in a few dinners and get-togethers with the consultant. As Pastor Lynn's overinvolvement with the congregational family continued, his wife became more depressed and finally left for her parents' home and, while there, was hospitalized for severe depression. After several weeks of individual therapy interspersed by periodic visits by her husband, she killed herself during a weekend visit to her parent's home.

The consultant had failed to seriously consider Pastor Lynn's family, operating as if there were a firm boundary between Pastor Lynn's marriage and his behavior in the church. For his part, Pastor Lynn had not been aware of his wife's increasing depression because of the depth of his immersion into his new congregation and his dogged pursuit of professional excellence.

Even in less tragic circumstances, trying to attend to the demands of both the congregational family and the home family is not an easy task for members of the clergy. Most achieve a relatively workable balance, but any consultation with the clergy should include an assessment of the dynamics of and changes in this sensitive turf between the home family and the congregational family.

5. *How are differences tolerated and conflict negotiated?* Members of the clergy and their congregations differ dramatically in how they tolerate differences within the church. Differences of opinion and theological belief may be labeled "unfaithfulness" and "heresy," or "healthy diversity." In more conservative congregations, where the range of tolerance is reduced, the clergy may tread carefully for fear of offending members. In other congregations, so much diversity of belief and behavior may be encouraged that the clergy and congregation will suffer from a lack of cohesiveness and mission. Although differences may be welcomed, there may be a set of core, nonnegotiable beliefs in the system that are like buried minefields, forcing a nearly paralyzed clergy and membership to be overly cautious in order to avoid potential explosions.

When conflicts do arise, as they will in the most peaceful of organizations, how are these conflicts negotiated? Some congregations have adeptly used their religious beliefs as resources to help them express differences and to negotiate problems. On the other hand, many clergy and congregations are uncomfortable when it comes to experiencing and expressing negative feelings. Williamson (1967) has suggested that religious people are concerned more than others with the problem of impulse control. Core beliefs that justify pushing conflict underground include: "To be angry or hateful is to fall into sin," "Turn the other cheek," "Think positively," or "Peace at all costs." Conflict that is pushed underground and expressed in forms of passive resistance and petty criticisms is debilitating for both clergy and congregation and results in depression and lifeless ministry. Rabbi Friedman (1978) has emphasized that clergy most effectively take leadership in conflict when they (a) stay in touch with the members of the congregation and (b) take a well-defined position without overfunctioning and trying to solve every conflict in the congregation.

6. *How are organizational roles clarified and power exercised by the clergy and members?* Clergy are powerful parental surrogates and need power to run the church organization. Nevertheless, while some members of the clergy command the power to fulfill their appointed tasks, others are apprehensive of power and may, in fact, deny their power as "servants of

God." In their efforts to be loving and helpful, are the clergy and other congregational leaders avoiding the use of power? Are roles clear or are they duplicating or unknowingly counteracting each other's efforts as they all respond to problems with "concern"? Are the clergy and members, in their efforts to be "all things to all people," overextended and too ambitious so that tasks are begun but never finished? Is leadership confined to the clergy or well distributed among members of the congregation? Has the power base within the church been shifting so that those who once had power now have little? A consultant may empower certain members in the church without being aware of the unintended withdrawal of power from other members.

"The risks of remodeling": A case example. Pastor Marty requested consultation to help her deal with the growing psychological needs in her congregation. In the initial planning stage, it was decided that the consultant would train a small group of qualified members to function as "pastoral assistants" who primarily would visit sick, shut-in members. Two older members of the congregation, who had been more informally assisting the pastors of the congregation in visitation for years, were not informed of this consultation and training until the news appeared in the church bulletin. Angry at being bypassed and intimidated by the apparently strict qualifications for "pastoral assistants," these two members did not apply for training. Instead, they continued their informal visiting without informing Pastor Marty and, furthermore, seeded complaints among the members about Pastor Marty and her new program. Fortunately, the consultant heard about these complaints and quickly recognized that he had forgotten to assess the risks of instituting this new program, especially how the program would shift existing roles and redistribute power in the church. The older visitors were immediately included in the training because of "their many years of experience" and served as co-consultants to the training program.

SUMMARY

The clergy historically have shaped, nurtured, corrected, and guided the lives of countless individuals and their families. Because of the wide diversity of their responsibilities, their primary presence in the midst of families, and their relative isolation from other professionals, they often are in need of assistance from family systems consultants. Usually members of the clergy will bring to consultants problems involving counseling issues, staff disagreements, or church–organizational conflicts. Regardless of how narrow the presenting problem is defined, systems consultation calls for giving careful attention to the following interlocking subsystems: the individual clergyman or clergywoman, his or her family of origin and family of procreation, the church staff, the church membership, the church administration, clergy groups in the community, the surrounding neighborhood, and the regional administration under whose auspices the church operates. Expanding the focus beyond the presenting problem is likely to lead to greater clarity and a more crisp and effective intervention.

For years, the gulf between the domain of churches and the behavioral sciences has remained wide, fueled by suspicion and misunderstanding on both sides. Now, as a result of the rise in mutual respect and the eagerness of many of these professionals to enter joint training and educational experiences, there are increasing opportunities for interdisciplinary cooperation.

ACKNOWLEDGMENTS

We wish to thank our colleagues, Roger Anderson, James Austin, Don Fahrenbrink, Steve Rice, and Connie Reece, for their most helpful comments on this chapter.

REFERENCES

Anderson, H., & Fitzgerald, C. G. Use of family systems in preparation for ministry. *Pastoral Psychology*, 1978, *27*, 49–61.

Bowen, M. *Family therapy in clinical practice.* New York: Jason Aronson, 1978.

Fairchild, R. *Finding hope again.* New York: Harper & Row, 1980.

Friedman, E. H. Leadership and self in a congregational family. *CCAR Journal*, 1978, *25*, 9–25.

Guerin, P. J., & Pendagast, E. G. Evaluation of family systems and genogram. In P. J. Guerin (Ed.), *Family therapy: Theory and practice.* New York: Gardner Press, 1976.

Kelley, D. M. *Why conservative churches are growing: A study in the sociology of religion.* New York: Harper & Row, 1972.

McWhirter, D. P. Consultation with the clergy. In W. N. Mendel & P. Solomon (Eds.), *The psychiatric consultation.* New York: Grune & Stratton, 1968.

Noyce, G. The seasons of a cleric's life. *Christian Century*, 1983, *100*, 90–93.

Penn, P. Circular questioning. *Family Process*, 1982, *21*, 267–280.

Selvini Palazzoli, M., Boscolo, L., Cecchin, G., & Prata, G. Hypothesizing–circularity–neutrality: Three guidelines for the conductor of the session. *Family Process*, 1980, *19*, 3–12.

Wynn, J. C. *Family therapy in pastoral ministry.* New York: Harper & Row, 1982.

Williamson, D. S. A study of selective inhibition of aggression by church members. *Journal of Pastoral Care*, 1967, *21*, 193–208.

21

SYSTEMS-BASED CONSULTATION WITH SCHOOLS

LAWRENCE FISHER
Veterans Administration Medical Center
Fresno, California
University of California, San Francisco

American society has undergone rapid and profound change in the years since the Second World War. This is clearly evident in its educational institutions that, in many ways, have illustrated the failure of our society to adapt successfully to alterations in values, beliefs, and behaviors. As population mobility, divorce, and fast-paced lifestyles have disrupted both urban and rural settings, schools have been hard-pressed to deal with the resulting problem behaviors of our society's children.

The school is a microcosm of community life. Suburban bedroom communities, comprised of upwardly striving professionals, contain schools in which competition is high and issues of college selection and attendance are noticeable even in the early grades. Likewise, communities where unemployment is high and the strains of poverty and alienation are pervasive contain schools that are, by and large, autocratic in their attempts to control the disillusionment and hostility acted out by the community's children.

Within this context, schools have become a public laboratory for experimenting with interventions in many areas. Starting with the community mental health movement in the 1960s, a national mandate was established to provide mental health consultation for the schools. The history of this process is interesting in its own right for it reflects the evolving interaction between idealism and cold reality. Initially, there was the hope that the sensitivities and skills of the clinician and of the clinical enterprise could be applied to the school setting. Training programs in child development, communication effectiveness, and behavior modification, and a host of new approaches in teaching basic skills were initiated. Even the term "classroom" became suspect and could refer to one that was self-contained, multigraded, open, closed, without walls, extended, or multiply taught.

Thus, the school as we know it became the setting for major input from a variety of extra-school personnel: demanding parents who wished the school to solve the problems of home and community life, idealistic clinicians who wished to extend the arena of clinical intervention, and educational innovators who wished to demonstrate the best way to teach Johnny to read.

I have been actively involved in school-related work from both clinical and research perspectives since 1968 when a valued supervisor led me away from the safety of our clinic playroom to a local elementary school for a teachers' meeting on curriculum development. About the same time, I became interested in the family as the unit of clinical treatment. My dual roles as family therapist and systems consultant to the school "leap-frogged" in their evolution over the years. Although the process has been unsettling, I have developed a more or less unified approach to systems-based consultation with the school. In this chapter I shall provide a subjective perspective of issues and models in doing school consultation from the viewpoint of a family therapist.

Two points of clarification may be useful at the outset. The word "school" needs to be viewed as a generic term representing some kind of educational setting. By and large, most intervention programs and some consultation programs have been aimed at the preschool or elementary levels. The Head Start and Follow-Through programs as well as the highly successful mental health intervention programs of Cowen (1980) and of Shure and Spivack (1978) are good examples. Because high schools are far different settings from elementary schools, and because schools for "special children" are equally different from specialty training settings (e.g., arts, technical, or academic), the term "school" can refer to many types of settings as well as to students of different ages. It is important to remember in this discussion that "schools" refer to a variety of contexts and settings as well as to the more traditional institutions that we may have encountered in our own educational careers.

A distinction between systems therapy and systems consultation is also useful to consider. A discussion of this topic could comprise an entire monograph, so I will restrict my comments to those issues that seem to have particular relevance for day-to-day practice. I use the term "therapy" to apply only to clinical settings, even though a similar systems-level intervention could be delivered to the system of a school. Beyond the specific content of the consultation request, clinical issues are always present in family or personal settings even when a "consultation" has been requested. This restriction in the use of the term "therapy" is based on the fact that psychopathology in one or more family members creates an immediacy of concern and a seriousness not experienced in a nonfamilial setting. There is a human urgency, a subjective pull, and a heartfelt compassion one experiences in working with a disordered family that is not experienced in the same way, for example, in a dysfunctional middle-management work group. With this somewhat limited overview, I will use the term "therapy" to apply only to family-based clinical situations. All other nonclinical evaluation and intervention programs will be called "consultation." One does therapy with a family, but one consults with a school, even though similar principles of intervention may be utilized.

THE CONTEXT OF THE SCHOOL

Schools are monolithic institutions constructed on an educational–political base. While there is a clear hierarchy within the structure from teacher to superintendent, most consultations are centered on the semiautonomous, individual school setting. Schools and families share several fundamental organizational similarities that make the family systems model particularly applicable to the school setting. First, like the family, one primary role of the school is the care and education of the young. Second, the school classroom is, in many ways, a maternal setting with the teacher (especially the stereotypic, elementary classroom teacher) assuming the role of a benevolent, loving, sensitive, and tolerant female who rewards and punishes with compassion. Although urban high schools stray far afield from this description, the ideal of what schools "should be like" remains.

Third, the frequency of encounters with males in the hierarchy increases as one goes up the administrative ladder. This is particularly the case within the preschool and elementary school levels, although less so in junior and senior high school where there is greater balance between the sexes in terms of actual numbers. Males are more frequently found in science, math, shop, and other "masculine" subject areas. Thus, there is a relatively clear sex role distinction among educators not only by content area of teaching but also by organizational power.

Fourth, schools are comprised of various subsystems that, depending upon grade level, serve to facilitate some functional tasks and to hamper others. As in families, schools contain both overt and covert subsystems. The overt subsystems may include administrators and faculty, teaching specialists, department heads and so on, whereas the more covert subsystems may include younger teachers versus older teachers, teachers of different races, teachers whose classrooms are in close physical proximity to each other, or teachers who are popular with students and teachers who are not. As in families, covert subsystems and alliances form the foundation for organizational distress, and their identification is a prerequisite for effective intervention.

Fifth, schools, like families, have well-articulated belief systems that strongly influence staff functioning. The community of parents may be seen as threatening and outspoken critics who create problems with their excessive demands. The myth of "at all costs do not cross a parent" may create a school-based atmosphere of appeasement at any price. Internal myths having to do with who is the principal's favorite teacher, or who is competing for resources and acknowledgement (tangible or emotional), all have parallels within the family system.

Sixth, repercussions of negative, stressful interactions at the administrative or parental level will be felt at lower levels of the hierarchy. A war between the senior building teacher and the principal, or conflict between the principal and district administration frequently leads to acting out or tension among maintenance personnel. When the parents argue or family stress is increased due to father's work problems, children often covertly manifest the disturbance. The marked intensity of interaction among staff members and the compressed high activity level of the school provide a setting in which organizational stress at any level is quickly reflected throughout the system.

In summary, the context of the school presents many characteristics similar to the family. It has levels of cohesion and rigidity or flexibility of role structure; it allocates power; it is divided into overt and covert subsystems; and it has a pervasive set of belief systems about its role in the district and in the community vis-à-vis parents and vis-à-vis students. The emotional charge created by its stated task and by the high level of activity within it creates a setting that is highly comparable to a family and to which systems concepts are particularly applicable.

FAMILY THERAPY AND CONSULTATION WITHIN THE SCHOOL

I shall make a distinction between family therapy and a family orientation to consultation. Our goal has *not* been to do family therapy with the "family" of professionals who work within the school. Rather, our goal has been to employ systems principles to both families and schools. A systems perspective can be operative regardless of the mode or form the actual intervention takes. For example, one can see an adolescent in individual psychotherapy and still be utilizing a systems outlook if the decision for this kind of treatment is preceded by a thorough study of the family. Likewise, one may meet regularly only with a school principal or individual teacher, or undertake traditional clinical case-consultation activities and still consider oneself as doing systems work if the context of the system is considered. A systems orientation refers to the utilization of a conceptual model and not to a specific form of intervention or treatment. Any form of consultation or intervention may use systems concepts regardless of the specific plan involved.

Under this conceptual umbrella, a variety of school consultation programs was devised as part of a school consultation training and research program at the University of Rochester Medical School through the 1970s. Classifying these programs by process or content (Caplan, 1970; Fisher, 1973, 1974) is a somewhat arbitrary task, for few projects ever seem to fit clearly into a specific category or heading. However, a nosology of approaches helps to avoid the pitfalls of ambiguity, to organize one's plan of attack, and to clarify one's thinking.

It has been particularly useful to classify our work into two broad areas of consultation, namely, program-oriented and agency-oriented consultation. These are not to be viewed as discrete categories, for there are occasions when a program model will be incorporated into a broader agency model. Rather, this dichotomy has served a useful purpose in organizing our thoughts and clarifying the consultation process. The following is a brief description of each model's goals, the position of the consultant, and the underlying assumptions of the approach.

PROGRAM-ORIENTED CONSULTATION

The exclusive goal of this kind of consultation is to provide the school with a specific program based on formal content. Although some knowledge of the system and its operation is useful, expertise in systems dynamics may not be as necessary in this kind of program delivery as it is in agency consultation. In program consultation, the consultant is seen as a knowledgeable expert who delivers a product without getting enmeshed in the inner workings of the system. Such programs may include case or referral consultation around certain students or a variety of in-service educational programs aimed at teaching or administrative staff.

The Case-Consultation Model

The case-oriented consultative role is perhaps the most traditional for the mental health consultant. The consultant brings his or her clinical skills and expertise to a case conference of pupil-services staff (psychologists, social workers, counselors, attendance personnel, and so on) and provides input on a case-by-case basis. The goal is to assist the school administration in (1) dealing with problem classroom behaviors, (2) creating a unified school–

clinic treatment team, (3) dealing with the family, (4) making an appropriate referral, or (5) facilitating school–clinic liaisons. The consultant is a clinical expert who advises the school on a course of action in a particular problem situation.

In-Service Educator

There is also a need for a variety of content-based programs for administrators, teachers, or mental health personnel. Examples include teacher in-service programs on dealing with children of divorce, programs for mental health personnel on dealing with problem parents, and programs for elementary school principals in designing and implementing in-school work group structures. The consultant is seen as having knowledge from which the school can benefit and is asked to create a formal, educational program for a specific unit or subsystem of the school or district.

Problems Encountered in Program Consultation

Program-oriented consultation, including both case and in-service work can pose major problems for consultants. First, entering a system as an "expert" opens the door to overt or covert competition from in-house staff. Most often, district or building administration requests an in-service training program for teaching or mental health staff. The system messages often behind such a request are (1) staff is lacking in some area, (2) appropriate school personnel do not have the resources or skills to "fill the gap," or (3) "we need to demonstrate to administrative superiors that we are working to improve." In all three cases, the covert message can frustrate the consultant's getting the task done. Resistance to the program may be expressed by scheduling and attendance problems. All staff are suddenly busy at the scheduled hour, or the number of regular participants drops substantially over time.

The reverse situation also can occur. The consultant can be embraced as a godlike rescuer who will meet all the needs of the system. Often there are attempts to ally with the consultant against an antagonist who could be an administrator or a covert subsystem of the staff. For example, consultants may find themselves surrounded by the younger, more energetic staff who are battling, and have excluded, the older, more traditional teachers. Or consultants may receive delightful invitations to staff social events only to learn later that the school administrator has been excluded. Interested and supportive consultants who are sensitive to the needs of their consultees may be inundated by calls for support that initially are flattering but, later, indicate major system deficits. Quite clearly, systems issues have a direct impact upon program-oriented efforts and they need to be taken into account in planning program consultation.

AGENCY-ORIENTED CONSULTATION

The goal of this type of consultation is to assist the school system in solving a problem, building a program, and so on. Unlike program consultation as described above, no content-focused product is delivered directly. Rather, consultants use their consulting skills to guide the system through program development. Consultants are viewed as issue specifiers, group process resource people, or more objective, externally based problem managers. They do not provide content or solve problems in a direct manner but facilitate the system in reaching its stated objectives. Examples include facilitating teacher–administration interchanges during weekly school meetings, aiding in the development of an organizational unit to handle teacher duty rosters, assisting in curriculum development meetings, facilitating school–community relations, or assisting in the development of a school-based educational philosophy.

Agency consultation implies a relatively long-term commitment in which the consultant "joins" the system without really becoming part of it. In fact, it is safe to say that the consultant's ability to remain outside the system yet be perceived as a safe and trusted advocate for the system are fundamental prerequisites for a successful consultation. The goals of agency consultation are not as clear and well-defined as in program consultation. The aim is to help the system to deal more effectively with its internal and external responsibilities, to advance its skills in managing group, educational, and administrative issues, and to help in the development of new programs to meet new needs.

Most agency-oriented consultation takes place prior to, or in conjunction with, program work. Agency-oriented consultation requires a degree of trust and familiarity between the consultant and the school personnel; it takes time to build and often is the result of a previously successful consultation in that setting. In a few circumstances, however, one may be asked at the outset to provide a vaguely defined service to a school. Below is an example of an agency-oriented consultation in a school established for mostly black, economically deprived youngsters in kindergarten through grade 3.

The school "family": A case example. An urban district school was housed in an old, large, and delightfully spacious, though drafty, building. A young male principal headed an all-female staff comprised of an assistant principal, nine classroom teachers, a part-time social worker, a part-time psychologist, and nine teacher aides. The principal was white, the assistant principal black, the aides black, and the teachers split relatively evenly by race. Three teachers were over 40 years of age, and the rest were relatively young; each had taught in other settings before.

The goal of the school was to provide intensive stimulation and training to a group of socially and economically deprived children and to involve parents and community leaders as much as possible in the operation of the school. Parents were encouraged to become teacher aides; evening educational programs on parenting were established; and a community advisory group was created. As part of a university-based consultation service, I was asked to become involved in the program at the beginning of the second year of the school's operation. The invitation came from the principal, who had heard of me through a colleague in whose school I had recently completed a yearlong, in-service program for teachers. His request was for aid in "reducing the stresses and strains" the school was experiencing so that "things would work more smoothly."

In an introductory meeting, it became apparent that this young, white, male authority figure felt extremely insecure not only about his ability to manage his racially mixed staff, but also about his relationships with a vocal and active community of parents. The staff was young and energetic, and held definite views on how the curriculum should be developed. In later meetings with the staff, the principal seemed to scurry among factions trying to keep peace and to prevent overt conflict. His request for consultation appeared to be a plea to reinforce his authority over a highly ambivalent staff. His assistant principal was a middle-aged, very attractive black woman who seemed allied with both her principal, with whom she had a social relationship outside of school, and the black community, with which she strongly identified. She also was the covert leader of the black teacher subsystem.

In addition, I learned from other sources in the system that the district had created the school in an effort to placate black parents who were active in the community. Although the district administrators thought that the school would serve a useful purpose, they were more interested in channeling the funds established for the special school back to the regular elementary school program in the community. While supportive of the new school in one sense, the district was not really enthusiastic.

After discussion with the assistant principal, teachers, and mental health staff, it became clear that the tension the principal experienced but could not talk about was pervasive throughout the school and was recognized at each level of the building's organizational structure. The assistant principal was somewhat jealous of the principal's position, frequently scowling at and quietly criticizing his activities. The principal tended to seek his assistant's maternal and social support by questioning her about her views and by pursuing their limited, but visible, social relationship outside of school. However, he generally felt unsupported and alone. Consequently, here was a young, white, male principal operating a program for blacks with a racially mixed female staff in a system that was only marginally supportive.

I met regularly with staff for 4 weeks before deciding if I could help and, if so, how. Since all members of the staff expressed a need for help (the staff voted positively on the principal's request to bring me in initially), and since it appeared that my previous work in the district was both known and respected by the school's personnel, I decided to make a formal agreement to provide consultation to the administration and staff of the school.

The 4 weeks of formal meetings and informal conversation permitted a broad systems diagnosis. The school personnel that "lived" in the building appeared to be functioning like a family with a frightened husband who had an ambivalently sabotaging yet supportive wife, and whose adolescent children were threatening to act out the insecurity and uncertainty of the family system. The unstable support of the district and community also reduced the husband's ability to establish appropriate and consistent internal boundaries and roles. Furthermore, the husband's attempts to keep the family operative by placating his wife and children and by being "sensitive," "listening attentively," and trying to "promote understanding," was ineffective against the varying views of his children and the competition of his wife. Thus, the school "family," because of the uncertain support of the district and the need to pacify its members and the larger community, had a need to keep their problems a secret and to present a calm facade while tension mounted and visible acting out among staff began to occur.

Since the contract was only with school staff, I decided to focus attention on the internal operation of the school, although discussion of strategies with the district and the community was not ruled out. My approach was to (1) assist the principal in solidifying structural roles within the school by creating a flexible, but definitive, staff structure, and (2) create the norm that internal differences of opinion could be expressed directly in a constructive manner without destroying a school that was facing district and community pressures.

The intervention was aimed at three levels. First, I joined the principal and his assistant at their weekly administrative meetings and, with a variety of "couple-focused" interventions, tried to defuse their seductive, yet competitive relationship. At these meetings, a more formal role structure for the school was created and implemented. For example, I fostered the assistant principal's identification with the organizational model she was helping to create, thereby reducing chances of later sabotage. I also regularly visited a number of classrooms, had coffee with teachers, and so on, in order to encourage vocalization of problems. Whenever a problem was discussed, I suggested a similar course of action: Take the problem to the appropriate person in the newly developed role hierarchy. In addition, I attended the staff meetings where I remained visible, but silent. I turned all questions and comments directed at me to the person designated by the principal and his assistant as the responsible staff member. At each point, I verbally noted differences of opinion among staff and directly facilitated a public interaction among the concerned parties.

Over the course of the next 6 months, internal tension decreased as many of the unexpressed anxieties and fears became public and were accepted as present although not always resolvable. Cohesion increased and a sense of mutual support developed as the school personnel came together to address their common problems. Both leaders and followers became better recognized and supported. Unfortunately, district and community pressure had intensified during this time, and budget changes by the spring of that academic year changed the school substantially. During the next academic year, major staff changes and a reduced number of students altered the program and its goals considerably.

A CONCEPTUAL MODEL

There is little question that there are many content and process parallels between schools and families, and similarities in modes of intervention with each. Both are powerful, intense, caretaking systems; with both, consultants require a knowledge of systems and system-level intervention strategies. Yet the dissimilarities between schools and families do need to be taken into account when one applies systems concepts to the school setting. For example, the school's extended family (district) has a powerful and controlling role in terms of budget and other forms of support. Schools also have relatively intact and stable membership boundaries only for the interval of one academic year. Decisions about staffing are often made by personnel outside the school and, consequently, programs and structures are unstable and unpredictable from year to year. Finally, the sheer complexity of the system—its size (especially high schools) and the variations in ages of students and staff—make comparisons with families more apparent than real. Perhaps it is safe to conclude that both families and schools *share* a variety of system properties but, at the same time, the differences in their goals, size, and complexity also indicate a considerable number of dissimilarities.

A GROUP RELATIONS MODEL

A need exists for a theoretical or conceptual tool that, when combined with family-based systems theory, will provide a more well-rounded model appropriate to the differences between the school and families. I have found the Tavistock model of group relations developed by Wilfred Bion (Menninger, 1972; Rioch, 1970a, 1970b) to be of great assistance in implementing systems concepts within the school. The combination of family systems concepts and group-oriented organizational theory has provided a broader base than either alone for understanding the structural and thematic differences between schools and families.

Briefly, Bion and his colleagues, for example, Turquet (1973), have articulated a theory of how work groups operate, as well as the patterns and styles that emerge as work groups veer from the task at hand in response to group pressures, myths, and fears. By describing patterns of group dependency, fight–flight, and pairing, Bion arms the consultant with tools for short-circuiting certain tendencies of task-focused groups. The theory also articulates issues of task definition and group leadership. Emphasis is placed on keeping the task of the group clear and understood among both leaders and followers so that the frequency of sidetracking and responding to covert issues is reduced. Tavistock theorists also have provided considerable material on the roles of leader and follower and their implicit contract with each other. Emphasis is placed on the leader's ability to provide task clarity and definition, to utilize group members' skills appropriately, and to foster the group's recognition of its own responsibility for completing the task.

The Tavistock model and family systems theory are complementary approaches in providing an orientation to consultation with the school. Below I shall briefly address a number of technical and procedural issues in both program and agency consultation using a family systems–organizational approach.

ASSESSING THE SYSTEM

Regardless of the type of consultation requested, program or agency, systems assessment is necessary, given covert agendas and covert needs, even when the request has been for a particular, well-defined program. For example, we have been forced to alter or even terminate a variety of teacher-oriented programs when attendance declined due to anger at a team leader or when dismay over certain school policies disrupted discussion. Systems assessment is also important in determining whether or not the system will permit staff to employ newly developed skills.

Receiving "parental" permission: A case example. In one junior high school where there were many children from single-parent families, the psychologist, social worker, and teachers requested a seminar on management of children and their divorced or divorcing parents. Specifically, they wished to develop skills for handling frightened, anxious, and often guilt-ridden single parents. School staff often were faced with having to respond to highly emotional parents who sought clarification of their personal and parental responsibilities. The staff personnel were interested in upgrading their abilities to act effectively in these situations. Midway through the program, however, it became apparent that the only personnel permitted by the district to deal with such "sensitive" parental issues were the mental health staff members who, unfortunately, were often overburdened and unavailable. School administration promptly limited the teachers' opportunity to respond to such situations even though teachers were willing to acquire the needed skills.

Content-oriented programs can also raise staff awareness of organizational and other problems within other components of the school.

The dangers of helping: A case example. I once was asked to teach group problem-solving skills to high school teaching teams in a suburban district. As a result of the program, the teachers' awareness of organizational issues within their own team sensitized them to existing problems at other levels of the school hierarchy. Their subsequent activities with administrative personnel led to a friendly but concerned call from the school principal about how our seminar program had led to difficulties at other levels of school administration. Needless to say, it was some time before we were asked to return to that high school.

In summary, systems assessment is a crucial aspect of any consultation, even those with a program focus. As in family therapy, where the reasons for coming to therapy often differ from the presenting problem, requests for consultation from a school often are multiply determined. The success of the consultation, however, depends in part upon a clear understanding of (1) what the requesting party is "really asking for," and (2) the impact that the program will have on the system as a whole.

THE CONSULTATION CONTRACT

A great many potential problems about role, termination, method of intervention, and focus of the program, can be prevented by the creation of a very clearly written letter of agreement between the contracting parties. Unlike family therapy, where distortions of agreements, sabotaged interventions, and "misperceived intentions" are grist for the therapeutic mill, such resistances in consultation can be deadly. Consultation implies a much more limited emotional interchange among the participants than is the case in family therapy; the investment in resolving emotional issues, as well as the consultant's leverage, is less in consultation than in psychotherapy.

There are several reasons for this state of affairs. First, the need for intervention is often less pressing in schools than in families. Even while stressed, schools are rarely in crisis, and the leverage created by acute family crises is rarely available within the school. Second, because of pressures of time and funding, there is often less opportunity to work through problems that emerge in the course of school consultation than is the case in family therapy. As mentioned above, changes in personnel and programming from year to year place a time limitation on problem appraisal, planning, and evaluation. Most schools begin the academic year in late August or early September and are heavily involved with start-up problems until late September. By mid-November, holiday activities intervene, and winter break in January or February and spring recess in March or April also reduce the time for effective intervention. By May, the school is again preoccupied with end-of-year teaching and evaluation issues. What appears to be a full academic year at the outset ends up with a series of 4- to 6-week periods. Such a limited time period does not give the consultant sufficient flexibility to assess the system and plan the consultation in as thorough a manner as might be possible in family therapy.

One method for countering this problem of reduced emotional energy and insufficient time is to obtain a written letter of agreement or contract between school and consultant. The letter I have used clearly outlines (1) the problem as defined, (2) the approach to problem resolution agreed upon by the participants, (3) the consultant's role, (4) the number of meetings or seminars that will take place, (5) the time limitations of the intervention, and (6) how the consultation will be evaluated. At first glance, this may appear to be an overly formal approach to intervention, but I have found it useful in clarifying both the consultant's and the consultees' commitments and responsibilities. Such a letter, according to Tavistock group relations theory, defines the task and the responsibilities of all parties. It makes it very clear that the consultee has an active role in the success or failure of the consultation and, as such, must demonstrate an investment in time and energy if a positive outcome is to occur. Written as a formal letter, it concretizes the agreement and short-circuits potential attempts at sabotage.

METHODS OF INTERVENTION

Over the years, requests for consultation have undergone considerable change. In the early years, agency-oriented proposals seemed to occur more often. In recent years, schools have become more sophisticated in agency-related content areas and, when needs arise, they now tend to ask for more program than agency consultation.

My early work was characterized by an unstructured consultation style that focused on issues of process and emphasized the consultee's need to seek resources and build knowledge bases independently, although with support and guidance from the consultant. The goal was to teach school personnel the skills for developing expertise in given content areas and skills in dealing with the processes of working in a school setting. While generally successful in this undertaking, limitations of time and funding have forced a rethinking of the approach. In more recent years, my philosophy has been modified to emphasize a content-based focus, one that serves to deliver a concrete product or package specifically developed for a particular setting. This approach has meshed nicely with historical changes in school needs. The days of sensitivity training and group encounter within the education system have passed, and the drop in student enrollment and reduced school budgets has increased competition for funding among schools. Clearly, it is far easier to request funding for teacher education than for organizational development.

I have tended to enter the school in recent years as an "expert" in given content areas and with programs centered on the mental health needs of given populations. Such programs tend to be time-limited and make use of lectures, readings, discussions, films, and so on. Videotaped skill-development exercises also have been well received and deemed highly useful. These programs tend to be structured and present a systematic review of relevant content areas. Where they touch upon administrative or school policy issues, the group must then address whether or not a change in contract with the consultant needs to be considered. Often this becomes a vehicle for shifting to a more agency-oriented model; but it is better if one permits the impetus for such actions to arise from school personnel exclusively, with the consultant remaining an interested but passive participant. Such a position places the entire burden of this more difficult area of intervention upon the consultee, and it also permits the consultant to delineate whether or not he or she wishes to enter this more difficult phase, and whether there is sufficient motivation, time, and funding to insure at least a partially successful outcome.

Another issue is the introduction of a school program that most likely cannot be supported once external funding stops. For example, many programs provide funding for teacher aides and other supportive staff to be used with special populations of students. The funds for these programs often are sought by interested extra-school personnel housed in university, business, or other governmental settings. Although frequently helpful to the students served, such programs most often do not become integrated into the system of the school. Because of lack of funding or interest, schools often are unable or unwilling to support them. An alternative approach is to focus on those programs that can be incorporated into the framework of the school and that emerge from the desire of the school to address particular problems. Such a consultative strategy more readily assures that continuation of the program following consultation will occur and that the staff will not view the program as something imposed upon them by the administration or a demanding community.

CONCLUSIONS

Schools and families share many similarities as consultees of a systems-based consultant, but there are a considerable number of differences as well. Systems theory generated from a family systems model and from a group relations model can be applied to a host of settings as long as the unique characteristics of each setting are taken into account. In addition, one needs to keep in mind that systems consultation in schools is not the same as family therapy. Although both share the need for systems assessment and systems-focused intervention, the methods and styles of intervention are considerably different. Most important in school consultation is an overall orientation that emphasizes the nature and structure of the interpersonal unit as it seeks to achieve its aims and complete its tasks.

REFERENCES

Caplan, G. *The theory and practice of mental health consultation.* New York: Basic Books, 1970.

Cowen, E. L. The primary mental health project: Yesterday, today and tomorrow. *Journal of Special Education*, 1980, *14*, 133–154.

Fisher, L. Training in school consultation. In L. Claiborn & R. Cohen (Eds.), *School intervention.* New York: Behavioral Publications, 1973.

Fisher, L. Cautions about mental health consultation from a mental health consultant. *Elementary School Journal*, 1974, *74*, 185–191.

Menninger, R. W. The impact of group relations conferences on organization growth. *International Journal of Group Psychotherapy*, 1972, *22*, 415–432.

Rioch, M. J. The work of Wilfred Bion on groups. *Psychiatry*, 1970, *33*, 56–66. (a)

Rioch, M. J. Group relations: Rationale and techniques. *International Journal of Group Psychotherapy*, 1970, *20*, 340–355. (b)

Shure, M. B., & Spivack, G. *Problem solving techniques in child rearing.* San Francisco: Jossey-Bass, 1978.

Turquet, P. *The Tavistock theory of group relations.* Paper presented at the University of Rochester Guest Lectureship Series, Rochester, NY, May 1973.

22

THE SYSTEMIC CONSULTANT AND HUMAN-SERVICE-PROVIDER SYSTEMS

EVAN IMBER-BLACK
University of Calgary
Calgary, Alberta, Canada

This chapter will discuss systemic consultation to human-service-provider systems. The systemic consultant, as defined herein, utilizes principles of the systemic model (Selvini Palazzoli, Boscolo, Cecchin, & Prata, 1980; Tomm, 1982) elaborated upon and tailored for the unique nature of public sector systems. Case examples will illustrate this approach.

THE CONSULTING CONTEXT

The consultant to human-service-provider systems, including child welfare, probation, mental health clinics, aftercare programs and projects for diverse populations, such as the handicapped, adolescents, and the elderly, enters a particular kind of labyrinth. While each of these various systems has unique mandates, all share certain common features of importance to a systemic consultant who enters their relational and organizational domains.

OVERT AND COVERT DEFINITIONS

The first feature of human-service-provider systems of significance to the consultant is the incompatible definitions that underpin such organizations. All human systems have a definition formed by history, current experience, and the views of others. Such definitions more or less match the day-to-day operations of the system. When they do not match closely, or when mutually incompatible definitions require participants to choose one and exclude contradicting data, the system increasingly operates with mystification and distortion. Further, these definitions are either more open or more closed to modification by new information, depending on the flexibility or rigidity of the system.

Human-service systems define themselves and are defined by others as caregivers for the larger society. An aura of altruism generally surrounds human-service systems, and they tend to embody those trends that represent humane reform and social concern for such minority populations as children, the elderly, and the physically and the mentally handicapped. It is this definition that is overt. At the same time, there exists a second, less acknowledged definition: human-service-provider systems are "big business." An increasing portion of city, state/provincial, and federal budgets go to support public human services. They are often expected by the larger community to turn out "successful products," such as "well-adjusted" foster children, reformed alcoholics, or better functioning handicapped adults. Such systems are the employers of large numbers of people, yet cost concerns and issues of efficiency frequently take precedence over the human needs of both staff and clients. Struggles with financial constraints are usual and result in employees facing a continual state of uncertainty regarding their future employment.

The first definition is generally more explicit and may be incongruent with the less acknowledged business operations. Very few, if any, people connected with human services would define their work as "big business." Most employees of such systems are initially drawn to their work because of their identification with the first definition. They often have little knowledge of the second definition and tend to flee from its implications, thus reinforcing mythical attributions to the first definition. An observable phenomenon in this realm of definitions is that as some employees gain more senior positions, they become spokespersons for the issues involved in the second definition, for example, budget cuts, cost efficiency, and production. They never actually define their work as "big business" because they would then become more distant from the belief system of the majority of employees and the human-service mandate. The difference in these two perspectives can result in the generation of further myths in which line staff is seen as "unrealistic, soft, and lacking accountability," and so on, and high-level administration is viewed as "harsh, out of touch with people's needs, and uncaring."

The consultant must attend to both definitions or perspectives and the tensions between them. Both are actual, and while they are seldom the overt issue of the consultation, they are crucial to the organization's ongoing interactions. Generally, the consultant will be invited to make observations from only one of the perspectives. To see one to the exclusion of the other is to support the system's patterns of alliance, inadvertently perpetuate myths, and miss the opportunity to introduce greater flexibility into the system through interventions that allow for the viability of both definitions.

ISSUES OF LEADERSHIP

A second feature of human-service-provider systems is that changes in leadership occur frequently with attendant periods of upheaval. At the local level, the staff must deal with changes in leadership style, issues of loyalty to the former leader, questions of attachments in a temporary sphere, and anxiety about one's own place; due to rapid turnover, one's peers may quickly become one's supervisors.

Such changes in leadership may or may not herald changes in policy and practices. Unrealistic hopes may be pinned on the new leader who must struggle with the same systemic constraints as had the prior leader, possibly without being able to initiate change. Workers who have been through several leadership cycles that did not result in any systemic change often view a new leader with pessimism or resignation and so contribute to a self-fulfilling prophecy.

At a more distant level, vast bureaucratic structures connect local agencies to many hierarchies that are frequently remote from the day-to-day functioning of the system and may have conflicting agendas. Such bureaucratic structures are invested with key, decision-making powers that engender a sense of impotence at the local level that is embodied in the frequently heard comment, "There's nothing I/we can do. It's the 'system.'" A sense of dependence on a shifting sociopolitical climate may breed apathy, cynicism, or despair in the very people whose job it is to ameliorate apathy, cynicism, and despair in clients.

Regardless of the specific consultative request, the consultant must consider these issues of leadership and must evaluate the actual limits imposed by this phenomenon, intervening in ways that clarify and demystify decision-making areas and increase possibilities for personal potency at all levels.

ISSUES OF STAFFING PATTERNS

Staff members in human-service-provider systems are usually drawn to their work out of desire to help others, to work with people, and to participate in making life better for a particular segment of the population. The staffing patterns in such organizations frequently utilize paraprofessionals or very recent graduates. These people are often placed in positions for which they have had little prior training. Given limited supervision and in-service training, they are expected to do the very difficult work of assessment, intervention, and rehabilitation with persons in the larger society who have been *defined by others* as being in need of services.

Human-service workers are the recipients of several mixed messages from within their own agencies, the state and federal bureaucratic funding sources, and the public. At one and the same time, they are to put clients' needs first and cost concerns first. Simultaneously, they are to work on issues of human autonomy and yet maintain social control. They are expected to both facilitate responsible behavior and serve as rescuer. Professed self-definitions of human-service systems are often at odds with the day-to-day functioning experienced by both staff and clients; they generate rigid myths, outdated interactional "rules," and distorted perceptions. Finally, in a manner similar to that found in the culture in which they are inextricably embedded, human-service workers reduce the interactional, organizational, and societal complexities described above by ascribing blame to clients, other workers, leadership, the anonymous "system," or themselves when dysfunctional behavior appears or when aspects of their work result in little progress or in failure.

DEFINING THE PARAMETERS

NEGOTIATING A CONSULTING CONTRACT

The discussion above leads to several issues for the systemic consultant to human-service-provider systems that need to be addressed prior to and during the negotiation of a consulting contract.

An initial crucial question regards the timing of the consultation. "Why now?" should be foremost in the consultant's thinking and early action because the answers to this question inform the consultant regarding overt and covert agendas. Questions provide the consultant's frame of reference. Is the invitation to consult someone's agenda for change or someone's agenda to maintain the status quo? Is it, perhaps, a mixture of these requests and hence an invitation to triangulation which must be carefully avoided? The consultant may wish to ask, "Who, of all the people involved, agree that the agency needs consultation now? For what purposes? Who disagrees with the need for consultation at this point in time? Who holds a differing point of view regarding the issues?" The consultant must discover if consultation is being sought on one issue in order to diffuse attention from more pressing concerns. A useful question may be: "If there were no consultation now, what do people imagine would happen?" The consultant wants to evaluate whether the act of seeking consultation is seen by the potential participants as an act of hope, an act of cynicism, or an act representing the exhaustion of internal possibilities. Is the consultation a new or relatively unusual action for the system or does the consultant join a long list of prior consultants? What have been the topics and the results of prior consultations? Is the request for consultation coming from those who intend to be involved or is it a request that the consultant "fix" some other, often lower in the hierarchy, part of the system?

The consultant should seek to meet with as many of the potential participants as possible while communicating clearly that no formal contract has been assumed. A variety of questions posed to participants prior to assuming that a formal contract will ensue may free the consultant from the role of inadvertent perpetuator of the status quo or, worse, contributor to escalating cynicism regarding the efficacy of change. The questions highlighted above frame the parameters of any possible consultation, immediately focus the consultant on interactional and organizational issues, and avoid systemic traps.

Precontract negotation: A case example. Consultation was requested by the director of a geriatric care facility to deal with problems arising in staff–patient relationships. As the consultant began to gather information in order to decide whether she could be useful, it became apparent that relationships between the staff and the director had deteriorated markedly in the last 6 months. A cycle of mutual blame was in process. The request by the director for a consultant to deal with staff–patient relationships was seen by the staff as further criticism of their work and as a distraction from recent errors they believed the director had made. If the consultant had immediately negotiated a contract with the director to deal with "staff–patient relationships," she would have formed an alliance with the director and the consultation would have failed. Instead, the information gathered was utilized by the consultant to offer a consultation to deal first with staff relationships, which included the director, as an initial step toward dealing with other issues, including patients. The consultant offered her opinions in a framework that did not utilize blame, and she was able to enter the system without taking sides.

CATEGORIES OF CONSULTATION REQUESTS

Human-service-system consultation may be divided into three broad categories. The first category is *case-based* consultation, in which one consults on a specific case on which an agency or more than one agency is working. The case is extremely problematic in some way and no progress is being made. The systemic consultant enters the case-based consulting arena assuming that the unit for assessment and intervention is not only the particular case but also the agency interaction vis-à-vis this case and others similar to it. The consultant does not assume that his or her job is simply to provide an answer for this one case, because that simply leads to future consultation needs along the same dimensions. Rather, the consultant seeks to use the particular case in order to expand the agency's options with future cases.

Multiple agency involvement: A case example. Consultation was requested by a child-welfare agency regarding a family case. The consultant was presented with the agency's ostensible dilemma of whether to return the children to the family. Upon investigation, the consultant discovered that no less than 13 agencies had become embroiled in this case and had expressed conflicting opinions regarding the children's placement, the quality of the family, and so on. Further, it was discovered that multiagency involvement in cases that bogged down was a familiar picture. At one level, the invitation to consult can be seen as an invitation to join preexisting alliances and splits. The consultant declined this invitation by not giving advice about the placement of the children and focusing instead on the complex relationships among the agencies and the family. In so doing, the pattern of adding one more opinion to the stalemate was blocked and the available decision-making hierarchy, previously hidden by a covert pattern of symmetrical escalation among the systems, emerged. Thus, consultation regarding a particular case was utilized as an opportunity to introduce new patterns into the total system.

The second category of consultation requests is *education-based.* The systemic consultant, because of her general expertise in systemic work, is invited to impart educational material to a staff, or more often, part of a staff. For instance, a probation department may request input about family assessment or a mental health clinic may seek consultation regarding the establishment of a family intervention team. The systemic consultant moves carefully in the area of education-based requests, remaining cognizant that the introduction of new ideas into a system will generally be handled by the system's typical responses to difference (Imber Coppersmith, 1983b; Sarason, 1971). In addition, general patterns of interaction within the system will be operative regardless of content. Hence, stable alliances or relationships of symmetry will respond to new content with old patterns.

Conflicting requests: A case example. A consultation request was made by a residential treatment program for adolescents. The consultant was asked to assist in the establishment of a family therapy unit. The agency expected that the consultation would involve imparting information and consulting on cases. Upon examination of the system, it became apparent that any new learning introduced into the system would be triangulated between segments of the staff who mirrored a pattern of competition and symmetry between two codirectors responsible for the agency. For the educational component of the consultation to succeed, the consultant had to design and implement interventions that required a pattern of cooperation among the staff and between the codirectors. Such interventions were proposed as a response to the education-based request but were executed at the relational and organizational levels.

The third category of consultation request is *relationship-based*, although the request is often couched in terms of personal blame. These requests concern such problems as an entire staff not getting along with one another, two staff members relating with a high degree of conflict, symptomatic behavior of one person, a fierce split between a staff and a manager, and so on. Generally, the consultant is asked to focus on the particular problematic behavior and "fix" it; this is not unlike a family's request to "fix" a symptomatic member. The systemic consultant assumes that troubled interaction or symptomatic behavior in an agency plays an essential function in that system as well as being supported by unfortunate patterns.

A special view from the top: A case example. Consultation was sought by a multiservice system because two supervisors were not getting along with one another. In this system, one supervisor was in charge of a mental health unit and the other was in charge of a child-welfare unit. Their relationship was rapidly deteriorating and their respective staffs were, as might be expected, taking sides. Personal blame was high and resulted in mutual accusations and recriminations. Client care was beginning to suffer. Most of those who assessed the situation from within the organization saw it as a "personality problem" and believed that one or the other of the supervisors would have to leave. Investigation from a systemic perspective yielded a very different picture. The two units had been separate entities until recently when, by administrative fiat, a multiservice organization was created. Most workers were very unsettled by this change. At the upper levels, far removed from this particular agency, battles ensued regarding the meaning of the merger, the future of each one's service mandate, and where power would reside. The two supervisors attended high-level administrative meetings but each chose to protect their staff members from knowledge of the current chaos. Thus, their struggles with one another were a metaphor for interactions in central administration and a distraction for their staffs during a highly unstable time. The consultant was able to reframe their alleged conflict as a cooperative effort to protect their staffs and an attempt to discover solutions that were not being found at higher levels.

All three categories of consultation requests provide opportunities to see the system. It is important that the consultant not get caught in the framework of the specific requests. They are merely entry points for the consultant, who will work to solve problems with the participants in such a way as to expand the options for future developments and creative solutions.

DETERMINING METHODS OF CONTACT

In establishing a consulting agreement, the consultant must examine and make decisions regarding the length and frequency of contacts and who will be involved. The length of contact may vary from one meeting to several; however, the consultant should arrange for at least a follow-up to determine effectiveness, even if only one session is held. When possible, it is best not to determine an exact end (e.g., "We will consult for one year"), because this can often preclude earlier solutions and may negatively affect the consultant's maneuverability.

Frequency of contact is often predetermined in education-based consultations (e.g., "We will meet weekly to learn this material"). Longer periods of time between contacts are preferable in case-based and relationship-based consultations; they give the organization time to respond to the consultant's interventions and prevent the consultant from becoming like a staff member. Since the aim of systemic consultation is for the organization to be able to elaborate its own changes after the consultant's exit, it is important that he or she utilize time effectively, enabling the organization to experience its own creativity and problem-solving ability.

The consultant needs to determine who must be contacted for the consultation to be effective. Thus, invitations to meet with only one part of a staff may well be invitations to triangulation that will handicap the consultant. Requests to "fix" one person or one relationship are best met with counterrequests for information broadly gathered from all who are affected by the problem. Education-based consultations to one segment of a system without careful analysis of the likely responses of other segments of the system run the risk of feeding into dysfunctional patterns. Participants in a consultation need to know with whom the consultant will be meeting and for what purposes, in order to avoid the suspicion of secret alliances.

METHODS AND ISSUES OF ENTRY

UTILIZING AFFIRMATION AND NEUTRALITY

The tone set by the consultant upon entry into the organization shapes and affects all that is to follow. Participants in the consultation need to experience the consultant as affirming their individual and joint efforts. The consultant communicates affirmation by a stance of openness, curiosity about the system, and noncritical interest. Regardless of how experienced the consultant may be with organizations, people must be informed that this is a new experience for the consultant and that the participants are the best source of information about the system. Many organizations are initially cynical about consultation because consultants may have entered and exited often with no evidence of change. In such systems, consultation has often become part of a larger homeostatic pattern, and participants view the new consultant with mistrust. In other organizations, the consultant may be viewed as a kind of distraction being offered by administration to obviate unrest and avoid genuine change. Low-key affirmation of participants' pessimism in these situations imparts a sense of their being heard and appreciated, and it enables the consultant to enter.

The consultant utilizes neutrality not only toward people but also toward ideas (Selvini Palazzoli *et al.*, 1980). In so doing, he or she is able to remain outside of competing points of view and remain neutral about specific content issues, while exploring the larger relational and organizational domains. Unlike the participants who may be caught up in specific content or blame, the consultant can attend to the message value of particular issues and patterned interaction in the system's functioning.

Neutrality enables consultants to avoid imposing their own preferred outcomes on the system and, hence, becoming either too central in the day-to-day operations or generating symmetrical struggles with the participants. It is not a consultant's job to become the organization's director but, rather, to assist the organization in getting unstuck from a repetitive, narrow, and no-longer-functional range of patterns.

UTILIZING COMPLEMENTARITY

Upon entry, consultants are burdened with a relational definition that places them in a "one-up" complementary position by virtue of being an "expert" called upon to solve problems. If, however, a consultant's opening moves within the system are to seek information, affirm participants as being their own best experts, and so on, then the consultant seemingly moves to the "one-down" position of one who cannot do the job without the participants' help. Momentarily, the organization experiences a creatively confusing complementarity vis-à-vis the consultant. Is the consultant "one-up" by virtue of being a consultant or is he or she "one-down" by virtue of asking for help with the task? Rigid definitions regarding "consultants" melt briefly, and allow the consultant to enter with some degree of flexibility.

AVOIDING THE "MIRROR EFFECT"

When a consultant enters a system, a common trap involves the consultant relating to the organization in those very ways that mirror the difficulties within the organization. Thus, a system marked by tentativeness and ultimate paralysis in decision making may engender similar tentativeness in the consultant. An organization beset by symmetrical struggles may soon find itself struggling with the consultant. An organization whose mandate is to "rescue" may soon find itself with a "rescuing" consultant. A crisis intervention service that is already mirroring clients' crises by operating in a highly dramatic, crisis-oriented fashion may find the consultant only responding when there is a crisis. Because information that the system requires in order to develop is "news of a difference" (Bateson, 1972), this apparent sameness in the quality of relationships within the system and between the system and the consultant will contribute to increased reification of patterns and a failed consultation. The consultant must be cognizant of the mirror phenomenon and move early to introduce difference and the unexpected into relationships.

ASSESSMENT

While assessment begins with the initial request for consultation and includes many of the issues discussed above, there are several other specific areas to assess. The consultant must differentiate between intrasystem issues and intersystem issues and then determine the correct level or system for meaningful intervention.

INTRASYSTEM ISSUES

Intrasystem issues pertain to what occurs within the boundary of the organization. Several dimensions inform this aspect of assessment. The first involves definitions of the problem and include the following questions:

1. Who in the system is defining a problem requiring consultation?
2. What are the elements of the problem?
3. For whom is it a problem?
4. For whom is it not a problem?
5. Who first identified the problem?
6. Who talks to whom about it?

7. Are there other problems that some people identify as more pressing?
8. How has the system solved similar problems?
9. How would things be different if there were no problems?

While these questions focus the consultant and the participants, they also begin to impart information to the consultant regarding alliances, splits, myths, and staff expectations of the consultant.

The second dimension involves examining the system's cherished beliefs and labels. The way a system views itself may be incongruent with interactional actualities, and this may result in a distorted perception of staff participation. For instance, an agency may insist that it is a "nonhierarchical" organization when, in fact, key decisions are being made by a small cadre that excludes the rest of the staff. While cherished beliefs will often become apparent, it may be useful to ask some of the following questions:

1. What is most important about this agency?
2. What do you most want to be known for?
3. How are decisions made or policies changed?
4. How do you understand your mandate?
5. How are you seen by clients?
6. How are you seen by other agencies?
7. How are you seen by the public?

As the agency's beliefs about itself, its functional purpose, its structures, and so on, are verbalized, the consultant is able to observe how well these match the system's actual operations. It may emerge that one or more members hold beliefs that are antithetical to the majority and hence may be getting squeezed to conform. The system may show itself to have little or no tolerance for difference, and it may require subterfuge to belong. Conversely, the agency may have no strong belief system at all, resulting in a lack of connectedness and loyalty among participants.

The third area involves determining the system's preferred focus of blame for its difficulties. Does the agency blame one person and see all solutions dependent on that person's exit? Is blame placed outside on some amorphous "system"? Do staff members blame themselves and feel demoralized? Are clients of the agency blamed for not performing according to the agency's mandate? Is blame static or shifting? Most often, staff members will not discuss blame directly, and the consultant must devise questions to elicit this information. Such questions might include:

1. How do you explain why this is happening?
2. What do you think needs to change for this to be solved?

The answers to these questions often reveal where blame is being placed. The tone with which such questions are answered may also indicate morale level and issues of self-blame.

INTERSYSTEM ISSUES

Human-service systems operate in relationship to many other systems. These other systems must be considered in the consultant's search for the meaningful system for intervention. Three major areas must be assessed. The first involves the agency's relationships with the clients it serves. Human-service systems exist by virtue of providing a service to clients and hence these relationships are crucial to agency functioning. The consultant's assessment should include the following:

1. Do staff view their relationships with clients as positive or negative, as generally successful or failing, as accomplishing the agency's mandate or not?
2. Do staff feel a sense of satisfaction from their work with clients or not?
3. Do staff feel angry with clients? If so, what percentage of the time?
4. Do staff appear interested in gaining new skills for work with clients?
5. Do staff worry about particular clients for great quantities of time when they are not at work?

Questions such as these will reveal patterns of overinvolvement, burnout, and so on, or conversely, such themes as optimism or hope.

The second area involves the complex relationships between this agency and other human-service-provider systems. In any given community, the mental health clinic, the probation department, children's protective services, and so on, all interact with one another. Such interaction is generally regarding particular clients but may also be about funding, the service mandate, or staffing patterns. It is not unusual for the consultant to discover very difficult and troubled relationships marked by mistrust, fear of scarcity of resources, blame for failed cases, frustration over lack of agreement, and so on. The consultant who ignores these complexities may inadvertently contribute to their escalation. Thus, the consultant must attend to the potential impact on multiple systems, even if only one system has a designated consultant.[1]

The third area involves the agency's relationship to the larger community, to the public that, in fact, funds the agency through taxation. The

1. It is beyond the scope of this chapter to describe a full assessment method for examining relationships among larger systems See Imber Coppersmith (1983a, p. 16) for such a method.

agency's relationships to the community are often ignored and yet this may be an arena of great stress. Often human-service systems are given a profoundly mixed message by the larger community that simultaneously desires that the job be done and yet shows a lack of respect for those who do it. Clients (e.g., probationers, the elderly, the handicapped, welfare recipients, and so on) served by human-service systems are often not highly regarded by the community. Hence, the public often regards success with these clients as a form of control rather than something that facilitates their development. The consultant must be aware of this often more hidden course of stress that involves a sense of being unappreciated and poorly esteemed for one's work.

In addition, specific human-service systems may have particular difficulties with the larger community; an example might be a chronic aftercare project that wishes to establish a group home in a residential neighborhood. In such a situation, the unit for consultation may well be the agency *and* neighborhood residents.

In examining the various aspects of intersystem relationships, the consultant seeks to discover how others see the agency, how the agency believes it is regarded by others, and the ways in which such relationships affect the agency's overall functioning. This information helps the consultant determine the correct level for intervention.

INTERVENTION

Just as the consultant is involved in assessment of all interactions with the organization, so he or she is also involved in intervention. The very act of engaging with a system in a consultation is an act of intervention. Entering the system, even with the goals of affirmation and neutrality, and seeking answers to some of the assessment questions are interventions. However, two more formal aspects of intervention may be identified.

The first involves the manner of interviewing and asking questions according to the principle of circularity (Selvini Palazzoli *et al.*, 1980). Questions are designed and asked that provoke interaction, and they impart information about the system not just to the consultant but also to the participants. Such questions reveal alliances and splits, triads, themes of overinvolvement, skewed hierarchical arrangements, symmetrically escalating struggles, myths, and so on. Questions and their answers may repunctuate the system's causal reality or reframe meanings. The method of questioning, in which all are invited to give their opinion, puts everyone in the agency on the same level vis-à-vis the issue of solving the agency's problem, and thereby introduces a sense of empowerment and mutual responsibility. It should be noted that this does not mean that the agency suddenly becomes a "democracy" or "nonhierarchical" in its day-to-day functioning but, rather, that participants gain a sense of their own effect on others in mutually influencing cycles of interaction. Individual blame placing becomes more difficult to sustain. Issues previously cast in narrow definitions expand in possible meanings.

The second aspect of intervention involves tasks, rituals, and opinions given by the consultant. Requests for certain behavior to occur between consulting sessions may be given. Experiments may be offered and, in fact, it is often useful to frame interventions as "experiments" because most people are more willing to try an experiment than to follow a directive. This is especially true in those systems where there is a high level of resentment toward administrative directives that are often experienced as out of touch with the day-to-day realities of the agency. In education-based consultations, the tasks given by the consultant (both learning and applying the requested information) should be designed in such a way as to facilitate development in areas assessed by the consultant. The consultant needs to avoid those systemic traps that will reduce the usefulness of the new material.

Interventions should be designed that use the agency's own "language" and familiar modes of communicating. The more familiar can then be utilized to introduce difference and change. For instance, one highly effective method of intervention with human-service systems is to put one's opinions, reframings, task requests, and so on, in the form of a memo *that is sent to everyone in the system.* Agency personnel are familiar with memos. However, a memo from the consultant with copies to everyone, and with an invitation to respond, is an unexpected event, one that highlights the possibilities of shared information and lack of secrets.

A systemic consultation: A case example. A case-based consultation was requested by an aftercare project. The project existed within a comprehensive mental health system and was mandated to provide residential services for deinstitutionalized patients. Twenty-five staff members, mostly paraprofessionals, staffed three houses and worked with difficult clients, a task for which they had little training. In-service training efforts were generally experienced by staff as confirming how little they knew, rather than as relevant opportunities to learn. The project director was directly accountable to both the local mental health clinical director and the state department of mental health. Staff members experienced themselves as less important than the master's-degree-level professionals in outpatient services, and were, in fact, looked down upon by segments of this group. Pressure was great to make clients behave properly because the larger community was not enthusiastic about group homes in their neighborhoods. Thus, the consulting context involved a beleaguered staff who were viewed poorly by others, but who worked very hard to do a good job. The consultant entered the system initially by obtaining a clear sense of staff's experience of their own context and worth. The consultant's comments affirming the difficult, almost impossible nature of their work, were met with great surprise because no professional had ever imparted that view to them.

The consultant was invited to help the staff solve the problem of one client, Karen, who was 40 years old and had lived for 25 years in the state hospital. Now in a group home for 1 year, Karen refused to cooperate, dressed inappropriately, would not participate in house functions, and took other clients' money. She threatened other clients and had struck a staff member. She refused to shower. Of immediate concern was the fact that Karen would go into restaurants in the community and would urinate and defecate on the seats. The staff imparted all of this information with a tone of urgency and great concern. At this juncture, the consultant was aware of the potential that she would be drawn into the aura of urgency and concern and thereby lose effectiveness through the mirror effect. Utilizing neutrality, the consultant inquired about all that had been tried with Karen.

During this discussion, several key elements emerged. Personnel at the upper level of administration were under attack from the community because of Karen's behavior. The aftercare director was under enormous pressure from both the clinic director and the state department of mental health to solve this problem immediately, without rehospitalization. Their suggestions for how to solve the problem differed, but both clearly blamed the aftercare director for not getting her staff to solve the problem. Prior to this interview, staff members had been unaware of the pressure on their director and had simply been experiencing her as cranky. Blame cascaded down the system as the aftercare director blamed segments of the staff and staff members blamed one another and Karen. A pattern of competition emerged regarding "who knew best" for Karen and who could solve the problem. Staff members formed secret alliances with one another and inadvertently undermined any effective action with Karen. Behind each other's backs, staff members would countermand each other's directions to Karen. Most staff members were exhausted and thought of little else but Karen and her problems, to the exclusion of other clients and program concerns. Finally, Karen, like all patients in the program, had a legal advocate who viewed staff with mistrust and who, in turn, was viewed as a troublemaker by staff.

The first session with the staff, in which the above information was generated by circular questioning, had the immediate effect of framing the participants as engaged in a collaborative, rather than a competitive effort. The sheer act of gathering everyone together in a format that made apparent the alliances, splits, cascading blame, and competition, with a consultant who refused to see villains and victims and remained outside the competitive struggle for immediate solutions, began to free the system to explore new options. An intervention was designed to deal with the overinvolvement that was seen as contributing to the lack of resolution. Staff was asked not to change anything in its work with Karen but simply to note what percentage of its time both at work and at home was devoted to solving Karen's problems. Staff members returned and reported that they were shocked at the amount of time spent on this issue, including much free time at home. Competition over who could solve the problem abated when staff members began to experience themselves as mutually caught up with Karen in their struggle to "cure" her. Soon Karen began to hear similar, rather than conflicting, messages from staff regarding her behavior. At this juncture, the staff, with the consultant's input, worked out a ritual of "growing up" for Karen, framing her as "young" because of the many years she had spent in the state hospital. Crucial to the success of the ritual were the cooperative efforts of the staff. As the ritual succeeded in modifying many of Karen's behaviors, it had the effect of uniting the staff in an experience of shared success, thus reinforcing the new collaborative, nontriangulated pattern. This case-based consultation was followed by a request by the entire staff for a content-based consultation regarding the design and implementation of effective interventions with an aftercare population. Ten sessions conducted at month-long intervals were held. Evaluation of the success of the consultation effort was seen in the staff's subsequent ability to handle difficult clients effectively and to remain free of the previous patterns of competition, overinvolvement, and triangulation.

CONCLUSION

The systemic consultant and human-service systems exist in a broader cultural context, one that defines segments of the population as clients of human-service systems and other segments of the population as providers of those services. Successful systemic consultation seeks to introduce greater complexity into the life of an organization so that participants can draw upon a wide range of options in dealing effectively with clients and with each other. It is possible, however, that the systemic consultants, as part of a larger system that they cannot see fully, may contribute to that very social control that a systemic perspective seeks to avert. The success of systemic consultation may ultimately lie in the contradictions and anomalies it is able to highlight.

REFERENCES

Bateson, G. *Steps to an ecology of mind.* New York: Ballantine, 1972.

Imber Coppersmith, E. The family and public service systems: An assessment method. In B. Keeney (Ed.), *Diagnosis and assessment in family therapy.* Rockville, MD: Aspen Systems Corp., 1983. (a)

Imber Coppersmith, E. The place of family therapy in the homeostasis of larger systems. In L. R. Wolberg & M. L. Aronson (Eds.), *Group and family therapy 1982*. New York: Brunner/Mazel, 1983. (b)

Sarason, S. B. *The culture of the school and the problem of change*. New York: Allyn & Bacon, 1971.

Selvini Palazzoli, M., Boscolo, L., Cecchin, G., & Prata, G. Hypothesizing–circularity–neutrality: Three guidelines for the conductor of the session. *Family Process*, 1980, *19*, 3–12.

Tomm, K. The Milan approach to family therapy: A tentative report. In D. S. Freeman & B. Trute (Eds.), *Treating families with special needs*. Ottawa: The Canadian Association of Social Workers, 1982.

Editors' Commentary on Consultation with Community Groups and Service Systems

The chapters in this section have examined systems consultation with community groups and service systems. Enduring and monolithic structures such as the courts, schools, churches, and social services departments have been settings for consultation, as have smaller, more impermanent community self-help groups, like the organizations serving the families of cultists. Although these chapters are replete with contrasts, common issues emerge within the general systems framework of consultation shared by all of the authors who work within the community.

HELPING MORE BY HELPING LESS

One consequence of the advancement and complexity of our culture is that social institutions gradually have preempted some traditional functions of the family. Schools, courts, social agencies, and churches all are community resources for people in need. These centers have become "homes" for guidance, socialization, and the mediation of domestic disputes. In times past, families were more inclined to resolve their emotional problems within the boundaries of the household or, possibly, with the aid of the extended family and compassionate neighbors. Now it is more likely that when a problem arises, the family will look beyond itself and turn to surrogate family members in professional institutions.

Social critics such as Christopher Lasch (1977) have argued that in appropriating many of the training and caretaking functions formerly carried out by the family, these community agencies and professionals have weakened the spirit of families and have instilled a mounting sense of incompetency. The professional agency may directly, or more often implicitly, say to the family, "We can do this better than you can." In the guise of providing more help and relief, community agencies may promote self-doubt and spawn new anxieties among those whom they serve.

The consultation models proposed in these chapters run counter to the model of community service that says, "We know better than you what you need and how to get what you need." Repeatedly the authors have emphasized that a central mission of the consultant is to help people recognize their own inner resources and their capacity for self-judgment. For example, Landau-Stanton's consultation model is founded on the principle of evoking the inherent competence in systems requesting help: "One should enter a consultation relationship with the belief that the system at hand is intrinsically sound and possesses the competence to right itself, perhaps with only a little help from a friend." The position the consultant communicates to the family is collaborative: "You must see these problems over and over again. I'm sure you've learned an awful lot about how to deal with them. What are the things you've managed to do and what are the problems you've run into?"

By beginning at the point of the consultee's competence, a consultant may underscore the competence of those who work within a community agency. The agency, in turn, may likewise render help by "helping less," accenting the resources of strength and wisdom in the community people who seek their services. These organizations then become better equipped to do what they were intended to do. Rather than sapping the self-confidence of families, these groups themselves become agencies of consultation, collaborating with families and maximizing their use of their inherent resources.

The concept of "helping less" involves taking less responsibility for decision making and implementation of change. It should be clear that this approach calls for a change in the focus of help and does not eliminate active engagement and help of another kind, namely, to assist in identifying the nature of a problem, the resources available for change, and the options and means of achieving change. The help provided by a systems consultant is active and creative work with the consultee.

THE CONSULTANT AS CONVENER

When any individual or family receives services from a community organization, they frequently become part of an intricate web of community agencies and organizations. For example, Anderson and Goolishian note how in situations of domestic violence, the family may simultaneously become involved with the legal system, a child-welfare system, and a women's shelter. It also is quite common to have several staff members from each agency working with the family. The most obvious problem is that communication among these organizations, and even between individuals within the same organization, is slow at best and frequently is nonexistent.

Even when communication does take place, each individual's or agency's view may conflict with the other views. One agency seeks to confirm its definition of "reality" ("Mrs. Jones is too impulsive; she beats her child, and she needs psychotherapy") while discrediting other views of the same "reality" ("Mr. Jones is not supportive enough. He's always working and never at home. Pity poor Mrs. Jones." Or "Mrs. Jones's religion allows for harsh methods of discipline. The church needs to be confronted"). Not only is competition and blame a likely result in multiagency systems, but, worse, individuals and families are decontextualized; by emphasizing the details, the whole is distorted (Minuchin, 1984). Further, as Anderson and Goolishian note, these differing views in and of themselves can escalate a family's problems.

The proliferation of community organizations has created a complicated cadre of professionals, each claiming to specialize in a part of the "territory" of human problems. Although people may receive more technical and specialized services in the system, the net result is that the cell is examined, but the person is missed. In his book *Family Kaleidoscope* (1984), Minuchin investigates the larger social patterns in which people are embedded and decries the "chopped ecology," a by-product of having more and more specialties:

> This process of parceling territory is essentially sound in a complex world where there is no place for the generalist. Yet as specialties have mushroomed, the result has been a skewing of reality. Each area deepens knowledge within its boundaries and develops specialized norms, but when all the exquisitely crafted pieces are put together, the whole is violated. Consider this United States Department of Health, Education and Welfare statement about the number of professionals required to help families in which child abuse or neglect has occurred: "The abuse and neglect of children is a problem that cannot be managed by one discipline alone. A single case may involve social workers from both a hospital and the public child protection agency, a public assistance caseworker, one or more doctors, a psychiatrist or psychologist, both hospital and public health nurses, police, lawyers, a juvenile or family court judge, the child's school teacher, and any of a number of professionals." Eleven different institutions, without counting the family therapist, claim expertise about some part of the family body and, of course, challenge the expertise of anybody else who enters the territory. The statement frames the quandary in which members of the field find themselves; in order to function we need to specialize, but when we specialize we chop the ecology. (p. 120)

In the midst of a multiagency community system, one very important task of the consultant is to convene the system in such a way that the different and often contradictory views of "reality" are allowed to merge into some integrated, working whole. Bringing the disparate parts into a whole not only fosters greater communication and efficiency, but also minimizes escalating battles and multiplies strength. Convening members of the larger treatment system may be the consultant's most important task within this complicated community network.

Imber-Black's consultation model emphasizes using strategies that will maximize the collaboration among the competing parts of the consultee system. These strategies include communicating affirmation through openness and curiosity about the system, remaining outside of competing points of view, and remaining neutral about specific content issues. This stance of affirmation and neutrality allows the consultant to develop a new framework, that of the patterned interaction within the whole system. Interestingly, this consultation model is markedly different from the conventional view of consultants as "advice givers."

Wynne and Wynne also assume the roles of consultant conveners when working with the legal system "at the center of family cyclones." It is very easy for professionals to take adversarial positions in the midst of legal entanglements and bitter court battles over custody and visitation rights. This co-consulting model, however, steadfastly avoids sidetaking and blaming. Instead, the consultants tactfully and tenaciously convene warring members of the family, supporting the contradictory views while helping to develop a collaborative plan with the family and court system.

THE CONSULTANT AS BROKER

Although the community multiagency system tends to decontextualize, favoring only partial views, there are advantages to this system having a network of specialists. Families and other organizations at times may need more specialized information and care that could not be provided efficiently by the generalist. But how do these groups decide what they need and who might provide the services that will be of greatest use to them? Is there a better way than scrambling through the "Yellow Pages"?

The meta position of consultants, overlooking the labyrinth of specialists, allows them to help people decide what they need and who, with the greatest range of vision, may best provide the needed help. In Singer's words, the consultant is often in the role of a "broker or triage person." Her work with the families of cultists, for example, centers on providing information, connecting families with assistance networks, suggesting readings, and referring families to specialized groups and agencies. The consultant then continues in that "brokering" role, being available at different junctures to help families in their problem-solving efforts.

As brokers, consultants may decide to provide specialized services themselves, moving back and forth between the more meta position of the consultant and some other role. In their consultation with the clergy and churches, Weber and Wynn assume an ongoing consultation role within which they each take on periodic, specific "missions" as teacher, supervisor, or therapist. The hazard in doing so is that the clarity of role definitions and boundaries may be blurred. The consultant assists the organization in determining what and who is needed, with the possibility that the consultant may render those services or may link the organization with other specialists in the community. Similarly, Fisher in his school consultations is faced with an array of requests including providing educational programs, therapy, case consultation, administrative consultation, and so on. Whether or not the consultant has the expertise to render these specialized services, at least he or she, as broker, is in a position to help the organization define its needs and locate assistance.

REFERENCES

Lasch, C. *Haven in a heartless world: The family besieged.* New York: Basic Books, 1977.
Minuchin, S. *Family kaleidoscope.* Cambridge, MA: Harvard University Press, 1984.

V

CONSULTATION WITH MILITARY AND BUSINESS SYSTEMS

The chapters in this section address the challenges that face a systems consultant in consulting outside the health care field with military or business organizations. Florence Kaslow begins by discussing her experiences, both patriotic and challenging, as a consultant to psychiatry departments and training programs in various branches of the armed services. Next, Edwin Friedman uses his brand of Bowen therapy in consulting with individuals and groups about their work systems. Finally, Irving Borwick, the only non-family-therapist contributor to this volume, reports on his work as a systems-oriented, organizational development consultant. In this chapter, he makes recommendations to family therapists about what should and should not be transferred from family therapy to the consultation enterprise.

23

CONSULTATION WITH THE MILITARY
A Complex Role

FLORENCE W. KASLOW
Florida Couples and Family Institute
West Palm Beach, Florida

Working as a consultant with psychiatric programs of the U.S. Navy and Air Force is a challenging and multifaceted experience. Since 1974 the military facilities with which I have consulted include the psychiatric residency training programs in three Naval Hospitals and the staff training programs in the Alcohol Rehabilitation Services (ARS) of the Naval Hospital in Long Beach, California, and at Wilford Hall Medical Center, Lackland Air Force Base, in San Antonio, Texas. None of these experiences is encompassed by a narrow definition of "consultation," although that is usually the term utilized on the contract or purchase-of-service order received from the Navy. More broadly, consultation in this huge system has included teaching, staff training, program planning, serving as a resource specialist, and much more. The unspecified aspects include functioning as a mentor, role model, and group rap session leader.

Given the vastness of the military community, one can probably only be a consultant to a small segment of the mammoth labyrinth. This chapter will describe some ongoing periodic consultation at several installations. The people who have grappled with and incorporated knowledge about families, family therapy, and systems have taken this perspective with them as they have gone to the far corners of the military network to set up or administer training programs and treatment services. These are described in more detail in another volume (Kaslow & Ridenour, 1984).

Webster's Seventh New Collegiate Dictionary (1972) defines the "consultant" as "one who gives professional advice or services," that is, an expert. In the mental health field, the consultant, unlike the supervisor or teacher, usually has no administrative authority or responsibility for consultees (Kaslow, 1977). His or her input is invited; those who request it and receive it are free to utilize all of it, a portion of it, or none of it. If the consultant is external to the organization so that his or her major source of income is not derived from the consultees, that consultant can remain relatively unentangled in the political machinations of the system and can make a more objective analysis and have more impact. Given that consultants rarely participate in decisions to fire, retain, or promote employees with whom they consult, staff members and trainees may feel less threatened by consultants than they do by supervisors and, therefore, freer to be more honest and to participate without feeling pressured. The success of the consultation will be facilitated if the consultant is not overbearing about his or her special talents and gives recognition to the consultees' areas of competence. Consultation is often problem- or task-oriented, with specific objectives established when the process begins. As a consultant to the military, this is the framework in which I have been operating.

ORGANIZATIONAL CONTEXTS

It is important for anyone consulting with the military to become conversant with the many facets of military life—the values, tempo, language, protocol, formal and informal channels of communication, chain of command, explicit and implicit rules—as well as with what key personnel expect the consultant to accomplish. The milieu of the military setting will be more familiar to someone who has served in the armed forces; for someone who has not, it will be like a first trip to a foreign country with a different language and culture.

By way of elucidation, my consultation and training activities have taken place in five separate settings representing three different kinds of subsystems in the military. Three have been in residency training programs of the Departments of Psychiatry of general Naval Hospitals at Philadelphia, Portsmouth, and San Diego. The residents in these programs usually have a fairly traditional adult psychiatry residency, splitting time between a base hospital and more rural outposts. They may also do a portion of their clinical rotation in a local civilian medical school, particularly in child psychiatry if their own program does not include this training. Where these programs diverge from their civilian counterparts is more in form than in substance. Core content is apt to be up-to-date and residents reportedly fare well in becoming certified by the American Board of Psychiatry and Neurology. But the programs are less likely to shift as rapidly with new currents as do some of the more innovative civilian programs that have outspoken, "young Turks" in their classes and on their faculties. The military residents are much more disciplined. They are required to come to class and the work setting in uniform. They are immaculately groomed and their carriage is erect and proper. They are already commissioned officers, and may be at any rank from lieutenant to captain. They carry their rank and position with pride. As a corollary, they respect the authority of those in command.

These residents have chosen to take their training within the military and expect higher ranking officers, including their instructors, to be experts in their own areas, to come to class on time, and to be well prepared. They accord the same respect to civilian visiting professors and consultants, until and unless they find them to be unprepared, slovenly in dress or manner, unfamiliar with or disparaging of the armed forces, lacking in expertise, or supercilious. This system differs from the comparable civilian programs in that the patients whom the residents treat, in inpatient and outpatient facilities, are service members and their "dependents." These patients are "entitled" to psychiatric services free of charge as part of the benefit package they receive. Thus, they are less likely than civilians to complain about services or to seek another therapist, for if they go outside the system, they will have to pay that portion of the fees that are not covered by the Civilian Health and Medical Program of the Uniformed Services (CHAMPUS).

The second setting in which the activities to be described took place is the Alcohol Rehabilitation Service (ARS) at the Naval Hospital in Long Beach, California. This is the government facility at which Billy Carter and Betty Ford were treated. This facility achieved acclaim because of its celebrity patients and has a special image to uphold. Originally, its patient population consisted primarily of members of the Navy and the Marine Corps who were alcoholics. Now the treatment program also encompasses drug abusers and the spouses of the chemically dependent patients, generally called "co-alcoholics" or "co-patients" because of their role in contributing to and sustaining the illness. Treatment staff are predominantly Navy personnel—some of whom are recovering addicts and alcoholics. The facility periodically runs an intensive 2-week training program on treatment of substance abuse for nonstaff military physicians, psychologists, and chaplains who are expected to incorporate their newly derived information and insights into programs with which they are affiliated. Thus, the Long Beach ARS is a major training and treatment facility that has often been in the limelight and wants to keep everything functioning in peak condition.

The third kind of facility at which consulting activities have occurred is Wilford Hall Medical Center, Lackland Air Force Base, in San Antonio, Texas. A huge, modern enclave, it may be best known as the facility at which the Shah of Iran was hospitalized. It is the major medical center of the Air Force and is staffed largely by Air Force personnel. The same rules prevail here about wearing well-pressed uniforms and highly polished shoes, keeping equipment and facilities spic and span, and saluting superior officers. It is assumed that everyone has undergone rigorous training and is a reliable team member who will shoulder all assigned responsibilities and be cognizant of the position he or she is to occupy. Military personnel are supplemented by civilian staff, many of whom are ex-military or members of service-connected families. They take on the erect bearing and other behaviors of their military brethren.

ROLE OF THE FAMILY-ORIENTED CONSULTANT

Apparently none of the Navy settings had had a family-oriented consultant prior to my involvement, but the Air Force at Wilford Hall Medical Center has used eminent local consultants including Alberto Serrano, MD, and Lewis Richmond, MD. There is a dearth of literature on such consultations. Given the great variations in facilities and programs under the auspices of the far-flung military establishment, generalizations are not yet in order. The role I played evolved differently in each of the facilities, in response to the specific request received, the needs and objectives defined by the officer in charge, and my assessment of:

1. the covert as well as overt goals to be achieved by my activities or interventions;
2. the personalities of the individuals with whom I was working;
3. the power structure;
4. the formal and informal communication network;
5. the patient population served; and
6. the larger societal–ecological context in which the military system was currently functioning.

My role changes somewhat each time group services are requested. The invitation can be fairly specific, as when I have been asked by the Long Beach ARS to talk about and demonstrate family therapy with a family involved in substance abuse at the Zuska Conference (1981), or it can be much more general and open-ended, as when I was asked to serve for several years as Distinguished Visiting Professor for a week each year at Wilford Hall.

CONCEPTUAL FRAMEWORK

For these various involvements, I have utilized an organizational development model (Schein & Bennis, 1965), similar at the macrosystem level to the perspective adapted with the family at a microsystem level. This model suggests attending to (1) what kind of assistance is being sought; (2) who is making the request and through whom it is relayed; (3) the nature of the problem to be resolved; (4) the extent of agreement and disagreement among those involved in the department about the consultation and the desired outcomes; (5) the intellectual, emotional, and ethical climate; (6) available financial, material, and personnel resources to support the endeavor; (7) the length of time for which the activity is projected; and (8) completion of activity, including evaluation and feedback. The approach parallels the scientific method of designating the problem or goal (diagnosis), collecting relevant data (history taking), generating hypotheses and proposing alternative strategies (treatment planning), implementing the agreed-upon activities or plans (intervention phase), evaluating what has been accomplished (assessing what changes have occurred), and concluding the training or consulting involvement.

THE ENGAGEMENT PHASE AND ASSESSMENT OF THE SYSTEM

In the Navy residency training programs, contact about consultancy has been initiated either by the chairman of the Department of Psychiatry or the director of training on behalf of a selection committee. The consultation contract for each activity arrives in the form of a military purchase-of-service order that specifies date, time, location, honorarium, and expense allocation. All of this has been previously agreed upon with whoever has requested the service. Likewise, my goals and the organization's goals for each visit are discussed when each new contract is drawn up and, then, again when I arrive. A high level of concurrence about my role and the objectives for these visits has always been reached. Perhaps the process of "joining" can be better depicted by recounting several actual experiences.

PHILADELPHIA NAVAL HOSPITAL

In 1974–1975, when I was on the faculty at Hahnemann University, the residents at the Philadelphia Naval Hospital came to Hahnemann for their child psychiatry rotation. One of the residents, Richard Ridenour, expressed interest in family therapy and began doing cotherapy with one of the psychology interns whom I had been supervising. He had rapidly become fascinated with the power and efficacy of family therapy and wanted to learn more about it.

After several supervisory sessions, Dr. Ridenour mentioned that they had no family therapy training in their residency program; he thought it was critical that it be included so they would be better prepared to intervene with the families of service personnel. As Chief Resident for the following year, he wanted to recommend inclusion of a 12-week (30 hours) family therapy course taught by me at the Naval Hospital. With my permission, he moved ahead to talk to the Director of Training and the Chairman of the Department. Since neither of them knew much about family therapy and the Department until then had been utilizing an individual psychodynamic model of therapy, he had a good deal of interpreting to do and groundwork to lay.

There were two potential stumbling blocks to moving ahead—difficulties other potential consultants might also encounter. They had never had a PhD "consultant" to the department and they were not sure this would be permissible (it was and is). Further, they had never had a female consultant and were uncertain how acceptable this would be in this male bastion. After the initial hesitancy on all parts was overcome, acceptance was contingent upon competence, not gender.

While details were being worked out, I found out as much as I could about (1) the kind of problems Navy families are likely to have; (2) the kind of men who take their training in a Navy residency program; (3) the size of the group expected to attend classes; (4) what facilities were available (there was a treatment room with a one-way mirror); and (5) whether any senior staff or faculty were sufficiently trained in family therapy to supervise the family cases the residents would begin to carry as one of the projected clinical requirements of the course (no one seemed to be). Then I drew up a syllabus and bibliography geared to teaching theory, process, and technique of family therapy specifically as it might be pertinent in this environment.

The sessions were attended by all the residents and several interested senior faculty and staff members who were to carry the ongoing supervisory responsibility. For the first week, I gave a lecture on history and theories of family therapy, and a lively discussion ensued. Each resident was to carry at least one family case, and they could do cotherapy. The men indicated they wanted to view a live family therapy session the next week; one resident volunteered to set up an intake interview that he and I would co-conduct. The format for the remaining sessions was that a family came in and the resident did the treatment while the group observed. My role could be to serve as an in-room consultant or observer; the choice was theirs. Several were ambivalent—they wanted the consultant in the room with them for backup support and guidance but were afraid of feeling overwhelmed. Consequently, I sometimes held children on my lap or played with them on the floor, a "one-down" position that enabled the resident to take charge without feeling threatened while still allowing me to intervene as I modeled playing behavior for parents. When need be, I could be confrontative with officer patients without being intimidating because of my special "nurturing" role with the children. This "one-down" position has proved to be a valuable strategy in subsequent situations because it has avoided power collisions and permitted the consultant to remain task focused.

After each live session, I led a discussion teaching concepts, dynamics, and intervention strategies based on the actual clinical material that had unfolded. The residents were perceptive and eager, they learned rapidly and undertook the challenge of applying this approach whenever it seemed warranted.

Several weeks into the semester, Lieutenant Commander S commented that therapy conducted by a male–female team (when the consultant was involved) seemed to have advantages over a therapy team of two males and asked if I thought they should involve some female staff. I said I doubted it would work (intending a paradoxical effect); next week we were joined by two female social workers. This led to new working relationships and friendships, changed the alignments in the department, and added a new dimension to the residents' work.

SPECIAL SITUATIONS IN MILITARY CONSULTATIONS

With regard to the issue of women in the military, the absence of high-ranking female personnel in training and consulting slots in the Navy and Air Force continues, although as more women enter and remain in the services, a few are being promoted to such key positions. I rarely, if ever, have raised the issue head-on. Rather the presence of a woman functioning well in this capacity speaks with a silent eloquence and does not antagonize. In the feedback, wrapup portions that typically are part of any sessions that run 3 hours or more, one of the women will invariably comment on how important it has been for her to finally have a woman "up front" as a leader with whom she can identify, saying that until then she lacked role models, and that this experience provided her with a new incentive. Frequently, some of the men will also comment on the novelty of the experience and their unexpected comfort with a woman who conveys gentleness and sensitivity blended with strength and conviction. Reportedly, some ripple effect ensues that is conducive to inculcating more positive attitudes toward women professionals. Since command personnel are also in attendance, they seem to be influenced in future personnel selections by comments made during verbal or written evaluations.

PORTSMOUTH NAVAL HOSPITAL

At the end of the year of consultation at the Philadelphia Naval Hospital, the residency program was shifted to Portsmouth, Virginia. Dr. James Sears, who had been Chairman of the Department of Psychiatry, relocated to take a similar position in Virginia. Dr. Ridenour, upon completion of his residency, joined him there. I continued to go to the Philadelphia Naval Hospital as a consultant several times a year for the next 5 years, speaking on a variety of family- and, later, forensic-related subjects. I also consulted with the chairman regarding ongoing inclusion of these activities in the department, how to incorporate them in a way that was compatible with other therapeutic approaches, how to generate research to evaluate effectiveness, and indications and counterindications for family therapy in this setting.

Meanwhile, I was invited to the Portsmouth Naval Hospital several times a year to do psychiatric grand rounds and teach the residents family therapy. Topics for grand rounds included areas of pressing import like "Understanding and Treating Families Following a Major Disaster." Grand rounds were open to all hospital staff and attendance was high, with people coming from many allied specialties like pediatrics, neurology, psychology, nursing, art therapy, and family medicine. For many, this was their initial exposure to family therapy, and it was intended to help make the climate more receptive and to broaden the base of appropriate referrals.

Hours were set aside for small-group discussions for the residents exclusively. A high level of esprit de corps evolved. In addition to the teaching activities, each visit included lunch with the residents and staff at the Officers' Club, and one or two social evenings—usually including a dinner party at someone's home. Several times the residents asked to restrict the party to just them, their spouses, and me, and the chairman gave his permission. The residents utilized these evenings to talk about their frustrations, dreams, social expectations, protocol, and discontents.

A case example. A specific incident may help to convey the central part that informal contacts play and the potential problems that are stirred up for the consultant. Evening plans were made for one resident to take me to a dinner at another's home. Spouses were invited to this potluck supper. Shortly after dinner, the light atmosphere shifted to a serious one. All the residents clustered in the living room with me, and their wives stayed in another room behind closed doors. What quickly emerged was that the residents had decided to use this as a group therapy evening with the consultant as leader. My efforts to say it was inappropriate, unfair to their wives, and uncomfortable for me, got drowned out. I decided to wait and see what evolved.

Legitimate concerns and angry feelings emerged about gaps in curriculum, friction between senior staff members, blunders residents and their wives had made because they were inadequately acquainted with formal Navy protocol and social decorum, difficulties caused by the program's relocation, and so on. Following their expressions of frustration, I asked if they were ready to formulate their issues and grievances and select a committee to meet with the Chairman or were they holding this meeting as a way of requesting that I play "go-between." Once what was happening was framed into terms of action to be taken, the residents were free to relax a little and move ahead. They recognized in some ways they would like to be taken care of and have someone else intercede on their behalf, but that for their own self-respect and maturation process, they had to carry this responsibility. They were assured that the content of the evening would be kept confidential, but not the fact that the "party" had been transformed.

Next morning I met with the Chairman and told him about the predicament that had evolved. He indicated that he was aware that something like this might be brewing when he was apprised that the residents did not want faculty and staff present. He had gone along because he realized that they wanted to ventilate their annoyance in the presence of someone they trusted and perceived as safe. Likewise, he thought I would cope well with the outpouring and help them move toward some resolution of the underlying dilemmas without further inciting them. I told him to expect a delegation from the class within the next few days and, because some of their issues seemed reality-based, I said that I knew (self-fulfilling prophecy) he would be receptive and attempt to make some of the modifications they sought. He concurred and warmly expressed his gratitude. This response, combined with the brightened affect of the residents in morning group, diminished my annoyance at having been covertly "set up."

I was aware that I was beginning to occupy a special position as confidante, friend, and mentor, in my consultant role. The staff realized that I thoroughly enjoyed what I was doing and had come to treasure my role and status. I continued to have much more to learn about military protocol, rank, vocabulary, life-styles, humor, family, and community structure. Asking questions, listening, and observing carefully were essential. The widespread adherence to values of patriotism and loyalty expressed in serving one's country in an honorable and dedicated manner is impressive. I learned to respect the willingness of these bright, competent men to accept assignments to duty stations they did not choose because that is where they were needed. All of this was an essential part of "joining" the system.

LONG BEACH ALCOHOL REHABILITATION SERVICE

When Dr. Theodore Williams, whom I had met in Portsmouth, was transferred to become Director of the ARS in Long Beach, he decided that the annual Zuska Conference, which he initiated, should focus on themes of substance abuse as these related to family dynamics and to treatment interventions. He has invited me to participate in various ways ranging from plenary speaker to seeing a family live in a demonstration treatment interview. On each visit there, I meet with staff in a case consultation and staff-training format.

Prior to 1980, family therapy had been limited to treatment of spouses on an outpatient basis at Long Beach ARS. Since then, the "co-alcoholic" program, to which spouses are urged to come as inpatients for several weeks, has blossomed. Family therapy is utilized when it is deemed to be the treatment of choice *and* when they can get family members, who may reside quite a distance away in other states or overseas, to come in. The government underwrites the travel costs.

My first visit there was a prolonged one as I wanted to become familiar with the setting, key personnel, current program and its aims, and philosophic milieu before deciding how to maximize the impact of my contribution. Here, as with the residency training programs, meetings were held with the director and his top staff to discuss introducing family therapy into the setting, what the likely resistances might be, how these could be minimized, how to create a receptive climate, and what disruptions of routine and changes in service patterns were likely to be entailed. Part of joining with this program involved taking part in the excellent, 2-week training program, Treatment of Chemical Dependence, that they offer to military health care personnel from susbstance abuse programs. (Another joining approach has been attendance at the Military Psychology Division of the American Psychological Association.) As elsewhere, lunching with staff and attending functions with staff and patients have been part of coming to know and enjoy the organization. It is quite probable that failure to do so graciously would be a violation of expectancies and would impede the consultation process.

SAN DIEGO NAVAL HOSPITAL

When the Navy decided to inaugurate a new residency training in San Diego, Dr. Sears was again appointed Chairman of the Department and Dr. Ridenour became Director of Residency Training. By now the latter had become an experienced family therapist and he instituted an ongoing family therapy course for interested staff. My services were retained as a consultant with the program; my responsibilities were similar to those elucidated above. In San Diego, the grand rounds lectures have been opened to professionals in the surrounding civilian as well as military community to enhance their ties with, and contribution to, the local scene.

Over the past 8 years, many of the men who took their family therapy training through these Navy programs have completed their residencies and gone to far-flung bases in countries like Guam, Spain, and Japan as directors of inpatient and outpatient psychiatric services. Many report back that the family orientation, particularly around issues of separations and reunions, dependence and independence, abandonment and intimacy fears, has proven extremely valuable in their clinical practice and supervision activities (Kaslow, 1984; Ridenour, 1984). Some periodically call for guidance and curbside family case consultations.

LACKLAND AIR FORCE BASE

My involvement at Lackland Air Force Base began when I was recommended as a Distinguished Visiting Professor by Alberto Serrano, MD, a San Antonio psychiatrist and family therapist. During my several visits there, I have done grand rounds, some workshop-style training sessions, and consultations to individual staff and programs on request. These consultations are quite diverse, for example, career counseling for retirement planning, family-oriented consultation with the drug and alcohol inpatient unit, and consultation on forensic issues such as incompetency and insanity. With the Air Force, as with the Navy, being with staff informally at lunch or dinner is an important and pleasurable aspect of joining the system.

ENGAGEMENT WITH THE SYSTEM

Involvement with the military as a consultant has been productive and gratifying. I accept as many of their offers as my schedule permits. Given that I have never served in the military, this has become a special avenue through which I can express my own patriotic commitment. This factor is juxtaposed with another that potential consultants should be aware of: The per diem when consulting for the military is substantially lower than for comparable activities in private sector consulting or than that paid on the usual workshop circuit.

Each of these systems is clearly structured and is fairly sophisticated developmentally. Each time before reentering, I try to get a briefing by phone, mail, or in conversation, in order to be brought up to date on subtle and substantial changes of personnel, philosophy, rules, and patient population. Generally, much power resides in the contact person, who has authority endowed by virtue of rank and position. Power is much more clearly accepted in the military than in business, industry, and academe, so it is easier to ascertain if the program in which one is invited to participate has strong backing and support. If credibility for the program is not forthcoming from the top level, it probably is not wise to accept a contract.

The formal or explicit values, beliefs, and rules governing the military consultee system can be learned by reading manuals of operation and policy statements, by tactfully asking questions, by sensitive listening and observation, and by attending ceremonies and absorbing the atmosphere and behavioral norms. During a visit to one military hospital base, I was invited to attend a "frocking ceremony" (and hastened to ascertain what this meant). Such an invitation conveys an honor *and* a definite expectation of attendance. This is the occasion when officers are formally promoted to the next higher rank and receive their new bars. It is a special celebration because rising in the hierarchy is considered crucial in an officer's career. Everyone, accompanied by family and colleagues, comes in dress uniform. Protocol is assiduously followed and one doesn't dare deviate!

Some rules and values of a military system are ambiguous, informal, and less explicit, at least until one violates an unspoken or unwritten taboo. Then the curtain of denial descends and one becomes aware of the inadvertent transgression. The topic of homosexuality is such an area. Official policy is that homosexuals are to be discharged from the military. Unofficially, if homosexuality is not identified or discussed, the problem of discharge is avoided.

A case example. In one training program, the homosexuality of one of the men was revealed during the discussion about a situation with a patient he was describing. His officer colleagues in the class were aware of his homosexual lifestyle, as he had at times brought his male partner with him to social events as a "date." After class, I approached one of the officers and queried whether senior staff were aware of this situation. I wondered how it had been handled, and if I had any responsibility to discuss or report what had been communicated. He quickly changed the subject. The next day I raised this issue with another officer/faculty member. His advice was that a good consultant should focus on the agreed-upon task and not exceed his or her function by "making waves."

One can assume that a parallel process is operative at many levels of the system. In this example, the officer's classmates and their spouses were aware of his sexual preference and of the fact that to report it would mean his discharge. They became part of a conspiracy of silence—loyal to him, yet also defying rules and regulations. His teachers, supervisors, and consultants also became involved in the mass avoidance of the subject. If and when the situation is finally revealed, all involved in the silent cover-up are likely to have their careers shattered. Any consultant who ventures into this terrain may jeopardize future contracts and incite the wrath of many valued associates.

Throughout activities with the military, a consultant must constantly monitor the following: To whom is one responsible, and where is one's primary loyalty and commitment? In all of the foregoing material, this decision had to be balanced between the trainees, the chairman of the department, the director of training, the patients they ultimately treat, the larger military establishment, and our government as the broader ecological context.

Related to these issues are concerns over confidentiality and boundary issues. How can one give feedback to a program director without violating the trainee's privacy about what has been revealed in class? Similarly, when a service person enters therapy with a military therapist, the clinician may be required to send a mental health evaluation to the commanding officer with comments on the effect of the person's dysfunction on the military's mission, and with recommendations about possible discharge. Clearly, limits to confidentiality must be established before treatment, training, supervision, and consultation are undertaken.

MAINTAINING CHANGE

Various measures are undertaken to insure the durability of change after consultation. Reprints of articles and current bibliographies pertinent to the focus of a visit or the topics of scheduled presentations are distributed. Relevant books for individual and base library purchase are recommended. Also, over the years, as the cadre of the military mental health personnel qualified as family therapists has grown, supervision within the ranks has become available to insure quality practice. I maintain ongoing contact with these programs and am available by phone as needed.

During the first 6 years of this consulting work, requests were frequently received for literature geared more specifically to understanding and helping the military family. Finally, when Dr. Ridenour and I were approached to prepare a book on this topic, it appeared that this would fill a definite gap in the literature. The resulting book, *The Military Family: Dynamics and Treatment* (Kaslow & Ridenour, 1984), covers many of the important issues that frequently arise in working with military families.

TERMINATION AND EVALUATION OF CONSULTATION

Inasmuch as each contract is initially negotiated for a specific time, such as a 12-session course, or a 3-day special training event, a termination time has been agreed upon and built in. When appropriate, a verbal feedback period is conducted during the last half hour of the final session. If I have worked with several different groups, this is done with each; the time frame will vary depending on the number of participants and the length of the session. The focus is directed toward what participants have found to be new and professionally useful, how the consultation fulfilled their goals and expectations, and what format and content they might wish to pursue during future sessions together.

The consultee system usually has its own standard written evaluation forms. After these are filled in, they are returned to the director of training or the consultation committee. We have found a high level of congruence between the verbal and written evaluations.

Given the usual assumption of regimentation and fixed structure in the military bureaucracy, I have found surprising openness, flexibility, and receptivity. The people with whom I have worked are bright, innovative, and willing to brainstorm to come up with options that are most likely to be productive and have far-reaching, positive influence on service delivery. They are accustomed to carrying out their commitments and, therefore, the follow-through on implementing agreed-upon changes is excellent. The only constraints and resistances encountered have revolved around discussing topics that are "touchy," like the status of homosexual personnel, alcoholism, and incest in military families. One becomes sensitive to certain cues and learns to observe the "No Trespassing" signs.

The excellent, unexpected opportunities these activities have afforded are manifold. As a consultant to the military, one periodically enters a world that is very different from the one he or she usually inhabits. Here one becomes aware of the high intellectual caliber, emotional solidness, and dedication of mental health personnel in the armed forces. It is revitalizing to meet so many people who have a fundamental moral commitment to the values of "duty, honor, and country." Most of all, one can make numerous wonderful friends and establish some fine relationships with colleagues to whom one would not otherwise have access. At the risk of sounding saccharine, it has become a privilege for me to make this contribution, albeit small, to the well-being of the families who help to protect and defend our country.

Those who might undertake activities with the military should remember that it is important to have an open mind and to learn as much as possible about the armed forces, its language, traditions, structure, mythology, and heart and pulse beat. All that one knows about systems theory and organization development will be applicable. It is important to realize that the "military family" should not be narrowly defined. It may include the service person's family of creation or nuclear family, the military base extended family, the battalion or squadron, or any unit that takes on family-like loyalties. To enter and join the military network as a consultant, one may need all of these skills as well as high energy, adaptability in coping with emergencies and their fallout, and a sense of humor and adventure.

REFERENCES

Kaslow, F. W. Training of marital and family therapists. In F. W. Kaslow & Associates, *Supervision, consultation, and staff training in the helping professions.* San Francisco: Jossey-Bass, 1977.

Kaslow, F. W. A diaclectic approach to family therapy and practice: Selectivity and synthesis. *Journal of Marital and Family Therapy,* 1981, *7,* 345–351.(a)

Kaslow, F. W. Profile of the healthy family. *Interaction,* 1981, *4,* 1–15.(b)

Kaslow, F. W. Training and supervision of mental health professionals to understand and treat military families. In F. W. Kaslow & R. I. Ridenour (Eds.), *The military family: Dynamics and treatment.* New York: Guilford, 1984.

Kaslow, F. W., & Ridenour, R. I. (Eds.). *The military family: Dynamics and treatment.* New York: Guilford, 1984.

Ridenour, R. I. The military, service families, and the therapist. In F. W. Kaslow & R. I. Ridenour (Eds.), *The military family: Dynamics and treatment.* New York: Guilford, 1984.

Schein, E. H., & Bennis, W. G. *Personal and organizational change through group methods.* New York: Wiley & Sons, 1965.

Webster's seventh new collegiate dictionary. Springfield, MA. Merriam, 1972.

24

EMOTIONAL PROCESS IN THE MARKETPLACE
The Family Therapist as Consultant with Work Systems

EDWIN H. FRIEDMAN
Private Practice
Bethesda, Maryland

The first time I began to realize that family therapists could be consultants to work systems was with the case of an extremely competent, highly placed government official. He had two teenage daughters and a wife in open rebellion, and the only response he knew was to grip tighter on the reins. In family therapy, he learned to loosen up, to delegate anxiety as well as responsibility, to overfunction less, and to enjoy his own solitude more. The family calmed down, the kids made wise choices about college, and the marriage began to breed intimacy. At no time during this period had he ever mentioned his work. Then one day he came in all concerned about his job. As far as his own "shop" went, those below him were functioning better than ever, but his superiors were beginning to have doubts about his commitment. He had been known as an articulate devil's advocate and could always be relied upon at subcabinet meetings to keep the participants on their toes. But the same process of change that had freed up him and his family, and that enabled those he supervised to "feel their own oats," had gradually made him more reflective than reactive. This increased circumspection was misperceived by those above him as loss of verve and will. Because he did not want to lose his job, and also did not want to lose his family, he was told to stay on his new course with everyone except with his superiors. With them, he should pretend to be as intense as ever.

Over the years, I began to realize that almost any family breadwinner who increased his understanding of emotional process in his own personal family (Bowen, 1973) soon made similar changes in his occupational arena. Eventually, I found that I was making suggestions for his behavior at work, drawing genograms of organizations instead of flow charts, and applying various aspects of family theory to the work situation. I also began to apply what I was teaching my clients about their work to my own personal work system as a rabbi in a small synagogue. Over time, many of my former therapy clients began to return for advice specifically on their work system, saying that they could not help but see similarities to their previous personal family issues, and they had been wondering if I had developed my theories any further.

Today I find it quite easy to switch these roles of family consultant or business consultant while working with the same client. Clients can often gain insight more easily into various aspects of family process by seeing them in the less emotionally invested area of work. Their grasp of triangles and of the problems of overfunctioning can be sharpened. I have also modified my supervision of therapists to allow them to bring in problems from their professional work systems (clinics, partnerships, hospitals) as well as from their therapy with patients. I have found that the same reciprocity of insight between work and therapy also exists there. My experience as a consultant to "work families" has included a diverse set of organizations: nursery schools, government agencies, hospitals, architectural and law firms, medical partnerships, small businesses, large corporations, religious institutions, academic systems, and mental health clinics.

In this chapter I will describe the various ways in which family therapists can serve as consultants to business and professional systems. When it comes to emotional process, work systems replicate and function like family systems. There is one modifying factor, however, that needs special mention. Work systems are rarely as chronically intense as family systems. Even if fellow workers spend more time with one another than with members of their own families, the emotional investment conditioned by genes, culture, race, and family roots, is usually not as deep. However, there are two types of work system that do approach the level of emotional intensity and investment of that found in family life: (1) work systems that are family businesses and (2) work systems whose product is human services: hospitals, clinics, schools, churches and synagogues, medical partnerships, and so on.

In the former case, a work system can become every bit as enmeshed as the family that is operating it, and there is a constantly open conduit for problems in either system to cross over into the other. Transitions are also especially difficult, and the onset of serious physical symptoms among family leaders can almost always be correlated with issues that surface in the organization. In one small town church, where every member of the congregation was related to one another, the minister died of a sudden heart attack during an intense crisis over proposed changes in the service. To prevent this type of occurrence, a very large business consulting firm in New York regularly advises its large, family-owned corporations that the majority of the board should never consist of family members and, as far as responsibilities are concerned, no family member should report directly to another.

With regard to the second factor, where the business product is human welfare, the constant emotional intensity in those work atmospheres seems to bombard the nerves of the workers more than is the case with a material product. When in an excited state, the workers are more likely to interact and overreact. For this reason nonprofit work systems tend to be extremely intense. But a life-threatening crisis in an organization can make any institution, whatever its size or purpose, "act like a family." During Watergate, for example, attorneys, media, and government representatives often found themselves thrown together for long, arduous hours in an atmosphere in which the "fate of the republic was at stake." They were surprised at their difficulty in maintaining a professional, interpersonal distance.

There are four major ways in which family therapists can bring their expertise to bear in work systems: (1) create a systemic way of thinking about relationships and relational problems, and identify who is prone to dysfunction; (2) foster a less stressful, more effective mode of leadership; (3) promote an approach to transitions that will ease the effects on newcomers, outgoers, and on the system itself; and (4) heighten awareness of the problems spawned by the emotional interlock between work systems and workers' own families (Friedman, 1985).

SYSTEMS THINKING

One of the major ways in which family therapists can aid work systems is to modify the thinking of people who work in organizations. Industrial psychologists, for all their concerns with the overall environment, think in terms of the individual model. When workers are not communicating, these psychologists assume that the way to solve that problem is to get them to sit down and communicate. When productivity has gone down, the specialists look for better methods of motivation or recommend changes in the physical environment. If someone burns out because of stress, they design exercises and programs to help with that *individual's* rehabilitation.

Similarly, individual-model counselors are always advising managers and leaders to delegate responsibility, an enervating task in itself. A family therapist would understand that such advice never really works because what must be delegated is anxiety! ("I just wanted you all to know that based on last month's productivity levels our corporation will probably not be around too much longer. So if you want to submit your resumé, I will be glad to give you all glowing recommendations.")

Individual-model thinking does not provide an adequate frame of reference for dealing with the systemic concept of family emotional processes. Whether it is a business system or a family system, emphasis on productivity alone will only bring symptomatic relief. Further, getting caught up in symptomatic issues will create misperceptions of the problem, ultimately recycling the symptom.

Four family therapy concepts can be helpful to business leaders, employers, managers, and the workers themselves in avoiding those pitfalls: homeostasis, process and content, triangles, and identified patient.

HOMEOSTASIS

Homeostasis is a basic notion that transcends individual-model dynamics and permits a systemic perspective, with a focus on emotional process rather than symptomatic context. The concept of homeostasis can be extremely useful to work systems in a variety of ways, one of which is that it can provide an understanding of why problems seem to come out of nowhere and why they resurface continually despite the best intentions.

Another curious fact of business life explained by the concept of homeostasis is the willingness of even the most ruthless corporations to protect incompetents who may make trouble for co-workers and who may be psychotic, but who are undeviatingly loyal to "the company" and to the way things have always been done. A bright, creative worker who makes waves with suggestions is more likely to be fired.

In families, I have found that the vast majority of symptoms, whether located in the marriage, in the health of one of the partners, or in a child, surface within about 6 months to a year after a major change in the family of origin of one of the partners. Similarly, a change at "headquarters" can be the forerunner of a crisis in some office out in the "extended field." With work systems also, significant issues and dysfunctional symptoms tend to surface within 6 months of a major change in the larger system. It can begin at the executive level and surface almost randomly in one of the lesser branches. The corresponding changes do not have to be obviously related, for example, relocation of a budget division and reduced efficiency elsewhere, a new VP for academic affairs and burnout in the nursing school, or conflict in a private school's board of trustees and severe acting out in one particular class or one particular child.

It is possible to list some of the major homeostatic changes that can almost always be found in the background of the suddenly appearing eruption of an organizational problem. These changes are:

- change of leaders, especially a founder
- change in the personal life of a significant leader (boss, owner, member of the board of trustees)

- merger or acquisition
- reorganization
- relocation
- moving headquarters
- creation of new branch
- decentralizing or recentralizing
- significant promotion or retirement
- new competition in the field
- change in the laws governing the regulation of its product

Being aware that a problem in a seemingly unrelated location could be the fallout of some major disruption in the overall homeostasis of the "family" can help members of the work system keep their anxiety about the focal content problem in check. This is a very important point when it comes to healing. Many, if not most, problems go away if they are not inflamed by reaction (see below on the importance of leaders maintaining a nonanxious presence), and reducing or lessening anxiety increases the potential for objective solutions.

PROCESS VERSUS CONTENT

But, if focus on content issues can increase anxiety unnecessarily, failure to focus on systemic process issues will allow pernicious processes to continue undetected. The total number of content issues that all the marriages in the world have ever differed over probably does not exceed 12. The differences themselves do not cause the "differing," but, rather, the homeostatic shifts that made the difference (which may have always been there) become the foci of unresolved emotional processes. It is similar with work systems; the total number of different issues that have ever surfaced in all work systems is probably not much larger than those that surface in marriages. Yet, as with families, when these issues arise, the tendency is to assume that these content issues are the problem (e.g., personality conflicts, personal habits, productivity, punctuality, efficiency, cost-effectiveness, communication, co-operation, motivation). Keeping in mind this tendency to focus on content rather than process and teaching these systems-principles to members of work families can help clients to shift their focus to emotional process and to be less content with symptomatic relief.

Lifting the embargo: A case example. Ann, a 35-year-old woman, had been hired by a large advertising agency to create and administer a nationwide program. One of the major benefits for her was the latitude for travel. Outspoken, she freely gave input at all staff meetings. Suddenly her immediate boss began to warn her that his boss had decided to restrict her travel. When she went to this man's boss directly about the matter, he accused her of trying to subvert his authority at staff meetings. She was totally befuddled because she thought this man generally liked her ideas. She thought maybe it had to do with traditional male–female hierarchies. She found, however, that toning down her opinion did not lessen his antagonism, and that her travel plans were being further restricted.

Investigation of the larger system showed that this man's own superior, the president's son, who had been away for a year, was returning to his post, and that these two men had never gotten along. I told Ann that this was a system in search of a symptom and encouraged her to "lay low" until the transition was complete. Next, she was to work more on an individual relationship with her antagonist, perhaps going to him for (unneeded) advice. Within a month or so the "embargo on her passport" had been lifted.

EMOTIONAL TRIANGLE

One of the family therapy concepts that can prove most useful for business organizations is the concept of the emotional triangle. Presented to those who are in great stress, it can help their soma as well as their psyche. Overall, it offers practical ways of making the aforementioned concepts of emotional process operational. When consulting with work systems, I like to introduce the concept the first time that a triangle issue surfaces in the discussion. With the aid of a blackboard, I diagram the basic rules:

1. An emotional triangle is any three persons or part of a system with a "problem."

2. It is not possible from the position of A to change the relationship of B and C.

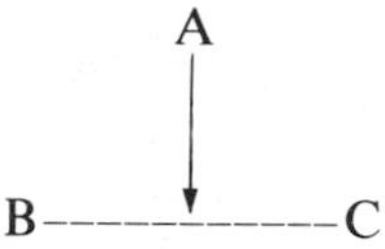

3. Continued efforts to change the relationship of B and C from the position of A will be converted by homeostatic forces to their opposite intent (pushing them apart will make them "fall in love," and trying to push them together will create polarized opposition).

4. Change in B and C can only come from changing one's own relationship with either or both, individually.

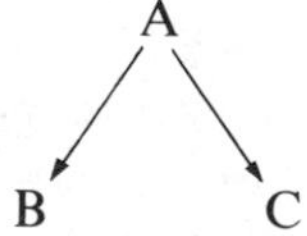

5. If from the position of A you become responsible for the relationship of B and C, then you will wind up with the stress for their relationship, if not for the entire system.

It is extraordinary the extent to which individuals in business systems who are somatizing severely are caught in such a position. I use as a teaching tale the experiment done back in the 1950s when, in an attempt to give them ulcers, monkeys were stressed in their efforts to get food pellets. This experiment was unsuccessful until a monkey was made responsible for getting food for the other monkeys as well. Even as an apocryphal tale, it captures some universal truth: Individuals are capable of handling enormous stress when they are doing it for themselves. Trying to handle stress for others is malignant, especially when the others are pulling from opposite directions.

6. Triangles interlock; an important triangle in one branch of an office or on the board of trustees can interlock with others, as can those involving romantic or personal family relationships. At one psychiatric hospital, a physician had ambivalent, romantic attitudes toward a nurse on a specific ward. He was responsible for one of the patients on that ward. The amount of psychotherapy that patient received in any month was directly proportional to the degree that the physician was moving toward or away from the nurse. Similar relational phenomena go on in every office.

The significance of interlocking triangles is that they are the key to plotting how problems in one system (or subsystem) can produce symptoms in another and, as will be described below, how unresolved issues in work systems and family systems can leap over into one another.

It is important to point out that triangles are not exclusively pathogenic. They are also the seat of power. We are all in triangles. What is stressful is to *be* triangled, to be caught as the focus of the unresolved relationships of others. However, the triangled position can also be the most powerful point from which to promote change once one understands the system. The following story is about a partner in a consultation firm who had had chronic back pain for a year, and who was thinking of starting his own firm because of his triangled position. The story exemplifies many aspects of the use of the emotional triangle concept to help bring change to a work system.

The flea collar: A case example. Harry Ford was one of four partners who created a consulting firm specializing in social science contracts. Each partner had specific areas of responsibility, but Harry's took him somewhat out of the executive level because his job was to see that the internal workings of the organization were coherent. Viewing himself as a sensitive person who was always willing to listen, he spent a great deal of time and energy trying to soothe ruffled feathers and reduce antagonisms between staff members. Nonetheless, he also found himself the target of animosity felt toward his fellow partners. Pained by the distance between his partners and the staff, he often suggested changes, but his partners came more and more to see him as not concerned with their own best interests.

Harry then heard that his partners had made several decisions, when he was not present, to expand the firm's business to areas that were not oriented toward social welfare. In addition, one of his partner's wives was to be brought in as a special consultant. She had a long-standing feud with the corporation's business manager with whom Harry worked closely and harmoniously. At this point, Harry became troubled by severe back spasms and took to bed for a week. As soon as he could walk again, he called for an appointment, having been in family therapy several years previously regarding the breakup of his marriage and a custody fight over his children.

It was suggested to Mr. Ford that he had to begin by giving up such unilateral responsibility for his firm. He saw himself as the only partner really interested in its original social goals. It was therefore suggested that he cease being so close to the staff and become an executive again. He was afraid the staff would think him a fink. I suggested that he tell his partners directly that he questioned whether he was right for the firm (not that they should change) because it had lost its original values, and that he also personally resented being left out of the decisions. Care was taken to prepare him for this meeting so that he could deal with the predictable complaint that "he had no business sense." We also discussed the fact that one of the junior partners and the senior partner were golfing buddies and so it was also suggested that he do nothing that might appear as if he were trying to put distance between them.

At the meeting everyone reacted predictably and tried to get Harry to feel guilty about his proposal. (In any system, if the symptom bearer tries to get out of that position, the others will uncomfortably respond to prevent change. A pack of dogs would not really like to see a flea collar put on the one with fleas.) Harry had been coached, however, not to counterattack on the content issues but to stay with the notion that perhaps he was not right for them, rather than that they should change and be like him.

Finally, the senior partner suggested that they have lunch, after which he asked Harry to be his right-hand man in handling all program and personnel responsibilities. Within a period of about a month, the other two junior partners grew closer; the wife who was going to be a consultant found something "more lucrative"; there were a series of efforts to triangulate Harry with his partner and the office manager, but this time he declined by being less "sensitive," though in other situations he volunteered to listen while they talked things out. Several staff members left, much to Harry's sorrow, but he managed to continue to abstain from his habitual efforts to rescue. Soon the anxiety over the future of the firm had shifted to his partners, particularly to the president who had decided to seek consultation himself! Harry was then coached to throw a party for all his partners and their wives in order to cement his reentry at the executive level. One day he found that his back pains had disappeared as mysteriously as they had arrived.

IDENTIFIED PATIENT

As suggested above, the symptom bearer in a work system is most likely to be an overfunctioner. People-people are far more likely to burn out than idea-people. Others likely to burn out, no matter what their expertise, are managers who are given insufficient control, or leaders who are unable to keep a system together, especially if they have a great deal of emotional investment in that system. This is particularly true in a family business where rifts in the family infect the work system, often killing the founder or president who is trying to keep the family (or the work system—he can't tell which) whole. (A particular aspect of this added stress regarding the family standard bearer will be discussed below.) Studies of burnout based on the individual model focus on the personality of the burned-out worker. Family systems thinking focuses on the nature of the system likely to burn out its workers.

For example, the following five criteria pertain to the likelihood that an executive officer will burn out. They were originally conceived for my book on the stressful factors in the position occupied by most clergy (Friedman, 1985), but they seem equally applicable to private business and large corporations as well. The notion is that to the extent that these following five criteria describe any organization (all do to some extent), then the executive officer, no matter what his or her personality, is likely to be severely stressed and will develop symptoms in whatever manner he or she is prone to when stressed. The criteria are:

1. the degree of isolation between the organization and the general community or other similar types of organizations in the field;
2. the degree of distance between the ruling body (board) and the workers;
3. the extent to which the leadership allows the work system to preempt its entire emotional life (no other friends or social network);
4. the degree to which the leaders have intense, interdependent personal relationships beyond their work system—in social clubs, churches, family, or other business interests;
5. the degree to which a chairman of the board or other executive is unable to take independent, well defined positions with clarity and vision.

Taken together, these five factors form a spawning ground for triangulation of whoever is trying to get the job done. They can be applied macrocosmically to an entire work system or microscopically to a small division.

LEADERSHIP

One of my first consultation experiences in a work system was with NASA. A family therapy client had noticed some similarities between what we were discussing in the breakdown of his family after the pioneer generation had died out and the breakdown in morale in the space agency after the United States had reached the moon and the space program was de-emphasized. He invited me to the monthly meeting of administrators from Canaveral, Houston, Greenbelt, and the other agencies. At that meeting, I happened to pick up a sheet of paper listing 10 rules of organization that the new head administrator had just presented. The very first one caught my eye and has been a basic premise of all my consultation with work systems and family systems ever since.

It read, "The character of any organization is determined primarily by one or two people at the top." This rather simple notion is itself a theory of organizations and leads to a specific set of interventions that any family therapist can teach to the leader of any organization or its divisions. The concept suggests that, when working with any type of relational network, the higher up the genogram (or flow chart) we can get, the more of the system we can affect. Implicit in the idea, however, is something much more profound: that when we obtain change in the functioning at the top, the entire organization is affected *systemically*!

Some of the strongest evidence for the vital importance of leadership comes from the sports world. On the one hand, no work system appears to be more dependent on individual performance; on the other hand, the most successful teams do not necessarily consist of the players with the best individual records.

The reason that the overall health and functioning of any organization depends primarily on one or two people at the top (whether the relationship system is a personal family, a sports team, an orchestra, a congregation, a religious hierarchy, or an entire nation) is not some mechanistic trickle-down, domino effect. It is rather that leadership in personal or work families is essentially an organic, perhaps even a biological phenomenon. An organism tends to function best when its "head" is well differentiated. A practical example: If the person at the top is weak, that is, will not take a stand, it erodes the position of anyone below who tries to take one. Those below any stand-taker will sabotage him or her by colluding with the weak boss, who will let it happen. The key to successful leadership has more to do with the leader's capacity for self-definition than with ability to motivate others. Here success is understood not only as moving people toward a goal but also in terms of the survival of the work family and its leaders. Ultimately, it is less a matter of how the "coach" manages his players and more a matter of how he manages himself.

Almost all leaders respond to lack of desired change by trying harder to push, pull, tug, kick, shove, threaten, convince, arm-twist, charm, entice, cajole, seduce, induce guilt, shout louder, or be more eloquent. Because the focus of such efforts is upon the follower rather than the self of the leader, it rarely occurs to the people at the top, at home or at work, that some threshold may have been reached. At this point, further efforts not only will fail to bring change, but also they will be converted by the developing emotional process into forces that stabilize the status quo. One major effect of this power conversion is that it gives leverage to the follower.

This paradox of counterproductivity is not the only form of resistance with which all "family" leaders must contend. Successful leadership must also be able to avoid being sidetracked by active resistance. A second paradox facing people at the top that it is an absolutely predictable fact that followers will work to throw them off course precisely when they are functioning at their best! This automatic, mindless sabotage of followers is so prevalent in human families that, if anything, it is usually evidence that the leader has been functioning well. It is as prevalent in Congress as in the Presidium.

Most approaches to leadership, based on the individual model, tend to fall along a continuum marked at one end by charisma and at the other by consensus. Neither tends to be very successful in resolving these twin paradoxes of resistance because they are essentially due to homeostatic phenomena rather than to "personality conflicts." As we shall see, leadership through self-differentiation does not view resistances as simply obstacles to be overcome. Rather, they are the keys to the kingdom. The charismatic concept of leadership recognizes that there is a magnetic quality exuded by certain people that is personally attractive. It does not seem to be a quality that can be taught, only cultivated if one already has it. If the evidence from ethology is relevant, it might even have a genetic component. The charismatic personality can unify disparate elements, inspire contagious enthusiasm, and galvanize a family into quick action. It seems to work best when the relationship system is despondent, helpless, confused, and hungry for change. Demagogy, whether it is political, religious, or therapeutic, is always most attractive in a depression.

Some of the problems with a charismatic approach are: (1) it can polarize as well as unify because of the emphasis on the personality of the leader; (2) the personalization of issues also creates polarization between the family and all other relationship systems; (3) leadership by charisma has difficulty with succession—families that become too dependent on their leader tend to lose their purpose after the loss; and (4) leadership by charisma ultimately is not healthy for the leader because he or she is perpetually forced to overfunction and constantly try to balance all the triangles. In the long run, such leaders paradoxically find that their functioning has become dependent on having a family or work system to lead.

A counterpoint to the charismatic philosophy of leadership is one of consensus. The basic emphasis in the consensus approach is the will of the group. The group is prepared to wait longer for results, being more concerned with the development of a cohesive infrastructure. It tends to value peace over progress and personal relationships, or feelings over ideas. In such a setting, undue individualism of a leader is more likely to create anxiety than reduce it. Since the will of the group is supposed to develop out of its own personality, rather than come down from the top, the function of the leader is more that of a resource person or an "enabler."

Basic problems exist with the consensus approach to leadership. (1) The family led by consensus will tend to be less imaginative. The world's most important ideas have tended to come to people in solitude. It is not that the consensus approach gives people less time to be alone but, rather, that it discourages idiosyncrasy and originality. (2) Leaderless groups are more easily panicked; anxiety tends to cascade. The circuit-breaker effect of self is missing. (3) Emphasis on consensus gives strength to the extremists because they can continue to dangle the carrot of unity as their price for cooperation. (4) Consensus is no guarantee against xenophobia or polarization. For instance, paranoia and other cultic phenomena of emotional interdependency are often a by-product of the charismatic approach. Ironically, as a consensus-based approach to leadership nears its goal, the degree of emotional fusion that results is likely to create the very problems its approach was designed to avoid.

LEADERSHIP THROUGH SELF-DIFFERENTIATION

In contrast, a family systems perspective does not create polarity between leader and follower. It focuses on the organic nature of their relationship as a constituent part of the same organism. Instead of viewing the interactions of leaders and followers in terms of the impact each has upon the other, a family systems concept of leadership looks at how they function as part of one another. In other words, leaders and the groups they lead are not considered separate entities but constituent parts of the same "colony of cells" (emotional system). Leadership, therefore, is not conceptualized in terms of how leaders should deal with their followers. Rather, the focus is on their own self-definition. The emphasis is on how the leader's own functioning within the system, his or her *self-differentiation,* will automatically affect the followers because of the organic nature of their connection. This formulation is at a different level of inquiry from the charisma–consensus continuum.

Like the charismatic approach, the family systems approach recognizes the importance of personal leadership but it emphasizes the leader's *position* in the system rather than his or her personality. The responsibility of the leader, therefore, ceases to be the entire family (a heavy load indeed) and becomes instead the position of leadership.

Like the consensus approach, a family systems theory of leadership does not belittle the importance of an organization's coherence, but it distinguishes between togetherness and stuck-togetherness, and refuses to purchase the integrity of the group at the cost of the self of its members. Consensus, while still an important goal, is not confused with a way of life.

The basic concept of leadership through self-differentiation is this: If a leader will take primary responsibility for his or her own position as "head" and work to define his or her own goals and self, *while staying in touch with the rest of the organism,* there is a more than reasonable chance that the body will follow. There may be initial resistance, but if the leader can stay in touch with others despite the tendency to pull away, the body will usually go along. The ability of a leader to be a self while still remaining a part of the system may be the most difficult task in any relationship system. Yet, to the extent it is accomplished, the process will transform the dependency that is at the root of the tendency to sabotage the leadership.

There are two distinct, but interrelated components to leadership through self-differentiation, keeping in mind that successful leadership means not only moving a system toward its goals but also maximizing the functioning, health, and survival of both the system and its leader. First and foremost, the leader must stay in touch. Since the system is basically organic, for any part of an organism to have a continuous or lasting effect, it obviously must stay connected with the other parts. Remaining connected, however, becomes increasingly difficult in direct proportion to the leader's success at defining his or her own being (the second component).

The second central component is the capacity and willingness of the leader to take nonreactive, clearly conceived, and clearly defined positions. Again, this is easier to accomplish when the leader is not in touch with (or beholden to) the rest of the system; it can be difficult even to think out such positions while attached. Yet, and this is crucial, the functioning of any organism, often its survival, and certainly its evolution, is directly dependent on the capacity of its "head" to do precisely that. *Define self and continue to stay in touch.* Note here that the leader is not trying to define his or her followers, only himself or herself. The issue of motivating the followers' "minds" or overcoming their resistance is thus bypassed; it is their need for a head that will move them. This phenomenon describes marriage, parenting, and organizational leadership.

The more self-defined followers will follow the lead of the leader and respond to his or her differentiation by taking their own nonreactive positions, which is not necessarily the same as simply agreeing. The more dependent followers, however, will at first respond reactively in an effort to pull the leader back.

Here is the moment of truth. Will the leader have the capacity to maintain his or her differentiated state, which is not the same as being unwilling to compromise, or to move back a little? A reciprocal "twitch" by the leader will return the organism to its previously undifferentiated state, and no evolution will result. Similarly, leaders can maintain a position by a rigid dogmatic stand or by cutting themselves off, but from that moment on, they are no longer leaders, only heads. It is in the capacity of the leader to maintain a position and still stay in touch (without being too anxiously helpful) that the organism's future resides. Many leaders have the capacity to stay in touch; fewer leaders have the capacity to define themselves; fewest have the capacity to remain connected while maintaining such self-differentiation. It is the most difficult part of leading any system, work, or family. Consultants who have observed this process in families are well prepared to coach its identical twin in work systems.

TRANSITIONS

Problems in a family can be the residue of emotional processes carried over from previous generations. The same transmission occurs within work systems, and such processes tend to be perpetuated or to originate during transition periods. In almost all traditions, demons and dybbuks enter and leave during rites of passage.

Two important family therapy principles concerning transitions are relevant to entering and leaving a work system: (1) incapacitating grief after loss is proportional to the residue of the unworked-out part of a relationship and (2) the capacity of any new relationship to "take" depends primarily not on the partners' own personalities or even the interpersonal transactions but, rather, on the residue carried over from the unresolved aspects of the previous relationships.

On the other hand, where previously unresolved issues are being transmitted from "generation to generation," this process can be modified during a future transition. Nodal events in work families, as in personal families, function like switchboards into which feed all the past and present emotional currents. Such moments have great power to determine the direction of their future flow, including whether they will be turned on or off. For example, it is often thought that people become "lame ducks" once it is known that they are leaving a post. This is as shortsighted as approaches that urge physical distance or minimizing contact as the way to reduce emotional intensity. Such all-or-nothing approaches to separation are far more likely to transfer the intensity than to reduce it. Cutting off totally can be far more pathogenic in the long run than hanging on.

The family model offers a third alternative. "Lame duck" periods can be among the most fruitful in the life of any work system because the nature of the separation always influences the lasting effects of all our previous years of effort. How individuals function during the end stage of their work relationships can prolong the effect of their previous efforts and be more important than the manner in which their ideas and programs were introduced in the first place.

A family systems approach to separation will enable the work system to be more objective in the selection of a new employee or partner so that the new relationship can have a fresher start. Also affected is the emotional interlock to be discussed in the next section. Often members of the work family are at the same moment going through some personal separation experiences (terminal illness, divorce, a child leaving home). During such coincidences, their anxiety over the work family breakup will be heightened, if not displaced. A family approach to transitions in the work system will minimize the effects of the residue left by the previous relationship.

STRATEGIES FOR SEPARATION

Here are four interconnecting elements in a family systems-based model for leaving work systems in a manner that minimizes pathological residue:

- Regulate one's emotional reactivity to others.
- Permit emotional reactivity in others.
- Be a nonanxious part of the transition process.
- Stay in touch *after* leaving; continue to detriangle.[1]

1. For a description of the author's own efforts to put these ideas into practice when he resigned after 15 years from a synagogue he had helped found, see Friedman (1985).

Emotional Reactivity

The most important factor that affects the resolution of intense bonds is the degree of emotional reactivity as compared to responsiveness. Reactivity promotes fusion. It inflames the wounds of separation rather than healing them.

The most intense forms of reactivity in divorce—for example, battles over property, visiting rights and support payments, kidnapping of children, refusal to let the other partner see the child, or lack of contact ever again—all are evidence that the couple has *failed* to separate. The continued struggle inhibits further separation. Property settlement struggles can also surface in any work-system divorce in which it is assumed that the material aspect is central because it is a business. What makes it difficult to control reactivity during transitional periods is that the other partner is often at last making changes one had sought to bring about for years. (This is much like the marriage partner who finds his sexless or frugal spouse has become the opposite after the breakup.) For example, one man, who had been a very dedicated member of his firm for 15 years, said the week after he left: "I have walked down these same streets for more than a decade and I just noticed some of the buildings for the first time." Such changes in attitude or perception are the natural result when fusion or enmeshment dissolve, and they reinforce the importance of self-defined leadership.

Naturally, in any relationship, the partner who is not initiating the separation will tend to be more reactive. In addition, in any breakup, the first partner who succeeds in finding a new partner will get a depressed or sabotaging reaction from the other. But even when the other partner is the "jilter," the capacity to commit oneself to a course of regulating one's own reactivity, while it is more difficult in such circumstances, can go far to facilitate the type of separation necessary for both to get on with their future lives. This is also beneficial for those further down the "flow chart" in any "split," marital or professional.

The person leaving can be prepared for this experience by having him or her list the types of remarks or behaviors most likely to cause reactivity, and develop strategies in advance for how to detoxify those situations when they arise. Parodoxical and playful responses are particularly apt here.

Permitting Reactivity in the Other

It is important to allow reactivity in the other. As most family members would prefer that their relatives die in the middle of the night rather than through a slow process of deterioration, and most marriage partners who leave would like to steal away nocturnally and never have to deal with their partner again, so members of work systems would like to have as little time as possible between the announcement of their resignation and the actual termination of their contract. Yet, in any kind of separation it is precisely such avoidance responses during the exit that "spook" the future.

Certainly, the shorter the period of the "interregnum," the less reactivity we have to deal with. But the ability to allow or even to make room for reactivity in the other, without reciprocating, creates the best chance for both partners to go on to their next relationships with the least amount of "baggage." Allowing the other to react while committing yourself not to react is what "dying with dignity" may really be about.

Engaging Actively in the Process

Parents often go to one or two extremes around the weddings of their children. Either they become overinvolved and interfering, or they remove themselves from the process as much as possible. Interference obviously hinders the separation, but so does distance. Where parents can become part of the leaving-home process without trying to influence its direction, more separation will be accomplished, and the new bond will have more flexibility than if the parents had just remained distant.

The same is true when leaving a work system. Certainly, trying to influence the selection process of one's successor is akin to trying to choose or nullify a choice of a mate for one's child. On the other hand, helping one's business partner during this period to become more aware of how the relationship looks from the other side can heighten the work system's objectivity in the selection process. Even though this engages the outgoing employee or manager more at the time, it ultimately promotes more disengagement. It requires minimizing reactivity, but also helps regulate it for both partners.

Staying in Touch after the Divorce

Just as in marriage, in which the other side of successful engagement is continued successful disengagement (from the families of origin), so the capacity of any work system or former employee to make a success of his or her next relationship is somewhat dependent on a continuing disengagement process after the "divorce." Indeed, some forms of disengagement are only possible after the separation. (Cemetery visits may serve the same disengagement process. Ostensibly for the purpose of remembering, they may really help us to forget better than when we try to carry our remembrances in our heads.)

Staying in touch after separation also exorcises the latent triangles. Where we allow former business associates to attack our successor, for example, but refuse to conspire in an emotional alliance against him or her (not too much more difficult than resisting the wiles of Satan), we further the disengagement with our separated partner. This will promote the process of a less fused engagement in our partner's new relationship as well as in our own. One effective response in such a situation is: "Everyone has their strengths and their weaknesses."

Are there dangers in this approach? Absolutely! But noncloistered virtues always involve more risks. Such moments of detriangulation foster more separation than if they never had a chance to occur. Playing it safe is more peaceful, but avoiding challenge is not what responsible leadership is about.

STRATEGIES FOR ENTERING A WORK SYSTEM

There is, of course, no guarantee that our predecessors have handled their leaving well. Even if they have, there will always be some residue. Each of us inherits the unresolved part of our predecessors' relationships with our business partner or employer. (Everyone marries the irresponsibility of their in-laws.) We must, therefore, ask what family theory has to say about entering a work family. Two major variables contribute to residue. One is the length of that work system's previous "marriages" and the leadership styles of its partners. The second is the nature of the previous separations and how those breakups were handled.

In any divorce, a highly emotional separation after a short-term relationship is more easily worked through than a less intense separation in a relationship nurtured by long-term, deep-rooted, emotional interdependency. The worst possible outcome is when both conditions are satisfied, that is, the nature of the separation was traumatic and the relationship had lasted many years, for example, as when a charismatic leader who built the business commits suicide or resigns without warning.

Taking all of these factors into consideration, family systems theory creates a threefold strategy for entering an established relationship system:

- Avoid interfering with, or rearranging, the interpersonal relationships.
- Be wary of efforts by members of the system to triangulate you with the "departed" or with other members of the system.
- Work at creating as many direct one-to-one relationships as possible with key members.

Avoid Interfering with the Interpersonal Relationship

The most applicable model is a "blended family" where two previously married partners, at least one of whom has children, set up house together. In any second marriage, both partners bring the baggage of some unresolved issues from their first marriages, and in proportion to the previously mentioned interdependent variables of the length of the relationship and the nature of the separation (as well as the degree of differentiation from their families of origin). One of the partners usually marries into the established relationship system of the other partner (though this also can be true in first marriages if one moves into the orbit or the house of the other partner's parents).

The partner marrying into the other's system must never try to rearrange the established pattern of relationships. If a new husband, for example, tries to change the relationship of his bride and her daughter, the process will sponsor an infinite variety of symptoms from physical problems to conflict over sex and money. The partner entering the other's system has a right to individual relationships with the new spouse, as do each of them with the other's children, but efforts to change the relationships of the new spouse with his or her own children will be at least ineffective if they do not get him or her expelled altogether. (Witness the number of American presidents who have entered office with enthusiastic resolve to change the civil service system, only to give up quietly by the end of their first year in office. Those most vociferous in this regard probably get the least amount of cooperation on other issues.) One woman who moved in with her new husband and his teenage daughters immediately went about changing the thermostat settings and the wattages of certain lamp fixtures. This "keeper of the thermostat" was out in 6 months.

This phenomenon does not mean that a new idea cannot be introduced. On the contrary, sometimes a relationship system is far more open to change during a period of transition. But expressing ideas or suggesting changes is one thing, and coming on as the fixer or the rearranger is another. It is also helpful to keep in mind that when there is a strong emotional reaction to an otherwise harmless suggestion for change, the content of the suggestion is not the problem, but rather it is what the suggestion portends for change in the emotional process of the relationship system. Therefore, when first entering a work system, trying to change the "thermostat" settings too quickly can have similar disastrous results.

Avoid Triangles with the "Departed"

Even when a partner marrying into a new system takes great care not to interfere with the existing pattern of relationships, there is no guarantee that other members of the family will accept such noninterference. The children, for their part, may try to triangle the new parent by complaining about or criticizing their own parent. The analogy to work families is obvious. To the extent that a work family contains unresolved issues among the various "sibs," the new "daddy" or "mommy" is going to be greeted with initiatives to get the new leader on one side or the other. The ambushes are various, subtle, and many. We might try to convey that we have allowed ourself to be triangled in an alliance, yet take care not to become emotionally committed to one part of the family. But to the extent that we form a new relationship based on the detriangulation of a third party, that new relationship has been built on pseudointimacy; later stresses will make the seams all too obvious.

A similar situation often found in second marriages is one in which the couple initially gains a calm togetherness by comparing the dastardliness of their "ex's." Thus, another type of triangulation that faces all when they first enter business systems is the negative remarks about the "ex," usually presented in a manner that praises the newcomer by contrast. All triangled remarks are residue. Because no relationship is ever totally worked through, there will always be such remarks. To the extent, however, that the person entering can resist the flattery, or the good feelings of togetherness that accompany such triangulation, the cleaner their own start will be. This is true not only because one is then less likely to become a replacement within old triangles, but also because, in refusing to become that replacement, one forces resolution of the residue left over from the previous partner.

Michael Kerr (1973–1974) has described a situation that occurred when it became his turn to take over the psychiatric division of a military hospital. On the first day, the administrative secretary greeted him with a barrage of comparisons to his successor, all complimentary of him and disparaging of the person he was replacing. Wary of his inheritance, he responded, "I'm surprised to hear you talk so negatively about the Major. He only had the nicest things to say about you."

Create One-to-One Relationships

The third element in a family systems strategy for entering a new work system is the creation of one-to-one relationships with as many members as possible, particularly those in positions of influence. This step follows logically from the first two and provides a concrete, positive approach for avoiding the pitfalls of the previously described separation dynamics.

In many ways this element feeds back to the concept of "leadership through self-differentiation," as well as to the importance of being connected. To become a leader of a new family, one must become its head. If it is an established family, one does not become its head simply as a result of the joining process. Time must be allowed for the "graft" to take. When it comes to top positions, if entering directors, managers, and others would make this joining their main priority for the first year, rather than hurrying to introduce new programs, not only would they increase their chance for a long-lasting "marriage," but they would be also more likely to see their program ideas accepted when they are introduced. And, to come full circle, to the extent that the entering person can function according to these principles, when the relationship is ultimately dissolved, less multiple generational residue will be transmitted to the next relationship.

Shooting the breeze: A case example. A very efficient new director found that members of her division were resisting her suggestions. She wondered if it was because she was from a different cultural background. It was suggested that she spend some time each day sitting on the desk corners of her employees and shooting the breeze. As do many efficient, no-nonsense types, she said she did not like to "waste time" like that. She soon found, however, that if she planned to devote 50% of her time to a project, taking 10% of this and putting it into the relationship system always potentiated the other 40% logarithmically.

Finally, family systems theory about the courtship period can serve as a paradigm for interviewing a work family before getting "hitched." Using the model of the genogram, whether or not one actually draws a schematic diagram, the following questions, would seem important:

1. How and when was the business (clinic, partnership) orignally created? To what extent did it form out of the natural coming together of the founders, and to what extent is it a splinter group from an established system?
2. To what extent are the founding members still in power?
3. In what ways do the articles of incorporation reflect the intensity of its origins?
4. How many different leaders has the system had? Is the average time span of these partnerships significantly different from the overall average for that type of business?
5. What has been the nature of the work system's previous separations from people who occupied a given position? To what extent have they been mutual, to what extent has the work system been the initiator, and to what extent has the employee been the initiator?
6. If any of the previous separations have been stormy or traumatic, what has been the nature of subsequent separations or relationships?
7. What major homeostatic changes have recently occurred in the overall emotional system? For example, has there been a geographical relocation, a completion of new plant or even a wing, any major changes in leadership, or any recent departure of other professionals (and administra-

tive secretaries) who have been there a long time? Has any other competition surfaced recently?

8. What is the relationship of the work system to the local community as well as to similar systems in the industry? What is its reputation in those extended systems and the extent of its involvement? Has there been any recent, abrupt change?

9. How do members of the work system talk about the person being replaced? To what extent is there clearly unresolved intensity, positive or negative, and to what extent do they immediately try to triangle you with that person? (How much and in what way do they mention him or her in the interview and early interactions?)

10. Test the emotional system. Take some stands about what you believe and observe the response of the system. To what extent do the interviewees respond with their own "I" positions, and to what extent do they try to engage you argumentatively?

11. Listen for the triangles (factions) within. Do they seek a well-defined leader or just someone to keep the peace?

A decision based on this information is probably more reliable in ascertaining the emotional system one is about to enter than is the hearsay of colleagues. At the least it will put that hearsay into perspective. This list will ferret out the homeostatic changes most likely to spawn content issues and the characteristics of a work system that are likely to burn out its executive officers. In personal or work families, entering really has to do with leaving, and the nature of new connections is primarily a function of the nature of previous separations.

THE EMOTIONAL INTERLOCK

The fourth way in which family therapists can effectively serve as consultants to work systems is with regard to the emotional interlock that often exists between family systems and work systems. Under certain predictable conditions, unresolved issues can be displaced from one into the other. This is automatically true in family businesses, small corporations, and partnerships. It is often so in nonprofit organizations in which the institution preempts much of the workers' social lives. It is frequently true in lifesaving organizations, but it can occur in any work system if the person involved is in a crucial position. The other factor, of course, is the degree of differentiation at home or at work, because the more enmeshed the system, the less capacity it has to resist the crossover.

It is important to emphasize that the emotional interlock concept is not simply saying that work systems have an "impact" on the family or vice versa. Obviously, if one loses a job or is made irritable at work, that event will affect his or her family. If someone has had a bad night at home, that can lead to a bad day at the office. The concept of "impact" might suggest two different, discrete entities that influence one another from outside each other's space, as might occur in a crash between two boulders, two trains, or two billiard balls.

The concept intended here is more analogous to electricity. The deepest effects that work systems and family systems have on one another derive from the fact that they both run on the same current, if not the same energy source. The influence is internal rather than external. They are plugged into one another and their respective states of homeostasis join to create a new overall balance.

The following example of a medical partnership shows how thoroughly interlocking professional and family functioning can be:

Always "on call": A case example. Four doctors joined in an obstetrical practice and one did not carry his weight. He failed to cover his assigned duty times, he did not bring new patients into the practice, and he was very rigid about the advice he gave his patients.

One of the other physicians took up the slack. As he became more stressed by the load, he seemed to change at home, and his wife began to blame the office. His response was that the poor colleague had a lot of problems at home with his kids and needed the income badly.

His wife became increasingly fed up, said in effect that she had to compensate for the other wife's failures, and continued to pressure her husband to change. He, however, resented her interference and seemed to respond by giving additional time to the practice, a position that his colleagues, especially the underfunctioning one, took advantage of. As the doctor's wife was taught about triangles, she pulled out of her husband's professional life. Then her mother become ill, creating a situation that fostered more opportunities for her to work on her own differentiation. The doctor began to stand up to his colleagues. The underfunctioning doctor become very depressed, went to a therapist, and learned to take a stand in his own family. Not only did he become a more responsible member of his medical partnership, but also the quality of his health care improved.

A more subtle, yet potentially far more influential, emotional interlock between family systems and work systems can be found in individuals who have been catapulted out of their families to achieve, and have become, in effect, their extended family's identified "standard bearer."

The "standard bearer" usually is the oldest male, or the only male, or anyone, male or female, who has replaced a significant progenitor two or even three generations back. Such individuals have great difficulty giving emotion or time to their marriage or their children. In my experience, every male and some females who get "cold feet" after a wedding date was set have been in this extended family position. Success has the compelling drive of ghosts behind it. They have too much to do in the short span of a lifetime. In addition, failure is more significant because it is not only themselves or even their own generation that they will have failed. Individuals who commit suicide after business failures often occupy the "standard bearer" position. If it had been only their own failure, they might have been able to "live with themselves." Such family members are trapped in a multigenerational cul-de-sac in which history is their destiny.

Where I find this type of emotional phenomenon in the family history of the clergy or the military, I ask, "Which of your ancestors really ordained (commissioned) you?"

The prince: A case example. The chief executive officer of a major American corporation committed suicide a few months after a new president took over. The new president had been moving very fast to make major changes in the corporate structure and one of the effects of this action was to overload this executive officer, who had been with the concern for 35 years. The only grandchild of his maternal grandparents, he had been "anointed" at birth by his grandfather who said, "What a prince!" and then died. He had been a generally quiet and gentle man, with no siblings or cousins, and his suicide came as a complete shock to everyone who knew him. The pressure had begun shortly after his mother died; his youngest child married and moved away, and his stepfather and wife came into conflict. His suicide note talked about the fear of failure, but the precipitating factor was that the corporation had become his extended family; he had no "option" but to leave, permanently.

The knowledge family therapists naturally come by in these matters of personal family systems can enable them to help enormously when important members of work systems are caught in the double bind of competing "family" loyalties.

SUMMARY

This chapter has tried to show how family therapists can serve as consultants to work systems by using their knowledge of emotional process. It is not necessary for the family therapist to be an expert in a work system's product. People are people, and their bonds and binds, whether in a work system or a personal family system, materialize and dissolve in response to identical processes. This universality, as I see it, benefits the family therapist. If my own experience and those of my clients are valid, family therapists can apply their knowledge of the dynamics of family systems to consultation with work systems and, in the process, should find their own understanding of emotional process deepened.

REFERENCES

Bowen, M. Toward the differentiation of self in one's family of origin. In F. Andres & P. Lorio (Eds.), *Selected papers, Georgetown family symposia* (Vol. I.). Washington, DC: Georgetown University Press, 1973.

Friedman, E. H. *Generation to generation: Family process in church and synagogue.* New York: Guilford, 1985.

Kerr, M. Application of family systems theory to a work system. In F. Andres & P. Lorio (Eds.), *Selected papers, Georgetown family symposia* (Vol. II.). Washington, DC: Georgetown University Press, 1973–1974.

25

THE FAMILY THERAPIST AS BUSINESS CONSULTANT

IRVING BORWICK
Management Executive Center, Inc.
Boston, Massachusetts

The theme of this chapter is that family organizations and business organizations are significantly different. Family therapists who consult to business must take up the role of organizational consultants rather than function as family therapists who happen to be working with business organizations. The techniques that are appropriate to use with families are not appropriate to use without modification with business organizations. Family therapists who, on the basis of applying systems theory to families, however successfully, attempt to apply the same techniques to business, will probably create significant problems for their clients. Consequently, family therapists who consult to business will have to develop new techniques and a new outlook in order to implement systems concepts into industrial organizations. A description of such techniques is outlined here.

BACKGROUND

In 1977–1978, Luigi Boscolo and Gianfranco Cecchin (Centro per lo Studio della Famiglia, Milan), Bruce Reed (Grubb Institute, London), and I (at that time Corporate Director of Management and Organization Development of International Telephone and Telegraph) formed a team with the expressed objective of applying the systemic theory and methodology of Drs. Boscolo and Cecchin to business organizations. We met in Brussels on approximately seven occasions in a 10-month period for 2 days at a time. Employing the systemic concepts and techniques of the Milan group, we worked with a number of management teams in the ITT organization. At the end of this period, we agreed to disband. What was patently clear was that applying the family systemic techniques without modifying them for the conditions of a business organization had proved unsuccessful. The anxiety level of managers was great and the fear for individual survival took precedence over organizational issues.

At that time, I set out to develop an entirely new approach to the implementation of systemic theory to business organizations that would also achieve the same remarkable results with business that I had observed in the work of Drs. Boscolo and Cecchin with families. It took another 2½ years before that was achieved.

The first task was to determine why our efforts at ITT had not worked, and what differentiated business organizations from families. What follows is (1) a differentiation of family and business organizations, (2) a differentiation of family system techniques from organizational system techniques, and (3) a description of a business systems methodology.

FAMILY VERSUS ORGANIZATION

One significant difference between families and organizations is that families are permanent relationships while organizations are temporary arrangements. An adopted orphan, three times married, is the child of her dead parents forever. A manager of IBM, employed his entire working life within that organization, is a member by sufferance and not by right of filial connection. Consequently, the relatedness of each to his or her respective system is unique and different. One may never be denied one's family relation as son, daughter, brother, sister, father, mother (however much at times one might like to do so), whether the relatives are alive or not. In an age in which the belief in equality and the self-made woman is endemic, too little is made of the biology of relatedness. The biology of flesh establishes a relational network with a boundary line that ensures permanent membership and influences all other relations.

This is not the case in organizations in which the network is established by the relation of the members to a common task. Organizations are temporary systems in which membership, regardless of the length of tenure, may be revoked at any time. Membership is a function of task, ideally, and each member is replaceable by another individual who is more or less competent to support the organization's task. Family members are singular, unique, and irreplaceable, no matter how devoutly one might at times wish to alter this law of nature. The consequences of this difference in the two systems has immense implications for managing and influencing behavior in both of them.

In business organizations, regardless of the affection or hostility engendered in any relation, the primary nature of the relation is established through the task system of the organization. I might never have met and would have had little interaction with a colleague, boss, or subordinate if we did not have a set of complementary work tasks to perform. Regardless of the degree of intensity of our emotional attachment, if the task were to disappear, then we must establish another organization or another relation.

This is not the case with families. The reconstitution of a modern family, which may consist of a married pair and three adopted children with no biologic connection, may well have more in common with a business organization than another family. But wherever there is a biological tie there is a boundary condition.

While biology and task are the differentiating principles of family and business organizations, each may take on characteristics of the other. Some families are clearly mobilized around tasks, particularly economic ones, and in the past, as well as in many underdeveloped countries today, a child is a form of indentured servant. Conversely, many subsystems within business organizations develop familial kinds of relations that bind its members to the organization. The greater the emotional attachment, the more difficult the reordering of relations. While all systems are mixed, the unalterable reality governing the system is whether it is a permanent (family) system or a temporary (business or other) system.

Both family and business organizations are hierarchical in nature. The family is hierarchical along generational lines, that is from elder to younger, from grandparent to parent, to child and to grandchild; industrial organizations are hierarchical along lines of organizational authority. The greater the formal authority, the higher the hierarchical position. Power is distributed according to either generational or authority position. The father is more powerful than the child, and the vice president is more powerful than the director. In reality, this is not always the situation, and wherever an individual occupies an inappropriate place generationally or hierarchically through the use of power, then we have what is called a perverse relation, which is intolerable to all systems. The system will either reject the perverse solution or adapt it into one that is functional but unconventional. Organizations can and often do resolve such a situation by removing the individual from the system. This alternative is not an option for families. The removal of a family member from the house does not remove him from the system, which is perhaps why the emotional life of a family is so much more intense. This option of removal from an organization makes life in the business world a somewhat fragile condition because organizational death is an imminent reality. However, death is usually final and, therefore, the emotional intensity is reduced.

ROLES

In a family system, one does not take up a role; rather, one is taken up by the role, the same role taken up by millions of others. One is born into the system and thereby acquires the role at birth; a sister is born and one acquires a sibling role; one gives birth and thereby acquires the parent role; and a child gives birth and one willy-nilly becomes a grandparent. The opposite is the case in business organizations. The role exists prior to joining; others may have occupied it and may still do so. One takes up the role and consequently one may also drop the role to take up other roles within the same system or outside it. As Arthur Miller pointed out, "A tragedy occurs when one cannot walk away from a situation and say to hell with it." One may not walk away from the family or the role in the family system so easily, which is why families are the sources of tragedy. Roles in business systems seldom become so compelling that one may not walk away from them.

ROLE AND PERSON

The role is not the person, and vice versa. Every individual has a potential for any kind of behavior. The potential gets worked out in roles. The danger occurs when people think that they are the role they act out. In families this is the greatest area for difficulty: To think that one is only the son or daughter, husband or wife, father or mother, is to get stuck in role. To equate role with person is to amputate the person and leave only the role. It is much more likely that members of families will get stuck in family roles, equating the permanence of the role with their own identity. This happens less often in organizational systems, but is not unknown. Successful persons in business often think that they are the role they play and confuse the trappings of the office with personal accomplishment. As with Nixon, who confused role and person and appeared to believe that Nixon (the person) and President (the role) were synonymous, business executives often exercise organizational authority as if they were managers only and cannot be held morally accountable.

On the other hand, some systems are purposefully designed to eliminate person and substitute only role. These are usually organizations of a religious or ideological (left or right) character that take their task from some "higher power." By erasing their person, they are free to act without personal responsibility, being merely the ordained instrument of some higher force. Thus, mild, kind, and meek individuals are capable of demonic acts as well as heroic acts.

AUTHORITY

Authority derives from the appointed tasks. In the service of some task, we are empowered to give authority or take authority to accomplish the task. The task of the family is to be a family; it is a process of being and not doing. The larger society defines the familial role and thereby influences the family's sense of task. Whatever task the family conceives of influences the authority that each member feels appropriate to carrying out the task. The authority of members within a family varies enormously, from feeling totally powerless to having full authority to act. Task is normally well-defined within organizations, and members who take up roles in such organizations are only members conditional upon their ability to perform the task. However, the overt task is not the same as the covert task, a subject about which I will speak later. Consequently, many members of organizations are disenfranchised of their authority at the covert level while expected to exercise authority at the overt level. The result is frustration and anxiety.

POWER

Power may be defined as the ability to influence. Power is partially independent of authority and may be exercised in support of authority or in spite of authority. In stable countries, successful companies, organizations, and families, power is used in support of the authority to facilitate the task of that system. On the other hand, there are many systems, familial and organizational, in which power is exercised without authority. In countries it results in civil war, for example, in Ireland; in organizations it results in subversion, for example, in slowdowns, wildcat strikes; in families it results in violent behavior, for example, in beatings, wife abuse, child abuse, or murder. This dynamic explains why most homicides are family affairs. Murder seldom occurs in organizations; rather, death is symbolically enacted through exclusion or removal from the system. The individual becomes "dead" to the system. The inflexibility of the family system makes it difficult to exclude members. Divorce is the only socially recognized system for uncoupling a family member, but this is because marriage begins as an act of volition.

Power used without authority in a family system tends to be anarchic and is directed toward no objective other than to resist the system. Power used without authority in organizations is a revolution directed toward overthrowing the real authority and replacing it with another authority, an impossible goal for a family, in which one can never become one's own parents (see Table 25-1).

TABLE 25-1. Characteristics of Family and Organizational Systems

ITEM	FAMILY SYSTEM	ORGANIZATIONAL SYSTEM
Boundary	Defined by relations	Defined by task
Task	To be family member	Achieve organization task
	Survival	Survival
Role	Individual taken up by role	Role taken up by individual
Authority	Based upon relations	Derives from task
Power	Anarchic when used without authority	Revolutionary when used without authority

INTERVENTION

Business organizations differ from family systems in terms of boundary conditions, tasks, roles, authority, and power. Interventions into a family system are frequently at the member level, that is, directed at one or more members of the system. This is not to overlook the work done with subsystems, for example, marital, dyads, children, or subgroups. These interventions frequently help the family members to differentiate their roles in the system and, when necessary, take up system activities appropriate to their roles. There is no need in such interventions to ensure or reinforce the membership role. A parent, son, daughter, sister, or brother cannot escape the role regardless of their anxiety about fulfilling it or their need to escape it.

The opposite is true in a business organization. Membership is always temporary, and members of the organization are aware of this fact. Interventions that single out organizational members, such as those used in family interventions, pose a threat to managers and employees. They threaten individuals in terms of their organizational membership and, consequently, their economic well-being, in addition to such things as status, belonging, recognition, and other such valued characteristics. For this reason, intervention into business organizations must ensure and support integration of the manager and employee into the system, rather than differentiation of these individuals.

This is *not* to suggest that differentiation in organizational systems is impossible or undesirable. Rather, such differentiation should take place at the sub*system* level and not at the *individual* level. A subsystem consists of at least two or more persons. The exception to this is the chief executive office (CEO) of the unit, who always comprises a system of one.

In summary, differentiation in family systems is frequently at the individual level as well as the subsystem level. Differentiation in the business organization should be at the subsystem level and only infrequently at the individual level. This is directly related to the fact that families are permanent systems whose members cannot, in the final analysis, be excluded, while business organizations are temporary systems in which no member is safe from exclusion. For this reason, the misuse of family therapy in business organizations is not only often ineffective, but also positively threatening to the system. Moreover, family therapists, lacking business organization experience, are not always able to differentiate the nature of the response to their intervention.

A case example. The work team of Drs. Boscolo, Cecchin, Reed, and Borwick, referred to above, consulted to the Beta Management Group, which is responsible for the management of 13 European companies. The presence of the two therapists was a threatening event, which is not unusual when consultants are also therapists. Drs. Boscolo and Cecchin are family therapists and consultants. Drs. Reed and Borwick are organizational consultants; they are not therapists. Using a model of two consultants and two observers, the Beta Management Group was interviewed and information solicited. After a session of approximately 2 hours, the work team retired to a private office to develop a prescriptive intervention.

After approximately 2 hours of systemic analysis, a number of hypotheses were developed. It appeared that the Beta Management Group, which organizationally reported to a more senior management group in New York, was operating in an inappropriately symmetrical relationship. In other words, they were competing with their own leadership to decide the policy for European operations, when, in fact, their task was to carry out policy as formulated in New York. It was clear to the work team that the pursuit of this policy would result in an inevitable debacle for the Beta management team.

In the afternoon, the work team returned to deliver its paradoxical intervention to the Beta management team. The Ten Commandments were not received with less reverence or respect than was our prescription for the work team; an aura of omniscience permeated the environment, and the management team fully played the role of the grateful congregation. On the other hand, the Beta management team also seemed traumatized by the experience. As a result of this intervention there was much discussion but little action. Six months later, the management group was disbanded, as had been foreseen by the consultants.

What went wrong? There are no easy or sure answers to this question. It is clear that the work team did in fact predict the outcome correctly, but the management team did not respond to the intervention and the consultation was unsuccessful. However, what dominated the actions and thinking of the consulting work team was the application of family therapy techniques to a business organization. It was assumed that a system is a system;

whether a family or business, it should make no difference. Regardless of the fact that two of the four work team consultants were *not* family therapists, the orientation of the collective work team was therapeutic, not organizational. In other words, the work team members used therapeutic models, therapeutic techniques, and therapeutic relations. The differentiations (outlined above) between family and business systems were unknown at the time and were only later developed as a result of observations made at these sessions.

One might suggest that the issue was one of consultant competence, not systems theory. However, the thematic anxiety, defensiveness, breakdown in group cohesiveness, and concern for individual job security that appeared in all four management teams, one after the other, suggest that competence was not the issue. Two years of additional work to develop a management and organization system model has resulted in a systemic intervention that yields highly successful results without the traumas experienced earlier. It appears, therefore, that it is crucial to differentiate between business and family systems.

ENVIRONMENT

Members of a family entering into family therapy expect that their behavior, relations with others, and so on, will come under scrutiny. That is their anxiety and their hope. Managers in an organization entering into group/team/organization development expect that their roles and role relations will come under scrutiny. They do not expect that they, as individuals, will be subject to examination, which is not to minimize the conscious or unconscious wish for individual therapy. Put another way, the "game" of family members is "The Family Game," while managers play "The Business Game." In the family game, members may display emotions. They have the "right" to be human, that is, to express what they genuinely feel, and they are linked to the family system by biological, social, and legal imperatives. The business game eschews personal emotions; managers have "managerial rights," the rights attached to getting the task done. They are linked to the system by task, financial rewards, status, and power relations. Many, if not most, managers differentiate self from role and try to act as if their private lives have no place in business. Family and business environments are entirely different. Therapists who struggle with family models within a business context frequently end up acquiring patients or creating them.

In three of the four departmental systems in which we attempted to utilize the Milan model, the managers reacted with frenetic anxiety. One manager called me up within an hour of completing the session and accused me of attempting to sabotage his department, and for the next 10 minutes he swore, cursed, and threatened me. The fourth department responded well because we decided to use our presence as an intervention and to make no formal, prescriptive intervention. For months afterwards I got calls asking if we were going to give them any feedback. Also of significant interest was the reaction of the two therapists, Drs. Boscolo and Cecchin, when they first entered managerial groups. They were surprised and pleased to discover such healthy groups, capable of coping, having "normal" defense mechanisms, and generally functioning well. The pathology of a family system in crisis was nowhere to be found.

PATHOLOGY VERSUS SYSTEM EFFECTIVENESS

In business organizations, the issue is system effectiveness. When individual pathology is identified, an outside referral is made to a therapist. A severely malfunctioning organization is not treated as pathological, but as a problem organization. It is not unusual for an organization to be restructured before a systems intervention is made. A new president is appointed, a manager in a key role is fired, the organization is restructured along new lines. On the other hand, families are never restructured by a senior authority. A new father is not appointed, nor is the son fired and replaced by a new son.

ROLE AND PERSON

Many managers distinguish who they are from what they do, and attempt to keep the two separate. This separation of the person from the role that he or she takes up is usually something that the manager is aware of at a conscious level. Most managers would feel that the work they do on behalf of a business organization is unrelated to their personal preferences, values, or their own human feelings. For most managers, the organization is a kind of machine or impersonal entity. One sells one's labor, energy, imagination, or efforts to this machinelike business and one is compensated accordingly. To introduce one's personal preferences or feelings of humanity into such an organization is not only a violation of the organizational norm, but a distortion of the "business" norm.

The behavior of managers within an organization is therefore influenced most strongly by the roles that they occupy rather than by the person they are. Shy, humble, or inadequate personalities can become rather ruthless, decisive, authoritarian figures. It is the role that is mobilized, not the person. For this reason, individual managers, who act primarily in a role function rather than in their individual function, attempt to avoid interaction with other managers. The minute one is confronted with another human being, one's own emotions, sensibilities, and human qualities are called into play. Therefore, such managers not only avoid personal interaction, they tend to emphasize the roles of other managers in order to deemphasize the person.

Nevertheless, the functioning of a healthy business system frequently requires some mobilization of the person within the managerial role, but this should be accomplished within the context of the business system. Therapists tend to mobilize the person and to treat the role as a simple adjunct, a job, something one does for a living. The result is frequently a denial or blindness to the issue that defines the relationship between managers, the very reason and probably the only reason that this group is gathered together.

THERAPY VERSUS EFFECTIVENESS

The family therapist in the business environment frequently brings in the family game, the intensity of relations with its attendant or inferred pathology, and the concern with person. All of these are a violation of the business system rules and send shock waves through the system.

This is in contrast to the systemic consultant, who is part of the business game itself and who focuses on system effectiveness and role awareness. The difference between these two approaches does not lie in the content or even the process, but in the definition of the relation, that is, in the metacommunication about the consultant role. In most cases, the consultant's communication about the communication in family therapy is about therapy by therapists and not about effectiveness. The organizational development model metacommunicates about being effective.

FEATURES OF CONSULTANT RELATIONS

The consultant's relation to a family or a business system is differentiated in four ways: by goals, tactics, results, and strategy (see Table 25-2). Describing the nature of a relation is akin to describing what sight is or how things smell. A relation is not tangible, but its impact may be. Nevertheless, the next section attempts to describe the differences between a therapeutic relation and an organization consultant's relation to a business organization.

TABLE 25-2. Systems Relations of Therapists and Organizational Consultants

	THERAPISTS	ORGANIZATIONAL CONSULTANTS
Goal	Member–system welfare	Organization functioning
Tactics	Person	Role
Results	Symptom resolution	Role resolution
Strategy	System–person relations	Role–system relations

GOAL AND TACTICS

The family therapist deals primarily with the relation between family members and how this relation facilitates the system, while the business consultant focuses on organization functioning. Both seek better system functioning, but one is defined by the welfare of individuals and the system, and the other by productivity of the system and not individual productivity.

Lange and Van der Hart (1983) list a wide range of techniques and interventions, from Minuchin's "tracking," "mimicry," and "support," through positive labeling, data recovery, behavioral exercises, role reversal, modeling, interaction feedback, topographic interventions, prescriptions, and paradoxical interventions. All of these techniques may be used with business organizations at appropriate times. In other words, the problem lies not in systems theory or in systemic techniques but, rather, in the different roles of these two very different types of social systems: families and businesses. Families create, nurture, and provide social members of society; business organizations provide their members with opportunities to produce, create, and maintain that society. These are decidedly different roles and the members relate to each type of generic system differently. Consequently, the consultant to each system relates accordingly, which is to say differently.

The family therapist relates to the member and the system. A family is usually in therapy because someone is suffering and the system is misfunctioning. Therapy is characterized by its goal of alleviating pain, suffering, anxiety, and sickness. An organizational development (OD) consultant relates to the organization, that voluntary group of members assembled and related to each other in order to produce, create, and deliver services and goods. A therapist and an OD consultant using the same techniques can achieve quite different outcomes. The difference lies in whether one relates to the person–system relation or to the role–system relation.

RESULTS AND STRATEGY

The results that therapists and the OD consultant seek are of the same order: a well-functioning system. In families, a well-functioning system will mean the reduction of symptoms, for example, of addiction, anorexia nervosa, schizophrenia, or phobias. In organizations, a well-functioning system means the resolution of role confusion and the reduction of "noise" in the system, that is, effective use of resources, improved strategy, reduced waste, increased productivity, and ability to change.

The strategy of therapy is nominally related to the relation between individual suffering and family functioning. System interventions are designed to improve the system relations so as to improve the individual–system functioning.

CLIENT RELATION

There is a contextual difference between therapist–client relations and OD consultant–client relations. The normal role for therapists is to supply service on demand. Patients come to the therapists and request help. Many exceptions exist, for example, patients required by legal authorities to take such services, therapeutic interventions to prevent suicides, or family members who resist participating in sessions. The norm, however, is service by request and the belief that the patient must take the initiative if therapy is to be effective.

The history of organizational development has been service by demand and/or by OD marketing and promotion. OD consultants frequently sell their services on the basis of results to be obtained. Many managers believe OD consultants have oversold their services. This has been detrimental to the profession and to the client–OD relation. Ideally, business managers would recognize the need for an intervention and request the services of an OD consultant. OD consultants would first determine if their services are needed before providing them. The sale of consultant services requires sensitivity. This dilemma is familiar to therapists, who have no accepted system for selling their services overtly, and do so covertly by selling to their potential referrers. (An interesting systems study might be to explore the informal relations and referral networks among therapists and related professionals.)

Therapists who undertake roles as business consultants create difficulties for both themselves and the client when they treat managers therapeutically, hooking them on personal issues and not their managerial roles, making patients, not clients of them. They can cause problems by selling personal health, not organizational health.

THE ORGANIZATIONAL INTERVENTION VERSUS THE FAMILY INTERVENTION

There is a significant difference between a family intervention and an intervention into an organization. After 6 years of research, development, and experimentation, three or four models of systems intervention into business organizations have been developed that deal with such issues as strategy development, team development, productivity, and large-scale communication issues. (Each of these has been described at some length in as yet unpublished monographs by this author.)

Some differentiations between family interventions and organizational interventions are outlined below in a series of hypotheses. Because no type of intervention is monolithic, any differentiation has some exceptions. It is hoped, however, that these hypotheses are more, rather than less, accurate.

HYPOTHESIS 1: ONGOING VERSUS RESIDENTIAL INTERVENTION

The first differentiation focuses upon therapist and consultant expectations of their relationship with their respective clients. The hypothesis is that therapists tend to expect an ongoing weekly or monthly relationship that may be open-ended or limited, while the organization consultant establishes a short-term, problem-related relationship that is usually residential. "Residential" refers to an intervention that takes place outside of organization territory, for example, a hotel or conference center where managers reside during the program that may last from 3 to 5 days or longer. Specifically, there may be one, two, or (at a maximum) three interventions in such a program. This does not preclude a long-term consulting relationship in which the client returns with additional organizational issues to be resolved and in which the consultant contracts for a new organizational intervention. On the other hand, a family, couple, or individual in therapy expects to return to the therapist for some period of time. Managers within an organization expect some form of short-term intervention that will be terminated as rapidly as possible, and with the issue resolved. There is no expectation of a long-term or even short-term helping relationship.

HYPOTHESIS 2: HOURS VERSUS DAYS

The second hypothesis is that family systems therapy tends to be bounded by short time frames. This can be anywhere from an hour to 2 hours, or perhaps just a morning session. Organizational interventions of a systemic nature are characterized by interventions that last anywhere from a minimum of a day to 3½ days, or even a week. Such sessions are residential in nature and sessions will continue from early morning to late evening.

HYPOTHESIS 3: THREE TO TEN CLIENTS VERSUS 12–34 OR 25–250 CLIENTS

A third hypothesis is that family systems tend to be of a limited size, anywhere from 3 or 4 members up to 8, 9, or 10. While some family therapists have worked with as many as 2,000 members of a system, this is the exception and not the rule. However, the working norm of organizational interventions is a minimum of 12 and an average of approximately 20 members of the organizational system. The norm changes according to the nature of the problem. Strategic problems limited to senior management groups fall with the category of 12 to 35, with an average of 20. On the other hand, those programs dealing with productivity are likely to include anywhere from 25 to 30, up to 150 or 250 people. Consequently, the number of individuals involved in a family intervention tends to be significantly smaller than that in an organizational intervention. Family therapists, however, when making interventions into organizational systems, tend to work with the same size groups within an organization as they do with a family. Many family therapy organizational consultants will end up working with anywhere from 5 to 10 members of the organization. The smaller the group, the more remote are the chances of success if one is attempting to influence the whole system.

HYPOTHESIS 4: PERSONAL SYSTEMS VERSUS ROLE SYSTEMS

The fourth hypothesis is that therapists in organizational settings tend to mobilize personal or family issues within the individual, and organizational interventions do not. I have more than once heard family therapists who have worked in business organizations marvel over the fact that a particular senior executive or vice president was able to confront a personal issue within the business context. It is almost as if they have brought him to an awareness of his own humanity. In part, one might hypothesize that this relates to the fantasies held by therapists that business executives are really human if you can break through the veneer. They seem almost surprised to discover that their hypothesis is correct. It is important to make this assumption; most organizational consultants know this is the case and have no need to verify it. This is not to deny that an organizational intervention may mobilize rather basic and sometimes primitive feelings in individuals. But the task of organizational development intervention is to mobilize the "person" parts of the individual in a manner that will aid him or her to integrate with his or her role in the organization.

HYPOTHESIS 5: PERSON SYMPTOMS VERSUS TASK SYMPTOMS

I have summarized below a 3-day organizational intervention based upon a systems approach. While the summary does not go into any great detail, it does provide the family therapist with some sense of a task orientation in such an intervention. It also illustrates the fifth hypothesis, which differentiates a therapeutic emphasis upon symptoms of personal relatedness from a focus upon organizational tasks and their relationship to various roles taken up in the accomplishment of these tasks.

An Organizational Intervention: Group Strategy and Action Program Synopsis

The process moves from individual to role to system and then alternates among them.

Introduction, Evening. The introduction establishes the rationale for the members' presence at the session, their relation to it, and their expectations of it until a kind of contract is defined.

First Day, Morning. The morning session focuses upon role relations through analysis of selected problem areas. It should be noted that all sessions have an overt, rational objective and a covert, emotional reframing objective. The overt objective is to define problem issues as related to role functioning. The covert objective is to educate members with regard to systems, role, and individual relations, to provide both skills and language to redefine these relations, and prepare members for the next stage.

First Day, Afternoon. The afternoon is dedicated to system analysis. Each member is offered an opportunity to define his or her relations to the others.

The overt objective is to understand the relation. The covert objective is to offer the opportunity to redefine the relationship.

Once the relations among groups are defined, each group is asked to prepare a set of hypotheses on how the system functions, how the subsystem functions, and how the groups relate to the larger system.

The hypotheses are exchanged at the evening session.

Second Day, Morning. The morning session is a repeat of the first morning session, with new issues to be worked on.

Second Day, Afternoon. During the afternoon, members are given a lecture on systems theory and how it operates. Immediately following this, they are provided with a series of staff hypotheses to explain the system. These tend to connote positively all system behavior, to identify the homeostatic nature of the system, the symmetrical and complementary relations that exist, and frequently to suggest a no-change strategy. They are designed to be of the "be spontaneous" kind, reflecting back the paradoxical reality that exists within the system, but not designed to shock or surprise.

The remainder of the afternoon is dedicated to the members reworking and integrating their various group hypotheses, the staff hypotheses, and any new hypotheses they may generate.

The evening provides an opportunity to exchange these new hypotheses and work out differences. No attempt is made to reach any kind of consensus.

Third Day, Morning. Members, working in groups, are asked to relate the hypotheses to their working situation and to identify issues they want to work on. Each group develops its own plans, which are subsequently presented to other groups. The overt objective is strategy development. The covert objective is the reframing of system relations.

Third Day, Afternoon. The last session is convened by the senior executive in charge of the system, for example, the president or chairman. The staff officially hands the organization back to him. The chief executive officer convenes the group with the explicit task of planning for implementation. Decisions are frequently made, plans agreed upon, and a new set of relations (already formed) now take on the protective coloring of the organization.

Follow-Up. A follow-up session normally takes place 4 to 6 weeks later. This session lasts about one hour and is designed to realign issues that are in the process of being worked out. Serious deviations or blocks may be identified and a further intervention agreed upon, if appropriate.

CONCLUSION

The first and perhaps the most significant conclusion of this chapter is that the family therapist who consults to business must take up the role of organization consultant and drop the role of family therapist. I have attempted to demonstrate here that family and business organizations are significantly different systems. Family therapists entering into business organizations may mistakingly bring their family therapy role with them, and with that role their own mental maps of family territories. If it is true that "the map is not the territory," it is even more true that the map of a family is quite different from the territory of the business world. Consequently, therapists who enter into business organizations must begin to develop new maps and new roles.

How does a family therapist go about taking up the role of organization consultant and developing new maps using systems theory to apply to business organizations? While all therapists have had primary experience in families, many, if not most, therapists lack exposure to and involvement with business organizations. Perhaps their first step should be to acquaint themselves with the culture of the business organization. There are numerous ways to do this, none of them very easy. They could include doing a research study of business organizations, taking part-time business jobs, consulting in nontherapeutic situations, becoming involved in educational programs for management trainees or executives, or actually taking a position within an ongoing organization.

A less direct but perhaps easier approach is to take courses in the business administration departments of universities. This method has the advantage of being readily available and, at the same time, of allowing therapists to mix with businessmen involved in these programs, and to learn specific business skills. This exposure will go a long way toward helping a therapist to understand the nature of a business and the business culture.

Another alternative is for a therapist to work in conjunction with an already established business consultant as a means of entering into the system and gaining the necessary exposure and experience to the ways in which organizations function. This is not to suggest that a therapist must become a business person in order to consult to a business organization. Rather, one must have some understanding of and experience within the territory before one begins to draw maps of what it looks like.

The second step, after one has developed some understanding of the organization and how it functions is to begin consciously to draw maps of the territory and to differentiate one's role as a consultant in that system.

Assuming some experience of the business organization and a relatively clear idea of one's role in consulting to it, the third step is to develop the necessary techniques for applying systems concepts to business organizations. One may either choose from the very restricted techniques that are readily available or begin to develop one's own. The practicing consultant will find that the techniques presently employed for families cannot be simply lifted from one system and implemented in another.

The family therapist utilizing a systems approach has a reservoir of knowledge and skills that is greatly needed and can add immeasurably to the effectiveness of business organizations. However, if the therapist is to make a difference in the business organization, it is first necessary for him or her to change before attempting to offer the opportunity of change to others.

ACKNOWLEDGMENTS

I express my thanks to both Dr. Luigi Boscolo and Dr. Gianfranco Cecchin, who have been instrumental in helping me to learn about systems, and whose truly "scientific" point of view helped us to recognize how much we had learned by not being successful. They have remained supportive throughout, and I am indebted to them. Most important, a public word of thanks to my wife, Bella Borwick, who introduced me to Drs. Boscolo and Cecchin and to systems thinking. She lives in both the worlds of therapy and business and helped me to differentiate one from the other.

REFERENCE

Lange, A., & Van der Hart, O. *Directive family therapy*. New York: Brunner/Mazel, 1983.

Editors' Commentary on Consultation with Military and Business Systems

In this section, more fully than in any other, our discussion of systems consultation moves outside of the health care field. In doing so, we recognize the vast areas of consultation that have not traditionally been within the province of family therapy. Certainly, we are not trying to generalize here about all topics involved in the broad fields of either military or business consultations. Rather, this section is limited to a brief consideration of those issues at the interface of military and business organizations, family therapy, and consultations. Most striking is the difference between the health care contexts described elsewhere in the book and the military and business contexts described in this section. This section most directly challenges a question that is further discussed in Chapter 26: Can a version of systems theory that is based in family therapy be usefully applied to consultation endeavors in other contexts? In our commentary, we also shall consider briefly the topic of family businesses—an issue not extensively addressed in these chapters but of interest to those working as family or business consultants.

SIZE OF ORGANIZATION

Unlike most other contexts, a consultation with the military or business offers the possibility of consulting with as few as one person in a small business or as many as thousands of people in a large organization. Determining the unit of consultation becomes a central issue for the success of the consultation. Each of our authors handles this issue somewhat differently. Florence Kaslow, in her work with American military forces, focuses on the training of psychiatrists. Her unit of consultation is the program directors, the supervisors, and the residents—a manageable group for someone experienced in family therapy and family therapy teaching. Edwin Friedman reports on consultation with individuals or small groups within businesses.

Whether working with an individual businessman, a moderate-size legal firm, or a large organization like NASA, Friedman advocates working with the leadership ("Where the head goes, the body will follow"). In this way, the unit of consultation may be large but the consultee is likely to be an individual or small group, again a comfortable size for the consultant who began as a family therapist. Irving Borwick observes that family therapists as consultants usually avoid working with large groups. As an organizational consultant, he believes that many business consultations are best accomplished by including the whole system, or at least a large subgroup of the system, in the consultation. He argues that organizational development techniques rather than family systems techniques are the most appropriate systems techniques for these consultations.

GOAL OF THE CONSULTATION

There seem to be two goals of business consultations: to increase productivity and, to some extent, to improve individual and group functioning. Productivity is clearly an explicit goal in a business organization, whereas productivity traditionally has not been a goal of social service and health-related organizations. Recent economic pressures, however, have led many health-related organizations to focus much more on productivity and to hire business people rather than clinicians to run their organizations. This pragmatic shift in goals sometimes conflicts with the traditional identity and values of the social service or health organization as a "helping" agency.

Irving Borwick reflects the values of the business community in his emphasis on increased production, whether the consultation problem is rooted in interpersonal conflict or in some other area. He contrasts therapy with consultation and warns therapists who become consultants to clarify the difference between therapy goals (improving individual or interpersonal functioning) and consultation goals (improving organizational functioning, especially increased productivity). In this same vein, Bella Borwick (personal communication, November 1984), a family therapist and systems consultant, said: "Clinicians do not make 'natural' consultants. If anything, clinicians may know too much about human pathology and not enough about organizational behavior."

While Irving Borwick highlights differences between the goals of therapy and consultation, Edwin Friedman emphasizes similarities. Friedman views the goals of a business consultation as quite compatible with family systems theory, regarding the goal of improved individual functioning as an important and even necessary route to the goal of increased productivity. This approach is based on Friedman's assertion that the family as the essential biologic group provides the pattern or rules for all other groups, whether business, government, or church congregations. Making this same point in other writings, Friedman says: "As you all know, there has been much analogizing of family process to what goes on in politics[;] . . . governments [do] act like families, for where else did the human race learn to function like that?" (1982, p. 61). In addition to Friedman, other consultants have also reported basing their business consultations on Bowen family systems theory (Bork, 1982; Gilmore, 1982). While a family therapist turned business consultant may feel most comfortable focusing on improved individual functioning within a business, Irving Borwick contends that this focus may at times be inappropriate because individuals are expendable in business whereas one cannot be "fired" from the biologic family regardless of how hard one may try (although divorce and disinheritance disrupt the sociologic family).

In the goals of the military, the emphasis is on productivity, individual, and group functioning. With training as her primary goal, Kaslow clearly works to improve the level of individual and group functioning, whether in her interactions with the head of a department or at a potluck-dinner-turned-confessional with the residents. Kaslow is hired as a consultant because of her skills and reputation as a family therapist; perhaps, in a sense, the military is seeking this kind of focus in their selection of a consultant.

WHO IS THE CONSULTEE IN A BUSINESS OR MILITARY CONSULTATION?

Closely related to the issue of clarity about the goals of the consultation is clarity about who is the consultee. Who really hires the consultant? Is the consultee the contact person, the person who pays for the consultation, the organization as a whole, the "boss," or some subgroup of employees? Especially in large organizations, the answers can be confusing.

Largely unaddressed in the chapters in this section, this unclarity might be illustrated by a recent request for consultation that came to one of us from the vice president of marketing for a high-tech firm. This vice president asked for a consultation regarding one of his employees who was having some difficulty with customers and regional managers. The vice president wanted an evaluation of how "healthy" and capable his employee was. The contact person was the vice president; he, not the employee, paid for the evaluation. A larger issue in the company at the time included the industry's being in serious financial trouble, necessitating a reshuffling of personnel. This example raises the questions: If a consultant is given a limited task (e.g., "evaluate my employee"), what leverage does he or she have to expand the inquiry or interventions to the larger systems level? In some ways, this problem may be similar to the request in family therapy to fix a problem regarding a child that is actually rooted in a larger marital problem. However, in most cases, the goals of a consultation and the role of a consultant are more delimited than that of therapy, in which people often give the therapist authority to operate in a broader field. Hence, keeping clear about the goals and the identity of the consultee is essential to the success of a business or military consultation.

ORGANIZATIONAL HIERARCHIES

In businesses and the military, the organizational hierarchy is usually clearer than in other contexts. Individual roles and organizational boundaries are well-defined, and rules regarding what one can and cannot do are evident. The regimentation of business and military organizations can be both an advantage and a liability to a consultant. Irving Borwick is clear about the care with which he maintains his own boundaries and respects the boundaries of the organization with which he is consulting. Edwin Friedman acknowledges structure and hierarchy by focusing his consultations on the leadership of the organization, where the power for change resides. In fact, when working with someone in a mid-level position, Friedman cautions about the limitations of what one will be able to accomplish in the larger system.

Most interesting is the effect of military hierarchies on consultation. Florence Kaslow is very careful to respect the hierarchies and the rules that characterize the military contexts in which she consults. While such clear regimentation allows one to know who is in charge, the many guidelines about permissible behavior can limit the impact of a consultation. This limitation was clear in Kaslow's example about a homosexual soldier who was the focus of some concern by other soldiers. Because of the prohibition against homosexuals in the military, Kaslow could not deal openly with this problem because she was told that to do so would exceed her role. As a consultant, it is important to familiarize oneself with organizational culture and hierarchies because their rules and taboos will affect the goals and the potential accomplishments of any consultation.

FAMILY BUSINESSES

Hierarchies can be confusing when it is a family that owns and operates a business. Rosenblatt, deMik, Anderson, and Johnson (1985), in their book on family businesses, state that more than 90% of the 15 million businesses in the United States are owned or operated by families. Consultation with family businesses, then, potentially accounts for a large proportion of all business consultations. While no author in this section explicitly addressed the issue of family business, it is an interesting phenomenon clearly situated at the interface of family therapy and business consultation, and likely to be problematic because of role conflict and role overlap.

Given the luxury of extrapolation, one might guess that Irving Borwick, with his focus on the differences between therapy and consultation, would apply these principles to consultation with family businesses as well, avoiding "personal" issues with individuals and focusing on role relationships, organizational group dynamics, and productivity. Edwin Friedman, on the other hand, would be likely to allow both family and business issues to emerge in consultation, treating the issues similarly in his attempt to coach his consultee to lower the anxiety in the system (business or family) and to function from a differentiated position in either context.

Applying ideas similar to those of Irving Borwick to family businesses, Bella Borwick (1984) has emphasized the importance of clarifying whether the goal of a consultation is family-oriented or business-oriented. She makes the point that many families who own businesses and have problems are not able to establish appropriate boundaries between the family and the business. For example, it may be difficult for a business executive to recognize the special skills and limitations of an employee if that employee is also an offspring or relative. Decision making in a dysfunctional family business can have more to do with family collusions and battles than with organizational structure; family members may attempt to resolve family relationships through the business rather than through the family. In family businesses, ambiguity about who really makes the decisions may be high—for example, is it the wife who inherited the business or the husband who is president? And, can one be fired for incompetence in a family business if one is a member of the family?

These characteristics of a family business lead Bella Borwick to suggest that a consultant must demonstrate appropriate boundaries and distinctions between family as a unit and the business as a unit. Otherwise, the consultant will be drawn into the same dilemma as the family in business: Where to focus—on the family or on the business? While Friedman or others may attack these problems together or in sequence, Bella Borwick recommends either choosing to do family consultation or business consultation, not both. If family members are quite enmeshed, and a consultant wishes to work on their business problem, she suggests first referring them for family therapy. After progress has been made in therapy, the family and the business consultant may effectively work on the business problem (avoiding the temptation to "therapize" rather than consult with the business).

Many approaches are likely to emerge for systems consultation with family businesses. We have only begun to discuss the issues and potential controversies involved in this work. To complicate matters further, it is interesting to contemplate how some large and long-standing business relationships, like those in the Japanese work system, can become more "family-like." And, on the other hand, contemporary marriages defined by explicit contracts and the increasing potential for dissolution may become more "business-like." The implications of these emerging patterns for systems consultation in either context remain to be explored.

REFERENCES

Bork, D. Using family systems theory in family and closely held businesses. In R. Riley-Sager & K. Crouse-Wiseman (Eds.), *Understanding organizations: Applications of family systems theory*. Washington, DC: Georgetown University Family Center Publications, 1982.

Borwick, B. Presentation to a study group of the American Family Therapy Association, New York City, June 14, 1984.

Friedman, E. Secrets and systems. In J. Lorio & L. McClemmathan (Eds.), *Georgetown family symposia 1973–1974: A collection of selected papers*. Washington, DC: Georgetown University Family Center Publications, 1982.

Gilmore, T. A triangular framework: Leadership and followership. In R. Riley-Sager & K. Crouse-Wiseman (Eds.), *Understanding organizations: Applications of family systems theory*. Washington, DC: Georgetown University Family Center Publications, 1982.

Rosenblatt, P. C., deMik, L., Anderson, R. M., & Johnson, P. A. *The family in business*. San Francisco: Jossey-Bass, 1985.

VI

CURRENT PROBLEMS AND FUTURE DIRECTIONS

26

CONSULTANTS AT THE CROSSROADS
Problems and Controversies in Systems Consultation

SUSAN H. McDANIEL

TIMOTHY T. WEBER

LYMAN C. WYNNE

University of Rochester School of Medicine and Dentistry
Rochester, New York

The preceding chapters have explored features of the existing territory of systems consultation. Theoretical issues have been raised and techniques in a variety of contexts have been described by family therapists, family consultants, and systems consultants. Together these ideas represent the current understanding of the application of systems principles to consultation. This chapter, as well as Chapter 27, will examine those areas that are in special need of future study. We will discuss here the problems we have encountered, both theoretical and technical, in developing our theory of systems consultation. We will also point to and discuss some controversies that have arisen as we and others have developed approaches to consultation from a systems perspective. The work of all the contributors to this volume is rooted in systems theory and they have used this framework in presenting their theories and techniques of consultation in a variety of contexts. Despite this similarity, there are striking differences in how systems consultation is conceptualized and practiced.

Some of these controversies reflect differing theoretical assumptions between contributors. Other controversies reflect differences in the contexts in which consultants work. For example, consulting with the military and consulting with a community self-help group may necessitate significantly different consultation approaches. Still other controversies relate more to the practical inexperience that is a fact of life when family therapists first turn to consulting endeavors. These problems and controversies warrant consideration and debate as they delineate both areas of difference and areas of ambiguity in the development of the thinking and practice of systems consultation.

In the following discussion, we will consider a series of abiding conceptual and technical problems and controversies as we compare the theories and practices of contributors to this volume with one another and with our own current thinking.

A SYSTEMS THEORY FOR CONSULTATION

Can systems theory as used by family therapists be applied directly as a model for consultation? The question of whether family systems theory can provide a model for the practice of consultation is central to the development of the ideas in this book. As family therapists we approach consultation grounded in systems theory, especially as it applies in our treatment of families. Many of the same systems principles that govern our practice of therapy also govern our practice of consultation. In the assessment phase, for example, we analyze the hierarchy and the effectiveness of leadership and its impact on subsystems. In reaching the goals of a consultation, we use many of the same techniques as are used in family therapy, such as joining, positive connotation, and paradox.

Several contributors to this book take the position that the practice of consultation is an extension of the practice of family therapy and that the principles of such therapy can and should be applied directly in consultation. Anderson and Goolishian, for example, view the two as differing only in the role of the person with whom they are interacting: "In our view, the practice of consultation parallels the practice of therapy and differs only in the point of application, that is, in who is involved in the direct consultative activity" (Chapter 18, p. 285). Specifically, a consultant may intervene with a consultee or consultees while a therapist intervenes with a patient or family. Landau-Stanton also subscribes to the view that consultation is the same game as therapy, only with different players. She describes her model of consultation as developing "in concert with" her model of family therapy, and states that they are "operationally inseparable" and "isomorphic" (Chapter 16, p. 253).

Although Anderson and Goolishian's theoretical orientation is strategic–systemic and Friedman's is Bowen family systems therapy, Friedman takes a similar position in favor of the direct application of therapy principles to consultation. Friedman even insists that a consultant does not need to be knowledgeable about a particular context or a particular work system's product but needs only to use knowledge of "emotional process" in consulting to a work system: "People are people, and their bonds and binds, whether in a work system or a personal family system, materialize and dissolve in response to identical processes" (Chapter 24, p. 421). Friedman clearly uses the same techniques and concepts with people on any issue they may present, whether it is a business problem, a family problem, or an organizational problem. The tenets of consultation, as we have described them, are used by these authors when they function as therapists. Perhaps they only do consultation, or perhaps effective consultation and effective therapy (following brief family therapy models) are becoming more and more similar.

We concur with these authors that family therapy and systems theory have much to offer the enterprise of consultation. However, as our own thinking has developed, we have focused primarily on the distinctions between the practice of psychotherapy and the practice of consultation. While systems theory provides a basis for our conceptualization of both therapy and consultation, in our view consultation is clearly a different enterprise from that of traditional psychotherapy (or teaching or supervision or administration). The consultant is basically an adviser to the consultee. Generally, as we discussed earlier, the goals of consultation are more clearly demarcated and circumscribed, the consultant joins the system for a brief period of time to accomplish these goals, and the consultant remains meta to the system so that the consultee retains primary responsibility for decision making and for any changes that may occur. This relationship is retained when a family, rather than another professional or agency, is the consultee. The family as consultee makes the decisions about what to do next, which may or may not be to proceed with family therapy. (See Chapter 2 for an expanded discussion of the differences between therapy and consultation.)

We agree that the newer brief family therapy approaches are similar in certain respects to systems consultation, yet they retain the language of therapy with its implication of illness and long-term caretaking. Therefore, brief family therapists must "work uphill" to undo the usual understanding by the public and professional colleagues about the nature of "therapy." Some consultants and therapists bypass these issues, or try to do so, by not labeling what services are offered: "Let us begin with a meeting of the whole family to see what the problem is and what could be done." In any event, these endeavors all require that the professional conceptualize clearly his or her own role, the goals and time frame of meetings, the limits and mode of sharing responsibility, and the linked systems that need to be taken into account in understanding the problem and options for change.

Several contributors think systems theory alone is not an adequate model for consultation. Both Kaslow, in her consultation with the military, and Fisher, in his consultation with schools, use an organizational development/group relations model in combination with a family systems model as a basis for conceptualizing consultation. Kaslow states: "I have utilized an organizational development model . . . [in my consultation,] similar at the macrosystem level to the perspective adapted with the family at a microsystem level" (Chapter 23, pp. 386–387). In explaining his use of a group relations model, Fisher states: "A need exists for a theoretical or conceptual tool that, when combined with family-based systems theory, will provide a more well-rounded model appropriate to the differences between the school and families" (Chapter 21, p. 351). Fisher believes that therapy and consultation often differ in their goals, in the number of people involved, in the complexity of the organization, and in the length of time that the contract calls for, and he believes that these differences necessitate the use of different techniques. Kaslow and Fisher interweave family systems and organizational development theory and techniques; however, neither discusses at length the compatibility or the pragmatics of the use of these two models for consultation.

Borwick takes a more extreme position regarding this issue in that he asserts that consultants, especially consultants to a business organization, *must* use an organizational development model and should not behave as therapists: "Family therapists who consult to business must take up the role of organizational consultants rather than function as family therapists who happen to be working with business organizations" (Chapter 25, p. 423). Borwick contends that families and organizations differ in terms of boundary conditions, tasks, roles, authority, and power. He states that a family therapist must drop the role of therapist and the mental map of the family territory. In contrast to Friedman, Borwick believes consultants must educate themselves about the business context and develop alternative techniques appropriate to this context: "The practicing consultant will find that the techniques presently employed for families cannot be simply lifted from one system and implemented in another" (Chapter 25, p. 440). Specifically, he encourages consultants to adopt techniques that emphasize roles, work groups, and productivity. He warns against using techniques aimed at individuals, personalities, or personal matters.

In summary, systems theory provides a broad, generalized framework for family therapists who work as consultants, but there are many variations in the details of how the theory is applied in relation to differing goals and diverse contexts.

THE META POSITION OF THE CONSULTANT

What is the role of consultant? In its popular usage, the term "consultant" is quite ambiguous because it is frequently and loosely used to refer to a wide variety of activities conducted by a person with some particular expertise.

The role of "systems consultant" usually is founded on either a person's knowledge and training in systems theory in general or in a special area, for example, consulting with community services or family businesses in which multiple systems come into play with one another. Consultants can find themselves in one of many different roles—that of evaluator who assesses, answers questions, and makes recommendations; that of facilitator who poses questions and allows consultees to discover their own answers; or that of trainer who helps consultees develop skills that will allow them to function without a consultant. Because of the many tasks that may be involved in a consultation, the boundaries between consultation and teaching, therapy, supervision, or administration can be blurred and may contribute to the failure of the endeavor. Many authors in this volume have commented on this problem; they focus on clarifying the goals and the procedure for consultation with the primary consultee early in the process as a way to clarify and negotiate the role of the consultant.

Whether or not one is publicly labeled a consultant, it is very often useful for "helping" professionals to conceptualize their work as consultation in order to gain maximum flexibility in shaping their role. Often a system that is in crisis or is highly stressed will request multiple functions from a professional. For example, a private school undergoing administrative changes may request that a family therapist evaluate its problem youngsters, treat many of these students, train teachers on special topics, facilitate faculty meetings, and be an adviser to the administration. In such circumstances, defining oneself as a consultant may allow time for assessment and help the consultant not to become overly involved or to accept an inappropriate role in the heat of a crisis. The consultant role can provide flexibility and authority while insuring that the primary responsibility and authority remain with the consultee system.

How does the meta position of the consultant influence outcome? Although the consultant is part of the "consulting system," the consultant is not a "member of the family," or of the therapy system, school system, or other context in which the consultant is functioning. The consultant's ability to stay meta to a system makes for successful consultations, as the work of Cecchin and Fruggeri especially well illustrates. We will explore in more depth three of the complex issues regarding the role of the consultant: Is a consultant more effective as an outsider or as an insider? Who has primary responsibility for a problem? Are consultants one-up, one-down, or peers?

Should the consultant be an "outsider" or "insider"? When the consultee is an agency, organization, or group practice, consultants typically are thought of as outsiders. In many situations, an outsider is needed to provide a fresh perspective on a problem. Some consultants see considerable advantage in staying outside the consultee system in order to clarify boundaries and spheres of responsibility and to increase leverage and maneuverability.

Landau-Stanton, for example, in her consultation to community groups and agencies, always defines herself as an outsider in order to increase leverage and maneuverability. In one of her examples, when she consulted with a group for mothers of twins, she minimized her insider identity as a mother of twins by denying that she or her twins had any problems that were different from those affecting families without twins. Fisher also advises an outsider position in consulting to schools. Emphasizing the outsider position as a consultant may help to keep clear the consultee's primary responsibility while still encouraging novel and creative solutions. Such consultants regard themselves as having facilitative skills, but expect the insider consultee to implement change.

While many advantages exist when consultees choose outsider consultants, the fact is that consultees frequently select insider consultants. The consultee may feel more comfortable with someone on the inside and may not want to pay for or take the time to educate an outsider. The joining phase can be easier and quicker for the insider consultant. Kaslow, in consulting with the military as an outsider, describes the risk of being cut off if her behavior does not knowledgeably conform to the military system. Military insiders do not have to acquaint themselves with military rules or rituals, and they can quickly focus on the problem. The danger, of course, is that the insider consultant, while more acceptable to the consultee system, may run the risk of having the same blind spots as others in the system. McDaniel and Weber, in consulting with a family medicine residency program, and Weber and Wynn, in consulting with clergy, discuss the advantages of being an insider in the joining phase of a consultation; however, they note the increased hazard later on of becoming regulated by the consultee system. An outsider's perspective as consultant may be "the difference that makes a difference" (Bateson, 1979), but the outsider will fail if the joining phase is not successful.

While consultees often seek consultants who have some knowledge of their particular contexts, controversy exists among consultants about how well a consultant needs to know a context to be effective. Friedman strongly believes that consultants should attend primarily to process rather than to content. He asserts that knowledge about a system, for the effective consultant and for the effective leader, is secondary to the ability to function in any context from a differentiated position. Other authors, such as Weber and Wynn, and Borwick, warn about presumptuousness, that is, the dangers and the misunderstandings that can beset consultants who do not gather enough data to familiarize themselves with a church organization, a business, or other consultee contexts. Certainly, in consultation as in therapy, a consultant must be able to speak the consultee's "language" but avoid becoming regulated by the consultee system.

Who has primary responsibility for the problem, the consultant or the consultee? Explicitly, the consultee retains primary responsibility for decision making and implementation, with the consultant acting as adviser, evaluator, or facilitator. A consultant may make recommendations, but the consultee may take them or leave them.

A variation on this principle is found in medicine when consultants agree to take responsibility for circumscribed treatment. For example, a radiotherapist may supervise specialized treatment for a cancer patient of a family physician. The radiotherapist has responsibility for this aspect of treatment, but the primary-care physician retains primary responsibility for the overall well-being of the patient, especially after this special treatment is concluded. In this situation, it is vital that the consultant, consultee, patient, and family clearly understand who is responsible for what. Many misunderstandings and inappropriate treatments have resulted from inadequate or unclear communication in such circumstances.

Are consultants one-up, one-down, or peers? Without directly addressing the issue, the authors seem to disagree about the nature of the consultative relationship, whether it is best described as collaborative or hierarchical. Tension may be generated over the issue of establishing a collaborative relationship between colleagues versus a hierarchical relationship of a consultant with those who are less expert. Particularly in medical arenas, consultation seems to be viewed as a hierarchical relationship in which the consultant with specialized training imparts knowledge and skills to the consultee, much like the complementary relationships of supervisor–supervisee and teacher–student. Weber and Wynn suggest another conceptualization in which the consultant is viewed as one-up with regard to circumscribed, specialized knowledge, and the consultee is viewed as one-up with regard to knowledge about the context of the work. In a sense, this balance of specialized skills and general knowledge may result in a peerlike, collaborative relationship.

THE REQUEST FOR CONSULTATION

What prompts a consultation request? Consultation requests often are viewed as resulting from destabilization in a system. Anderson and Goolishian describe consultations as being requested when the consultee system is "stuck" in trying to solve a systemic problem. Perhaps such systems are overstabilized rather than destabilized. Bloch subscribes to the view that consultations emanate from destabilization, but he cautions against the view that these changes have been necessarily negative; some consultation requests are prompted by "growth" that has destabilized the system. For example, a couple may request advice from a family consultant before expanding their life by adopting a child. At the organizational level, a medical group may be quite successful and may want to hire a family systems consultant to expand their services and increase their productivity.

Other consultations clearly do eventuate from turmoil or power struggles. A director chooses a consultant who will back his or her view of the organization against a threatening assistant director, or a consulting physician is chosen to verify a primary physician's medical approach to treating a heart patient when the family favors surgery. In many situations, consultants may find themselves asked to choose sides. As long as the consultant consciously chooses to take a side or not take a side, consultation has a chance of succeeding. The consultant who unwittingly joins a fight may be knocked out.

Whether consultation requests are a result of "stuckness," organizational growth, or turmoil, the requests all surface because of some change or some need for a change. This fact makes Imber-Black's emphasis on asking "why now?" essential to a good assessment and understanding of any consultee's request.

What are the goals of consultation? Much as they differ on the appropriate goals for psychotherapy, so do people differ on the appropriate goals for consultation. Some of the authors, such as Todd with mental health professionals, Landau-Stanton with community groups, Anderson and Goolsihian with domestic violence agencies, and Imber-Black with human-service-provider systems, advocate that consultation goals be specific, concrete, and problem-oriented. Also, medical consultations, like those of Munson with pediatrics, Wellisch and Cohen with oncology, and Sluzki with family medicine, traditionally are very problem-oriented. The medical consultant may be quite specific and circumscribed in his or her goals, often only communicating with the consultee through medical chart notes or letters.

All these consultations may be contrasted with the growth-oriented consultation approaches of Friedman and Whitaker. While the approaches of these two consultants are very different, they both view the fundamental goal of any consultation as an increase in the general level of functioning of the consultee, regardless of the presenting problem or request. As in psychotherapy, growth, not problem solving, may be the goal. For problem-oriented consultants, growth during consultation may take place but not be an explicit goal. Clearly the consultant's theory or belief system regarding the goal of consultation will determine his or her framing of the problem, approach to the consultation, and evaluation of its success.

Another dimension relevant to defining the goal of consultation is the primacy of either content or process in a consultation. Traditionally, consultations result in some advice about a plan, diagnosis, or strategy given by the consultant to the consultee. In this approach, as in many medical consultations, content is primary. All consultations do involve some process dimension, however, and many consultants, such as Anderson and Goolishian, Friedman, and the medical group of McDaniel, Bank, Campbell, Mancini, and Shore give process primary attention.

TECHNIQUES OF CONSULTATION

How does the consultant connect with a system? How does the consultant both join and stay meta to a new system? Certainly it is important to meet everyone relevant to a consultation, gather information, and agree on clear goals with the consultee. More than does therapy, consultation emphasizes a focused, collaborative relationship, an exchange of services, and it does not carry the burden of a caretaking role. Because of its connotation, the connecting or joining phase of a consultation may be brief, though it needs to be effective enough to draw on the relationships during the implementation phase of the consultation. Joining in consultation may be quite informal, such as a business lunch arranged to discuss needs of the system and contract arrangements. Other joining may occur while trying to familiarize oneself with a context. Borwick suggests taking courses or observing a particular business or organization for one day. This show of interest may help both the assessment and joining processes.

Therapists, especially those who see themselves as caretakers, may tend to join too quickly or intensely when they are functioning as consultants, making it difficult to remain meta to the system Being an outsider to the system helps to avoid this problem. Therapy requires more affective joining, whereas connecting in consultation may be established in a less personal, more relaxed forum. Arranging a lunch together or participating in a course may lessen the tendency to "come on like a shrink" when the task is consultation.

While therapists may tend to join too much, subspecialists in the medical world may tend to join too little with both the consultee and the patient, relying on their special knowledge and technical skill to make the consultation successful. While technical skill and expertise are important, clear and direct communication between consultant and consultee deserve careful attention so that the consultant's expertise is not wasted.

How can a consultant avoid de-skilling the consultee? No one likes to feel inadequate. Often a consultation request is motivated by the recognition of some inadequacy in a leader or an organization, some need that cannot be filled by a person inside the system. One of the first problems a consultant faces is how to provide the needed expertise while supporting the strengths of the system. This task must be accomplished without increasing any feelings of inadequacy that might have motivated the consultation request, and without de-skilling the consultee.

Many physicians, especially those in primary care, view consultants as necessary evils to be used only in extreme circumstances. They fear that consultants may complicate relations with patients and disturb the recovery process. Bloch, though not endorsing this perspective, does warn against the invalidation and de-skilling of physicians by consultants. Whitaker discusses both the negative and positive effects of an "invasion" by a consultant. While we believe a good consultation can improve an outcome and increase everyone's sense of competence, the addition of an "expert" to any system can certainly backfire. Demonstrations by expert therapists who consult on others' cases often are criticized for having diminished the stature of the therapist/consultee who then has to carry on with the family.

Consultants have found a variety of strategies useful to diminish this negative effect of de-skilling the consultee. At recent consultative demonstration interviews, neither Whitaker nor Cecchin made any recommendations or prescriptions directly to the family. They only interviewed the family and later made their recommendations to the therapist/consultee.

Perlmutter and Jones recommend strategies in which the consultant is deliberately "one-down." These consultants purposely expose and use their own mistakes for teaching purposes. These strategies make their expert role more palatable and also indirectly help the consultees to recognize that they are neither powerless nor unskilled. Anderson and Goolishian also discuss the importance of a consultant not "taking over" for a consultee. Toward this end, they limit their interventions to those that overcome impasses to effective treatment or productive organizational functioning. Other issues are left to the consultee and the agency.

The conceptualization of consultation as a relationship between colleagues based on mutual respect points toward the necessity of developing techniques that avoid de-skilling the consultee. Limiting the goals and the arena for the consultation as well as limiting the time of the consultation and the role of the consultant all help to prevent any overfunctioning by the consultant that might encourage underfunctioning by the consultee. This issue must be given special consideration at the time of terminating the consultation, when it is important to focus on the integrity and competency of the system that will continue functioning.

Should a consultant give advice? That there should be a controversy about this is interesting. *The American Heritage Dictionary* defines a consultant as "a person who gives expert or professional advice." This traditional view of advice as central to consultation is particularly appropriate in some settings. For example, most medical consultants render an opinion to another health care provider about specific issues regarding an individual patient. Some systems consultants such as Landau-Stanton and Imber-Black eschew the medical model of advice giving. Some consultants also view advice giving as potentially de-skilling the consultee. These consultants view their job as helping the consultee to find his or her own adaptive solutions. These consultations are not focused on information—or advice giving; rather, they focus on process, particularly on removing any blocks to successful functioning.

Clarifying the goal of consultation may provide an obvious answer to the question of whether advice is appropriate. For example, if the consultee has requested information about the relative merits of two treatment approaches, advice about these approaches may be sensible. But even in focused, information-seeking (lineal) consultations such as often occur in medicine, a *systemic* understanding of the context may assist consultees in making their own comprehensive treatment plan. The skillful consultant will be able to help the consultee reframe his or her goals and consider factors that were not considered initially but that may prevent a successful outcome.

Are insight and education necessary to successful consultation? Many consultations involve primary educational components, such as teaching specific skills like desensitization, teaching systems theory, or educating ex-cult members and their parents. Even with an educational emphasis, teaching must be balanced with the needs of the system so that the information giving becomes a vehicle to energize rather than de-skill consultees. An important distinction needs to be made between "insight" about motivation and dynamic relationships and "education" about facts and behavior. As discussed in Chapter 2, a psychoeducational component is now commonly introduced in meetings with families of schizophrenics (Anderson, Hogarty, & Reiss, 1980; Falloon, Boyd, & McGill, 1984). Meetings that are not called "therapy" but are labeled "consultations" or "educational workshops" usually are much more acceptable to families because such meetings do not carry the connotation that the families are blamed or regarded as sick. These meetings constitute a means of joining with families. Subsequently, such families often decide that they do have enduring difficulties for which they request therapy, but a therapy that is not experienced as imposed or prescribed. Often they then engage in a therapeutic relationship with an enthusiasm that is in striking contrast to the skepticism and negativism that prevailed before psychoeducational consultations were held. On the other hand, consultations based on structural and strategic approaches usually do not have a primary teaching component and are not concerned with facilitating insightful understanding in consultees. Rather, these approaches to consultation are more concerned with behavior change and decision making (as with Borwick, Anderson and Goolishian, and Landau-Stanton).

What is the best kind of contract for consultation? Several authors address the issue of formal contracts. Fisher, in working with the schools, recommends a letter be written by the consultant to the consultee, after an agreement has been reached, summarizing in black-and-white the goals of the consultation, the logistics, the expectations, and the financial agreement. This letter may prevent misunderstandings that can lead to consultation failures. Imber-Black, in her work with health service agencies, emphasizes the importance of a clear, concrete contract early in the consultation. An appropriate contract, from her point of view, is one that can succeed and one that does not unintentionally side with some covert consultee agenda. Negotiating such a contract may prevent the consultant from becoming what Imber-Black terms an "inadvertent perpetuator of the *status quo*," and from contributing to "escalating cynicism" of the staff about the prospects of change.

While many consultants thus favor clear and concrete contracts, Friedman prefers not to negotiate a specific contract early on, but to leave the consulting process fluid and somewhat vague. This flexibility purposefully allows the consultee to move back and forth from family to work, or to other issues if the client so desires. And this approach does not lock in the process on some early issue that might be much less important than another issue that eventually emerges. Friedman's wide-ranging approach may be most appropriate in long-term consultative relationships but not be as suitable to brief consultation models.

From our own perspective, contract or no contract, it is crucial to clarify one's own role in working with any system. A contract may make this process more explicit.

How long is a good consultation? Most consultants would answer, "Not very." The time-limited nature of consultation helps the consultant to maintain an outside perspective and introduce new "information" into the consultee system. The success of this approach depends on well-defined, concrete, short-term goals.

Several contributors to this book presented consultations that were not time-limited. Wellisch and Cohen presented an ongoing, 10-year consultation relationship with oncology at their hospital. In what might be termed a "continuous consultation," Wellisch and Cohen provide consultation services to a variety of health care providers whenever they are needed. The consultation is primarily case-focused and may be similar to ongoing consultations provided for family therapists who present many different cases for consultation. McDaniel and Weber also discuss a continuous consultation with a family medicine residency program in which education and case consultation are primary components. Wynne and Wynne describe their long-term consultative relationship with the courts. It is important to note that these consultants may still view their position as "impermanent," to use one of Landau-Stanton's definitions of consultation, vis-à-vis the particular case with which they are dealing. The overall relationship with the larger system may be readily renewed, while the specific consultations that constitute the work may be intermittent and be guided by brief, problem-focused principles. Landau-Stanton prefers the term "liaison" for such relationships.

Information regarding the general work system is usually more accessible to these long-term consultants as they straddle the boundary between being an outsider or insider to the consultee system. The danger with these consultations, of course, is that they will become blocked, stale, or stuck, much like the consultee system, due to the longevity of the endeavor.

What is the most effective size for a consultee unit? This technical issue revolves around the question of how many people are necessary to reach a consultation goal effectively. Borwick challenges family therapists who consult by saying that family therapists often only consult with three to six people in businesses, regardless of what number might be more productive, because this is the usual size of families to which they are accustomed. Borwick contends that if increased productivity is the goal of a business consultation, a consultant most often needs to work with most of the organization, however large. Borwick's challenge is well taken and deserves the same consideration that is given to determining membership in family therapy. Whether it be an individual, a couple, or a family, it is important to identify those who are relevant to the problem and who could contribute usefully to treatment or consultation.

One may also focus on the point of most leverage in accomplishing the consultee's goals. Friedman, in his work with businesses, aims his consultation at leadership, believing in a "trickle-down" phenomenon in which the organizational functioning will follow that of its leadership.

Whatever the skills or comfort level of the consultant, the issue of who should be involved in a consultation and who the initial consultee will allow to be involved may be crucial to the success of a consultation. For example, a consultation that involves teaching family systems theory to residents but has no forum for sharing ideas with faculty is unlikely to succeed. In some cases, widening the unit of consultation may require the use of a consultant team rather than a solo consultant.

What are the advantages and disadvantages of a consultant team? One strategy that can promote great flexibility is the use of a consultant team, rather than an individual consultant. If a team is affordable, the consultee then benefits from the multiple perspectives and potentially greater creativity that can emerge from a team.

Many formats exist for using multiple consultants. Wynne and Wynne discuss their teamwork in consulting to the courts. Their co-consultation seems to parallel cotherapy, possibly providing a special advantage when a consultant couple works with warring marital couples. McDaniel and Weber also report a co-consultant model in their approach to consultation in a family medicine residency program. In this consultation, with one consultant in-house and the other outside, both vantage points can be used to implement educational goals. Penn and Sheinberg use a team approach to consultation much like the "systemic" approach to therapy, with one consultant observing the consultation from behind a one-way mirror. This approach is, in effect, consultation to a consultation, and it introduces greater complexity as well as the potential for greater leverage with the consultee. McDaniel, Bank, Campbell, Mancini, and Shore report on a consultant group, a situation in which the consultants usually outnumber the consultees. No unified plan is dictated by the consulting group. Rather, the range of views is solicited as a strategy to introduce more complexity into the consultee system, allowing consultees to select or formulate their own solutions.

Other than cost, the disadvantage of using consultant team techniques is that they necessitate a well-matched team with some compatibility in approach and theory. The consultants also need to have the energy to communicate with each other during the process. The cost-effectiveness of such consultative groups is difficult to assess, but may well improve efficacy and reduce cost in the long run.

CONCLUSION

We only have begun to touch upon some of the major problems and controversies that have arisen in the field of systems consultation. Some are a matter of consultant preference or style, some reflect theoretical differences, others point to lack of clarity in the current conceptualizations of systems consultation. All of these issues deserve further thought and research as we work to increase our effectiveness as consultants.

REFERENCES

The American heritage dictionary. Boston: Houghton Mifflin, 1981.

Anderson, C. M., Hogarty, G. E., & Reiss, D. J. Family treatment of adult schizophrenic patients: A psycho-educational approach. *Schizophrenia Bulletin*, 1980, *6*, 490–505.

Bateson, G. *Mind and nature: A necessary unity*. New York: E. P. Dutton, 1979.

Falloon, I. R. H., Boyd, J. L., & McGill, C. W. *Family care of schizophrenia: A problem-solving approach to the treatment of mental illness*. New York: Guilford, 1984.

27

FUTURE DIRECTIONS FOR SYSTEMS CONSULTATION

LYMAN C. WYNNE

SUSAN H. McDANIEL

TIMOTHY T. WEBER

University of Rochester School of Medicine and Dentistry
Rochester, New York

In our consideration of future directions for systems consultations, there are a number of topics that trouble us: (1) present-day economic realities and the political context of psychotherapy and family therapy within health care systems; (2) research on consultation that will be relevant to these pragmatic concerns and to broader scientific questions; (3) the problems of integrating value orientations with systems concepts; (4) direct consultations with families as a precursor to decisions about family therapy or other options; (5) the selection of persons to be included in a consultation, that is, the definition of the boundary of the consultation system; and (6) the limitations and hazards for consultative and therapeutic endeavors in terms of societal needs and goals.

ECONOMIC IMPLICATIONS

In the current health care scene in the United States, a great deal of economic and ideologic pressure is being applied to shorten treatment. The brief contacts of most consultations fit today's economic ambience. However, almost any modification of health care practice in the United States is now greeted with suspicion by third-party payers. Payment for marital and family therapy treatment, which does not fit traditional health care formats, is currently reimbursed in most areas of the United States only if a traditional individual diagnosis is given. Also, third-party payment for consultation beyond a single session is often challenged, especially if the consultant does not see the patient and only works with the consultee. On the other hand, this perspective may be economically shortsighted because consultation as an alternative to therapy may well reduce overall medical care costs. And, with the increase of health maintenance organizations that require designation of a primary physician, referral for short-term consultation may become more attractive than referral for therapy, as a means of cost containment. Thus there are realistic, unsettled problems in establishing the merits of different formats for professional care, formats that must fit into economic patterns even before their efficacy is evaluated. In adapting to these changes, the traditional medical system already includes consultation roles and therefore may be more attuned to the viewpoint presented here than are current systems of community services. In many community programs, services are provided directly but consultation, as an indirect service oriented to evaluation and decision making, may not be available.

THE PLACE OF FAMILY THERAPY IN HEALTH CARE AND SOCIAL SERVICES

Economic considerations are compounded by the marginal place of family therapy in interdisciplinary politics. In the "real world," family therapy is still peripheral to general health care and even to mental health treatment, given the predominance of individual psychotherapy and pharmacotherapy in many settings. When family therapists get together in their own organizations, training programs, or workshops, they enjoy their camaraderie and easily forget the facts of life in the outer world. The continuing, limited acceptance of family therapy can be documented, for example, by the currently low level of family therapy input into the American Psychiatric Association, which has rejected the concept of a council on families and recognizes (as of 1985) no official liaison with any family therapy organization. A Division of Family Psychology of the American Psychological Association was established in 1984, but the kind of impact it may have remains to be seen. Social work, a field that called for contact with families long before "family therapy" was recognized, was enamored of psychoanalytic therapy in many clinics and training programs for a number of years. More recently, some social work programs have staked out family interviewing as their special turf—with the result, in at least a few settings, that staff members who are not social workers are actively discouraged from seeing family members together, while *only* social workers are approved to do family therapy. How far from a truly systemic approach can the family therapy field have moved?

As the identity of being "family therapists" brought advantages for some mental health professionals, many family therapists, like psychoanalysts before them, have gradually cut themselves off from other professional disciplinary roots and branches. Family clinics and private offices all too readily become scheduled sites for specialized practice. Many of us now attend family therapy conferences more regularly than meetings with colleagues from such fields as psychology, psychiatry, social work, and medicine. There is now a debate among family therapists about the optimal route of entry into the family therapy field. Some students now want to choose a doctoral program in marriage and family therapy so that they can surround themselves with family therapists and not be contaminated by anyone else.

Ironically, by overfocusing on a family therapy perspective, we may lose touch with other systems of health care and become less systemic, rather than more so. At this time we feel that family therapy is stable and secure enough to try to have a larger impact. Consultative roles offer the opportunity to do so in a variety of contexts. It is now time for us to reconnect with our roots as well as to venture forth into new settings. We need to have more of a dialogue with those whose points of view differ from our own. The roles of consultant and consultee offer opportunities to have such an exchange and not to perpetuate reciprocally isolationist positions.

However, the more visible and effective family therapy becomes, in comparison to other approaches, the more turf issues are certain to arise. An example of these problems occurred when a family therapist was asked by a psychiatric resident to consult about a case of anorexia nervosa. The attending psychiatrist went along with the consultation request in the belief that the consultation would be a teaching exercise that would not affect the inpatient treatment plan. This inpatient unit was organized around pharmacologic and individual psychotherapeutic approaches. Past proposals to introduce family therapy into this setting had been rejected. However, a family-oriented consultation took place and stimulated staff discussion of alternative ways of relating to the families of these patients—arrangements, however, that would only be acceptable in that setting if the family as a unit were *not* engaged in "family therapy." Even though one cannot be too hopeful about a collaborative approach over time under such circumstances, the introduction of family-oriented *consultation* was more feasible here than proposals for family therapy had been. Family therapy is still viewed by others in the mental health professions as a competitive modality, despite protestations and attempted clarifications by family therapists.

The family therapy literature has repeatedly made the point that family therapy is not just another modality for doing therapy, but that it is a whole new paradigm, a way of thinking, a way of orienting ourselves to the universe. While that may be true on a conceptual level, we should recognize the political consequences of taking a stand in which we intentionally and directly distinguish ourselves from everyone else. The claim that "family therapy" is not just a modality because it embodies a systems paradigm is almost always misunderstood both by professional colleagues and the public. The idea of family theory as a paradigm for systems theory is usually interpreted as the expression of an overreaching imperialism. On the other hand, if family therapy is viewed "merely" as a treatment modality, it can be readily dismissed as having very limited applicability within our culture's individually oriented health care thinking. In an era of shrinking funds for health care, the concept of family therapy is readily perceived as competitive with whatever other treatment approaches are available. In short, the family therapists' belief that they are systems-oriented and offer a new paradigm, rather than one more treatment modality, is not generally accepted or understood by other health care professionals.

To correct this difficulty, there have been suggestions from time to time that a term other than family therapy be used. For example, Virginia Satir some years ago commented that the generic term "therapy" would be preferable to the more constricting terms family therapy or individual therapy. Alternatively, we have considered the term "systems therapy" as a conceptual improvement over "family therapy." Although "systems therapy" may be more accurate in many circumstances, it seems to us that it is premature to expect other health care professionals to find this concept understandable. They probably would question the relevance of this approach and would doubt that it would add much to what they think they are already doing. The concept of "consultation" at least has a more familiar ring.

Consultation is a concept that offers more flexibility and leverage, particularly if we retain special competence in understanding families while also surveying larger systems. If we do so, then we have something to offer as consultants without getting into an either/or turf struggle. Consultation is a meta position from which one can take a broad perspective of problems and potential solutions, a position that is not identified as promoting any one particular way of working. It is a position of choice and opportunity.

At a family therapy meeting in 1984, Paul Dell stated that he felt that family therapy, from a conceptual point of view, was in a state of stagnation and that there are no really new paradigms or ideas coming onto the scene. Consultation and dialogue with other contexts and points of view may offer opportunities for family therapists to move, to grow, and be challenged. Practice in the consultation field may then help shape and inform a new conceptual framework.

RESEARCH ON THE PROCESSES AND OUTCOME OF CONSULTATION

Only in relatively recent years has there been a solid recognition that research on any form of psychotherapy is both possible and desirable. Some of the current pressure for this research comes from the unscientific desire that such research might help to persuade third-party payers that psychotherapy is worthwhile. While research on individual psychotherapy research has grown, research on the processes and outcome of consultation has languished. In 1972, Mannino and Shore comprehensively reviewed research in mental health consultation. The studies that were considered were mostly descriptive—the characteristics of consultants and consultees, the problems for which consultation is sought, and the uses of consultation in program development and management. There appears to have been no recent update on such research efforts. Neither before nor since has there been research that compares the goals and efficacy of consultation and therapy.

Considerable research has been conducted in consultation–liaison psychiatry that has capitalized on many opportunities for collaborative clinical studies. Topics from clinical psychophysiology to psychological coping with disability have been investigated (e.g., Byyny, Rudd, & Siegler, 1978; Dunbar, Rioch, & Wolfe, 1936; Kaufman, 1965; Lipowski, 1970, 1973; Mendelson & Meyer, 1961. Evaluation of the clinical and teaching aspects of consultation–liaison work is less well developed and has not incorporated attention to the family (Beckhardt & McKegney, 1982; Cooper, Richards, Ullian, & Weinberg, 1981; Goldman, Lee, & Pappius, 1983; Krakowski, 1973).

The very brevity of most consultative relationships poses practical problems for research design. The amount of background material needed to assess the characteristics of clients for research may take more time to assemble than is needed for a whole consultation. On the other hand, if consultation (with the family as consultee) is conceptualized as assessment leading to a decision about therapy, it may involve better data collection than much therapy that begins with only vague documentation of the presenting problem and its context. Consultation provides an explicit framework for assessing the crucial, but neglected, process of reaching a decision about therapy. Research could usefully be directed to the comparison of programs in which "therapy" is offered beginning with the initial contact versus programs that start with consultation and may or may not continue with therapy. In such studies, the issue of cost-effectiveness could become an important topic for research. Kornfeld and Levitan (1981) have conducted a relevant study of clinical and cost benefits of liaison psychiatry on an orthopedic ward. Studies of the cost-effectiveness of consultation are possible and clearly should be carried out.

A closely related, researchable question concerns referral sources: How and when are clients, patients, or families referred for one type of service rather than another? Recipients of referrals who respond by providing an initial consultative assessment, examining the context of the problem and working with the referring person, can be in an excellent position to study health care patterns and needs. For example, under what circumstances is someone sent to a family therapist rather than to a psychiatrist or a psychoanalyst? How the referral source has defined or framed the problem will be directly related to the type of referral or request for consultation that is made.

In the realm of physical illness, a great deal of potentially fruitful research from a consultative viewpoint is timely. Here the targeted issue may, for example, be the longevity or comfort of a seriously ill family member and/or the quality of functioning of the family unit and individual family members in the face of threatened loss of life or changed role of the patient. Often "family therapy" is not what families with a physically ill family member are prepared to accept. Family-oriented assistance in such circumstances may be easier for referring physicians to propose to families under the umbrella of "consultation." Consultants are a familiar component of medical settings; family therapists are not. Family consultations may be highly therapeutic in their effects, certainly more so than family therapy that is rejected or viewed with suspicion. These benefits of a family orientation could, in many medical settings, be studied without fanfare in consultation research.

SYSTEMS THEORY AND VALUE ORIENTATIONS

In the preceding chapter, we considered the problem of whether the version of systems theory adopted by family therapists is adequate for a consultation framework. There is the even more serious question of whether general systems theory (Bertalanffy, 1968) can be pitched at a level of practical, middle-range hypotheses that link observations and theory. Many consultants and therapists who subscribe to systems theory in a loose form find that systems concepts are only useful starting points because of their high level of abstraction. On the other hand, more lineal and narrowly defined hypotheses are usually inadequate for understanding complex problems involving a family or network. Thus, systems consultants as well as therapists will need to do much more work on formulations that can readily be grasped, preferably are testable in research, and to step back from such abstract concepts as homeostasis and system coherence.

There is a very real problem of how to integrate ethical and value-laden issues into systems theory. Ivan Boszormenyi-Nagy and David Ulrich (1981) and Bunny and Frederick Duhl (1981) have expressed misgivings about the adequacy of systems theory because of its content-free and value-free emphasis. Also, other authors, for example, Bograd (1984), have criticized systems theory for being neutral about such issues as battered wives or child abuse. Clearly, as systems practitioners, we necessarily infuse our values into our work. Cecchin and Fruggeri (Chapter 8) have described their use of the consultant role to make deliberate choices between such options as family therapy, social control of deviance, and use of medication. In the Milan approach, and with other consultation formats, the meta position of the consultant is advantageous in providing the appropriate distance for making wiser choices among a variety of value-laden options.

CONSULTATION AS A PROLOGUE TO THERAPY?

Willingness to enter any kind of psychotherapy carries with it certain implications. Many therapists implicitly, sometimes explicitly, assume that everyone who comes to them is saying, "I can't handle my life. Please help mc with therapy." A consultation framework makes no such assumption, and it puts no pressure upon the prospective client or family to behave in a dependent, needful, childlike manner. The widespread public belief that seeing a therapist amounts to a confession that one is incompetent, crazy, or childish, often interferes with seeking assistance (Selvini Palazzoli, 1983). Although many psychotherapists and family therapists, especially those involved in brief therapy, will categorically deny that they make such assumptions about individuals or families, the beliefs in our culture that surround the notion of "therapy" should not be ignored. The good intentions of therapists are not enough to set aside belief systems that fuse the concept of therapy and the concepts of disease and disorder.

The clinical and research literature on therapy and supervision are replete with concerns about how one can best start quickly in therapy, join with the patient or family in a therapeutic alliance, and find ways of insuring that this alliance will be sustained. While praiseworthy as efforts toward efficiency, many of these endeavors may crash soon after takeoff. The therapy-outcome literature often includes data on dropouts—those cases that are regarded as constituting premature termination. What therapists regard as a "premature" termination or a "dropout" may involve a failure to recognize what kind of goal or relationship has been sought by the patient or family. To be sure, patients and families may stop coming when the relationship has been unproductive and unsatisfactory, *or* they may do so when all the help they want or need has been achieved. The concepts of premature termination and dropout do not take into account this important distinction. Many prospective patients and families, we believe, are understandably hesitant to confront therapists with their decision not to seek therapy after all. If the relationship begins as consultation rather than as therapy, these issues can be much more easily discussed forthrightly and thoughtfully, bringing to light the alternative options and needs of patient or family. When a therapist uses the term "premature termination," this means that the therapist wanted the relationship to continue, but the family has unilaterally decided not to do so. The discrepant views have not been reconciled and probably have not been discussed. At present the therapy research literature reads as if therapists think that everyone they see should end up in therapy, and if they fail to do so, either the family is "resistant" or there must be a shortcoming in the technique of therapy. We contend that therapy is not always the game that many clients (who are not yet "patients") wish to play, need to play, or are willing to play. Consultation, with the family or client as consultee, offers a framework for consideration of what is needed and what could be helpful.

The existence of a presenting problem, even those problems that meet DSM-III diagnostic criteria, does not mean that individual clients or family members have understood, accepted, or agreed to the implication that the solution is therapy. During the exploration of such situations within the framework of consultation, a decision to proceed with therapy *may* result, but reaching agreement about what problem, if any, deserves therapy is often difficult. Especially with conflicted couples and families, this clarification often takes more than one session. By the time that the communication difficulties that impede clarification of the problem have been overcome, many couples and families need no further assistance. Beginning with consultation, they can start to acquire or reclaim skills in communication that they can apply to other problems. In our experience, framing the relationship as consultation enables many family members to experience themselves as part of a "normal family" wrestling with ordinary difficulties, and not as a pathologic or pathogenic, disturbed or disturbing family. The latter view of themselves stimulates reciprocal scapegoating, heightens defensiveness, and, ironically may make therapeutic *effects* more unlikely with therapy than with consultation.

Despite our concerns and strictures about the overexpansiveness that has overtaken the field of therapy, we hasten to make clear that we are not attempting to abolish the field of individual psychotherapy or family therapy. As we have indicated in this volume, we see ourselves as continuing to be family therapists, but therapists who take consultative roles *before* we establish a therapeutic alliance (if any is needed). Our position is actually conservative: Therapy is only one option among many alternatives, which may include *not* proceeding with any professional help. Training and research programs in therapy usually begin with the assumption that therapy will take place if "resistance" can be overcome. The public by and large cynically expects professionals will push their own product and will not insist that other alternatives should be carefully considered.

NETWORKING AND BOUNDARIES

A central pragmatic and conceptual question that urgently needs investigation is how to select the boundaries of the network to be included in therapy and in consultation. We have found that consultative assessment greatly enhances the chances that peripheral members of a network will attend meetings at which broader understanding and input about a problem can be gained. For example, in problems of divorce and remarriage, many persons who would refuse to engage in "therapy" together may be quite willing to come for a "consultation" to take stock of a shared problem, especially a problem that involves parenting. Often, stepparents and grandparents are crucially involved in these problems. There are various ways in which such network meetings can be conceptualized and presented to participants. A common way is for the professional to be a consultant to the whole network; another procedure is to ask newly introduced persons, such as grandparents, to come "as consultants" to an ongoing therapeutic group. Whitaker particularly uses the latter approach.

Furthermore, consultation enhances community and interdisciplinary work: A consultant is not "in charge," but is a collaborator. To be sure, working in consultation as a colleague with another professional may be difficult for those who prefer to remain hierarchically superior and relatively autonomous. However, a consultation framework usually can provide a relatively nonthreatening means of obtaining collaborative assistance. Systems-based consultation gives attention to understanding and treating problems within a comprehensive, ecological framework beyond the patient; it includes not only the nuclear family but also the extended family, community resources, and the key persons in the health care delivery system.

THE LIMITATIONS OF CONSULTATION

We have emphasized that consultation is not a panacea; it does not eliminate the need for other forms of professional relationships. Rather, consultation can be a precursor and a supportive adjunct to other relationships. Here we wish to note a few of the circumstances when consultation is inadvisable or inappropriate:

1. When it is impossible to become meta to the system, for example, when the proposed consultant is an enmeshed member of the system in an ongoing, insider role; when past, emotionally charged relationships are likely to produce a carryover of entanglements; or in some emergency situations in which one does not have the resources or the distance to hold

the system still for a consultation (though, in these situations, a *brief* consultation with quick referral may still be possible).

2. When another role better suits the situation—for example, when a beginning student asks for consultation but needs directive supervision and/or teaching, or when a presenting problem involves major-league, well-defined difficulties for which a particular form of therapeutic care is urgently needed, for example, when an actively suicidal patient without family support requires inpatient care.

3. When there are already other consultants and the designation of a case manager or a primary physician is needed first. Sometimes a systems-oriented consultant can negotiate by taking an overall, coordinating role to sort out if the consultants, therapists, and assorted "helpers" are working together or getting in each other's way.

AUTHORITY AND SELF-HELP IN THE THERAPEUTIC SOCIETY

Rieff (1966), Kittrie (1971), and Lasch (1977, 1982) exemplify a group of articulate social critics who have castigated helping professionals for contributing to a psychology and a culture of dependence upon therapists and other so-called helpers. In this view, "medicalization" in the West is the "triumph of the therapeutic" (Rieff, 1966). These critics contend that our spiritual center has shifted to the spectrum of health and well-being, of sickness and disease; sin and religion, crime and punishment have given way to sickness and therapy; religious and political authority have yielded to therapeutic authority.

These authors actually are joined by many psychotherapists who share a concern that people increasingly have become dependent upon therapeutic experts not only to satisfy their needs but also to define their needs. To a considerable degree, therapeutic authority depends upon defining illness and patient status. One consequence is that therapeutic practice can be construed as a demand that therapeutic services be accepted. Thus, a consequence of a therapeutic ethic may be the expansion of professional control at the expense of older traditions of family and community remedies and supports, as an expansion of the conditions labeled as "sickness" that require professional "treatment," and as heightened difficulty in resisting therapeutic dominance when it is disguised as "help." As a net result, many critics fear that the personal sense of responsibility for using one's own resources and the capacity for self-help have been undermined. They contend that sickness is represented as if it were an "invasion" of forces outside personal control or at least outside conscious control. If the concept of sickness includes not only individual misbehavior but also marital and family difficulties, critics fear that people will become increasingly incompetent in managing their interpersonal relationships and need to be enduringly in the care of therapeutic specialists.

Critics also charge that psychotherapists become too fully and enduringly surrogate parents. Until recently, the care and nurture of the young took place largely within the family. Increasingly, institutions, agencies, and professionals are appropriating many of the rearing functions formerly carried out by the family. Consensus among many helping professionals is that the family can no longer provide those needs. Schools, courts, social agencies, and therapists appropriate earlier familial functions and assume responsibility for guidance and socialization. The eventual goal of family therapists may be to help the family help itself, but sometimes they start by documenting the family's failings in terms of the latest principles of family communication, marital interaction, and child care. Thereby, it is claimed, parental authority and confidence are undermined, not strengthened.

From this perspective, mental health professionals are regarded as having inherently expansionist ambitions to usurp self-determination by families, to determine family needs, and to provide solutions for problems, instead of helping families to trust and enhance their own inner resources and judgment. Such therapeutic "help" may perpetuate needs for assistance and generate new anxieties instead of allaying old ones. At every stage of the child's life, some modern-style agency may say to the parents: "We can do this better than you can."

In summary, in our consultation model, a professional as consultant meets with another professional or with a family or client as consultee. As in all consultations, the consultee retains primary responsibility for decision making. The consultant assists the consultee to clarify the problem and its context, but depends upon the consultee's initiative. The consultee does not turn over authority to the consultant, but retains responsibility for accepting or rejecting the consultant's recommendations, if any. The consultant pushes authority back to the consultee and thus underscores the consultee's competency. The paradigm is *not* helplessness before a therapeutic authority. Rather, the consultee is defined as competent to handle these problems; retains responsibility to define the need for help; and is free to use, modify, or reject the consultant's advice. Consultation most often is brief, time-limited, and problem-focused. Within a consultation framework, "medicalization" is limited to aiding a system move beyond an impasse, with prompt retreat after the impasse has been resolved sufficiently, not necessarily completely. Instead of an expansion of conditions labeled "sickness," which create an ever-greater need for "treatment," skillful consultation minimizes the need for treatment. The application of the concept of systems consultation can go a long way toward tempering the real hazards of zealous advocacy of therapy by professionals and its acceptance by a dependent public. Consultative systems, we believe, can impair minimally and enhance maximally the ability of people to use their own resources.

REFERENCES

Beckhardt, R. M., & McKegney, F. P. Evaluative research in consultation-liaison psychiatry: Review of literature, 1970–1981. *General Hospital Psychiatry,* 1982, *4,* 197–218.

Bertalanffy, L. von *General system theory*. New York: Braziller, 1968.

Bograd, M. Family systems approaches to wife battering: A feminist critique. *American Journal of Orthopsychiatry,* 1984 *54,* 558–568.

Boszormenyi-Nagy, L., & Ulrich, D. N. Contextual family therapy. In A. S. Gurman & D. P. Kniskern (Eds.), *Handbook of family therapy*. New York: Brunner/Mazel, 1981.

Byyny, R. L., Rudd, P., Siegler, M. Preoperative diabetic consultation: A plea for improved training. *Journal of Medical Education*, 1978, *53*, 590–596.

Cooper, P., Richards, W. D., Ullian, L., & Weinberg, A. D. Informal advice and information-seeking between physicians. *Journal of Medical Education*, 1981, *56,* 174–180.

Dell, P. Presentation at "An Institute on Theory": Meeting of the American Association for Marriage and Family Therapy, San Francisco, October 19, 1984.

Duhl, B. S., & Duhl, F. J. Integrative family therapy. In A. S. Gurman & D. P. Kniskern (Eds.), *Handbook of family therapy*. New York: Brunner/Mazel, 1981.

Dunbar, F. H., Rioch, J. M., & Wolfe, T. P. Psychiatric aspects of medical problems. *American Journal of Psychiatry*, 1936, *93*, 649–679.

Goldman, L., Lee, T., & Pappius, E. M. Impact of inter-physician communication on the effectiveness of medical consultations. *American Journal of Medicine,* 1983, *74,* 106–112.

Kaufman, M. R. (Ed.). *The psychiatric unit in a general hospital.* New York: International Universities Press, 1965.

Kittrie, N. N. *The right to be different: Deviance and enforced therapy*. Baltimore: Johns Hopkins University Press, 1971.

Kornfeld, D. S. & Levitan, S. J. Clinical and cost benefits of liaison psychiatry. *American Journal of Psychiatry,* 1981, *138*, 790–793.

Krakowski, A. J. Liaison psychiatry: Factors influencing the consultation process. *Psychiatry in Medicine,* 1973, *4,* 439–446.

Lasch, C. *Haven in a heartless world: The family besieged.* New York: Basic Books, 1977.

Lasch, C. On medicalization and the triumph of the therapeutic. In M. W. de Vries, R. L. Berg, & M. Lipkin (Eds.), *The use and abuse of medicine.* New York: Praeger, 1982.

Lipowski, Z. J. New perspectives in psychosomatic medicine. *Canadian Psychiatric Association Journal,* 1970, *15,* 515–525.

Lipowski, Z. J. Psychosomatic medicine in a changing society: Some current trends in theory and research. *Comprehensive Psychiatry,* 1973, *14*, 203–215.

Mannino, F. V., & Shore, M. F. Research in mental health consultation. In E. Golann & C. Eisdorfer (Eds.), *Handbook of community mental health.* New York: Appleton-Century-Crofts, 1972.

Mendelson, M., & Meyer, E. Psychiatric consultations with patients on medical and surgical wards: Patterns and processes. *Psychiatry,* 1961, *24,* 197–220.

Rieff, P. *The triumph of the therapeutic.* New York: Harper & Row, 1966.

Selvini Palazzoli, M. The emergence of a comprehensive systems approach. *Journal of Family Therapy,* 1983, *5,* 165–177.

NAME INDEX

SUBJECT INDEX

D

E

F

G

H

I

J

L

T

V

W